STP 1104

Skiing Trauma and Safety: Eighth International Symposium

C. D. Mote, Jr. and Robert J. Johnson, editors

ASTM Publication Code Number (PCN)
04-011040-47

ASTM
1916 Race Street
Philadelphia, PA 19103

ISSN 1050-7582
ASTM Publication Code Number (PCN) 04-011040-47

Photocopy Rights

Peer Review Policy

Each paper published in this volume was evaluated by three peer reviewers. The authors addressed all of the reviewers' comments to the satisfaction of both the technical editor(s) and the ASTM Committee on Publications.

The quality of the papers in this publication reflects not only the obvious efforts of the authors and the technical editor(s), but also the work of these peer reviewers. The ASTM Committee on Publications acknowledges with appreciation their dedication and contribution of time and effort on behalf of ASTM.

Printed in Baltimore, MD
May 1991

Foreword

The Eighth International Symposium on Ski Trauma and Safety was held in Riksgräsen, Sweden, on 15–21 May 1989. The symposium was sponsored by ASTM Committee F-27 on Snow Skiing and The International Society for Skiing Safety. Ejnar Eriksson, Karolinska Hospital, Stockholm, Sweden, served as chairman of the symposium, and C. D. Mote, Jr., University of California, and Robert J. Johnson, University of Vermont, are the editors of this volume. The papers in this volume were presented at the symposium, and they were subsequently accepted for publication following rigorous peer review.

Contents

Introduction

The papers in this volume address injury as a result of snow skiing and, to a limited extent, the skiing process. The topics discussed include biomechanics and injuries of the knee; epidemiology of skiing injury and the changing and persistent patterns of injury; the ski boot, behavior and risk factors; and one paper analyzing ski turning. These papers were presented at the Eighth International Symposium on Skiing Trauma and Safety held in Riksgräsen, Sweden, 15–21 May 1989. The meeting was sponsored by ASTM Committee F-27 on Snow Skiing and the International Society for Skiing Safety (ISSS).

ASTM undertook development of standards in skiing in 1972 when the formation of a subcommitee, F8.14, to the ASTM Committee on Sports Equipment and Facilities. The interest in skiing standards was sufficiently strong that F8.14 was uplifted to full committee status, Committee F-27, where it continues standards work under the chairmanship of L. R. Young.

In 1974, the ISSS was founded and the first symposium was held at the Laplandia Hotel in Riksgräsen, Sweden, the location of this Eighth Symposium. The ISSS provides a forum for the presentation and discussion of original findings, studies, research, observations, and experiences relating to safety in skiing in the broadest context. The participants in the symposia include both skiing professionals and amateurs whose interests concern equipment manufacture and distribution, engineering, medicine, academics, biomechanics, epidemiology, entrepreneurship, ski area operation, ski area design, ski instruction, ski patrol, and ski retail and others who enjoy skiing and want to work to improve safety in skiing. Only through regular international symposia can current ideas and progress be adequately discussed and the changing patterns of injury problems be clarified so that our common goal of making skiing a safer and more satisfying activity can be achieved.

Eight symposia were sponsored by the ISSS between 1974 and 1989, and ASTM cosponsored the fifth through the eighth. The first one was held in Riksgräsen in 1974 which is located 240 km north of the Arctic Circle. At the time, Riksgräsen was accessible only by train, but now both rail and road transportation are possibilities. The proceedings of the first symposium were published by *Orthopedic Clinics of North America* in January 1976. In April 1977, the second symposium was held in the Sierra Nevada Mountains near Granada, Spain, and the proceedings were published by University Park Press, Baltimore, 1977, in a volume titled *Skiing Safety*. The third and fourth symposia were held in Queenstown, New Zealand in July 1979 and in Bormio, Italy in June 1981. The proceedings of those symposia, titled *Skiing Safety III* and *Skiing Safety IV* were published by the Technischer Uberwachungs-Verein Bayern in Munich in 1982. These volumes can be purchased from the ISSS Secretary-Treasurer, W. Hauser, in Munich. The fifth through eighth symposia volumes were published by ASTM in the Special Technical Publication Series under the titles *Skiing Trauma and Safety; Fifth* (or *Sixth* or *Seventh* or *Eighth*) *International Symposium*. The corresponding symposia were held in Keystone, Colorado, May 1983; Naeba, Japan, April 1985; and Chamonix, France, May 1987.

The four ASTM Special Technical Publication volumes contain refereed papers presenting what is known about skiing injury. We believe that there exist no more authoritative single sources on the current thinking and standards for research and development in the skiing injury field.

The symposium in Riksgräsen and the publication of this book celebrate 15 years of ISSS dedication to reducing the risk of snow skiing injury. Throughout this short but important history the ISSS has continued to meet its goals set forth in 1974 by continuing to bring forward programs at the leading edge of the skiing injury field. Credit for the technical achievements of the ISSS, and great thanks to skiers everywhere, is due to Dr. Ejnar Eriksson of the Karolinska Hospital in Stockholm. Dr. Eriksson was the founding father of the ISSS and its President until he stepped down at the Riksgräsen symposium. His enthusiasm, leadership, and breadth of interest bound the fabric of the Society during this critical period. Great thanks is due him by the Society and skiers everywhere who have, and will in the future, benefit from the work of the Society.

The articles presented in this book represent the considered opinions of the individual authors based on their studies, investigations, and sometimes conjectures. The reader must be aware that these are research papers on topics usually under development. Each paper has been reviewed by peers of the author, meaning that the standard of the presentation and the technical work supporting the discussion are sufficiently high to merit presentation of the author's work, conclusions, and opinions. Publication does not mean that the substance and conclusions represent the opinion of the reviewers, ASTM, or the editors. Most opinions and conclusions expressed in these papers should be expected to evolve and be clarified in future work.

This volume and the former ISSS-ASTM STP symposia volumes are excellent places to start if one wants to discover what is known about skiing injury and safety. They represent the most substantial body of literature in the field.

C. D. Mote, Jr.
University of California
Berkeley, CA; editor.

Robert J. Johnson
University of Vermont
Burlington, VT; editor.

Overview

Over the last two decades studies on skiing injury have witnessed a continual growth in the number of issues being addressed and in the sophistication required to tackle them. At the beginning of injury research, design of the ski release binding was thought to be the key element in the injury problem. Today, it is widely recognized that the likelihood of injury to an individual is determined by perplexing relationships between many factors, some of which not yet identified. Some relate to design of skiing equipment to be certain, but standards of equipment maintenance and adjustment, education of skiers, design of ski boots and skiing areas, control of exposure to cold and ultraviolet, age, sex, and skiing skill, and other issues determine the likelihood of injury for the individual. Surprising to many is the realization that the biomechanical mechanisms of injury are still not very well understood. For instance, knowledge gained from two decades of study of skiing injury does not permit prediction of the forces defining the threshold of injury and even the part of the body that will be injured by them. Empirical evidence provided by injury statistics determines progress made in reducing the risk of some injuries and the needs for continued attention to others.

Skiing Injury Statistics

Studies of the statistics of skiing injury, identifying the changing patterns of serious injury, remain an indispensable part of the skiing injury field and a substantial literature continues to develop. Seven papers in this volume are devoted to *Skiing Injury Statistics*.

Young and Lee, in their update of skiing injury patterns at the Waterville Valley, New Hampshire ski area, report an injury rate of about 3 injuries per 1000 skier days and a further decline in lower leg injuries (to 5%) and a trend toward reduction in knee (to 25%) and thumb injuries (to 10%). Their data support the slightly upward relative trend in injuries to the upper body, first noted a decade ago, particularly to the head (to 10%) and the shoulder (to 6%). The types of injury are virtually unchanged over eight years with sprains to the knee and thumb accounting for more than half the total. They also note, as previously, that a high frequency of injury exist despite the release of one or both of the ski bindings. Ekeland et al. compared injury rates between Danes, Swedes, and Norwegians and concluded that notable differences in injury rates are caused by differences in skill and experience. They believe the education of skiers about the risks in skiing is probably associated with the different rates observed. This view has been expressed by Danielsson et al. in *Skiing Trauma and Safety: Fifth International Symposium* and following education campaigns in Sweden.

Johnson et al. discuss femoral fractures rates over a 15-year period and found them occurring at a constant rate of 1 per 80 000 skier days. The type of skier experiencing femoral fracture is taller and heavier, more experienced, and more often had a ski binding release and properly functioning bindings than the skier sustaining tibial fractures. They also found that fracture was usually due to bending of the femur rather than twisting and concluded that twisting femur fractures are not likely ski release binding related because the femur is about 40% stronger in torsion than the tibia. Implantation of the knee in the snow and twisting the upper body during the fall is proposed as a likely mechanism for torsional fracture of the femur.

Shealy and Miller show that sprain of the knee in alpine and cross-country skiing is the dominant injury (about 26% in both sports similar to Young and Lee) despite the differences in skiing equipment used. They believe this further supports the apparent independence of the rate of knee injury in both sports from the specifics of the release binding design. Cross-country injuries may not be as benign as many believe, they remark. Lamont reviews injury rates given by different authors over a 50-year period. He notes the rates vary from 0.8 to 9.1 skiing injuries per 1000 skier days. While the types of injuries have changed, he concludes the rate of injury of about 3.5 per 1000 skier days has not changed significantly since 1939. He urges improvement in the use of statistical methods to measure injury so that the true improvement in safety can be reliably determined. Oliver and Allman surveyed risk factors in a closed population of skiers in an Atlanta ski club and reported 24 injuries per 1000 skier days. This high number probably occurred because they accepted less severe, self-reported, injuries into their classification of the injured skier. This is similar to the 17.3 injuries per 1000 skier days reported by Hauser in *Skiing Trauma and Safety: Seventh International Symposium* (*ASTM STP 1102*). In an injury measure similar to those used by others, the Oliver and Allman rate became 3.6 injuries per 1000 skier days.

Sandegaard et al. reviewed the national skiing injury registration started by the Swedish Ski Lift Areas Organization. The registration provides a basis to trace trends in injury patterns because the organization represents about 90% of Swedish skiing areas.

The Knee

The knee has always been relatively frequently injured in skiing accidents, but for at least the past decade, injuries to the knee have generally been considered the most serious of the common skiing injuries. The factors controlling knee injuries have yet to be fully identified precisely, stimulating research on both the biomechanics of the knee and the treatment of injury. Five papers in this volume are devoted to the knee.

Mills and Hull reported results of a biomechanical study of the combined varus/valgus and torsional properties of the human knee in vivo. They showed the existence of large variations between the pain tolerance levels of subjects and decreased stiffness of the knee at 45° compared to 0° flexion. They call for methods to predict ligament strains under general loading conditions. In their second paper, Mills and Hull report on the design of a system to test the flexibility of the human knee in vivo by applying forces to the foot and studying combined twisting and valgus loading behavior of the knee. They also observed the importance of the mechanism of foot restraint to the prediction of the flexibility of the knee and recommend the foot remained unconstrained during testing. This finding confirms the results of Quinn et al. reported in *Skiing Trauma and Safety: Seventh International Symposium* on that subject. Berns et al. described the development of an automated system to test cadaver knee specimen in combinations of axial force and twisting. The test machine described can apply a wide array of loading combinations to specimen while permitting natural deformation across the joint.

Quinn and Mote present two papers concerned with the development of instrumentation for studying the knee. One reports the design of an acoustic instrument for measuring the complete displacement and rotation across the knee using no mechanical linkages. All stiction, friction, range, and alignment problems of linkage goniometer systems are eliminated in this design. The second paper presents optimal design procedures for a new class of six-degree-of-freedom dynamometers that have been found to be excellent in skiing injury research. Linearity and uncoupled output in all six components are its distinguishing features.

Two papers on the treatment of knee injuries are in the volume. Jarvinen and Kannus report that the long-term outcome from conservative treatment of Grade II tears of the anterior cruciate ligament (ACL), medial collateral ligament (MCL), or lateral ligament compartment (LAT) was acceptable, but the results for conservatively treated Grade III tears was poor in every respect. Yamagishi and Yahashi discuss a new technique for ACL repair. They believe that ACL repair using synthetic material leads to early motion, rapid recovery, and creates a stable knee immediately.

The Boot

While the principal function of the ski boot is to permit the skier to control the distribution of force between the ski and the snow, it is also an important element in the injury problem. The same mechanisms that permit the skier to move efficiently the center of force forward and backward along the ski running surface also transfer efficiently forces to the knee and bend the leg. Changes in boot design and the patterns of injury have corresponded remarkably in a number of instances. Four papers in this volume address the boot.

Two papers discuss the pain caused by pressure between the leg and boot. Schaff et al. concluded that a general measure of pain tolerance for all skiers could not be found because of large subject differences in pain tolerance. They recommended that pain avoidance required nearly uniform pressure distribution on the contact surfaces of the leg and boot and avoidance of pressure on the tibialis anterior tendon. In the second paper, Hall et al. measured the pressure generated by the tibia against the boot tongue and found that experienced skiers can generate higher pressure than inexperienced ones. Given the range of ankle flexion needed for skiing, they concluded that the inexperienced skier required a boot with greater anterior-posterior rotation for a given pressure. This may be the principal reason that beginning skiers are more successful with "softer boots," their conclusion implies. The testing of boot stiffness requires the use of human leg models for consistency and repeatability and for comparison of test results of different testers.

Early attempts to model the human leg for the purpose of testing ski boot stiffness showed that reproducing the behavior of the human was not easy. Stiffness and hysteresis behavior of a boot with a human tester flexing it and with a prosthesis flexing it can be remarkably different. Senner et al. discuss the design of a prosthetic leg that more closely reproduces the pressure measurements found in human subject tests. The size and shape of the leg and the location of the ankle joint were concluded to be key variables in the quality of the prosthesis produced. In his paper, Zucco addressed the problem of temperature control in ski boots particularly with regard to comfort and proprioception. He evaluated the thermal efficiency of ski boot designs using infrared thermography to measure temperature and both human and artificial heat sources in the boot.

Education and Behavior

The existence of a strong link between behavior and education and the likelihood of injury has long been a widely accepted truth. Improvements in education of the skiing population about injury is probably the most effective short-term means to reduce the likelihood of injury. Recently, definition and quantification of the effectiveness of such programs have risen to an area of research focus in skiing. This volume groups three papers on this topic under the heading *Education and Behavior*. Damoiseaux et al. studied how skiers could be convinced to adjust their ski release bindings properly. The most effective method found was to send information a few weeks before skiing, preferably by cassette tape, and emphasize the *fear factor*. Adjustment of the bindings was most effectively caused by a high degree of fear elicited by the message, irrespective of the time it was sent and the medium used to send it. Bouter and Kok present a theoretical framework for planning and evaluating health education for skiers. This important paper outlines the issues to be addressed by behavioral studies, pointing to the errors of omission and commission common in available studies. The paper emphasizes the necessity to pretest education material for its efficacy and the need to address behavioral issues relating to skiing injury. Bouter and Knipschild discussed a case-controlled study of Dutch skiers to investigate the importance of their behavior risk factors. They found that risk underestimation by the skier may be a risk factor.

The Ski

Finally, the volume contains one paper on the ski. Being the most fundamental and complex piece of skiing equipment, understanding the mechanics of the optimal turning ski is important to improving technology and enjoying skiing. The paper by Renshaw and Mote addresses *conceptually and quantitatively* a new theory delineating the mechanical efficiency of the skiing turn and the ease of turning for skis of general design. This is the first general theory relating ski design to the turning speed and the *skiability* of the ski. The predictions of the theory satisfy truths garnered from experience and laboratory experiments.

Conclusion

The state of the art presented in this book covers a short list of current topics in skiing research. Areas not covered include: national and international skiing standards; release binding designs and adjustments; ski poles; first aid techniques and apparatuses; safety organizations; ski area design; snow boards, mono-skis and other types of skis; injuries to the thumb, eye, spine, tibia, and ankle; competition safety practices and injuries; eye wear and clothing; fatalities; and other winter sports injuries such as impalement, collision, sunburns, and hypothermia. In short, there are no closed topics and many are not represented here. We urge all who are interested in skiing safety to contribute to increasing our knowledge in these areas. Among the common injuries the most serious is injury to the knee, as it has been for a decade. Explanations of the injury mechanisms and methods to reduce the injury remain at the conceptual stage with little solid progress. Evidence that does exist continually points to the independence of the knee injury from the skiing equipment specification, which is particularly frustrating for those trying to improve safety through advances in skiing technology.

The boot continues to receive attention for its contribution to skiing injuries. Attention to shaft stiffness and pressure distribution along the tibia move steadily towards quantification of the safety and comfort of the boot design.

A promising development in recent years has been the study of skier behavior and the understanding of risk in conjunction with quantitative evaluation of the efficacy of educational methods. Excellent opportunities exist to open some new avenues to reduce the rate or severity of injury.

The good news from all of this is that the injury rate is down to about 3 injuries per 1000 skiers per day, and the bad news is the injury rate is still about 3 injuries per 1000 skiers per day. There has been little change in this rate, possibly because we have neared the limits available with current technologies. A new idea, that will probably not be a perturbation of what we have been doing, is needed to move us off this injury rate asymptote. When this happens, it will be the most significant contribution to skiing injury prevention.

C. D. Mote, Jr.
University of California
Berkeley, CA; editor.

Robert J. Johnson
University of Vermont
Burlington, VT; editor.

The Knee

Oliver S. Mills[1] *and Maury L. Hull*[1]

Flexibility of the Human Knee as a Result of Varus/Valgus and Axial Moments in Vivo: Apparatus Design and Performance Evaluation

REFERENCE: Mills, O. S. and Hull, M. L., "**Flexibility of the Human Knee as a Result of Varus/Valgus and Axial Moments in Vivo: Apparatus Design and Performance Evaluation**," *Skiing Trauma and Safety: Eighth International Symposium, ASTM STP 1104*, C. D. Mote, Jr. and Robert J. Johnson, Eds., American Society for Testing and Materials, Philadelphia, 1991, pp. 11–34.

ABSTRACT: The contributions of this paper are twofold. One is the design and performance evaluation of new equipment to determine the rotational flexibility of the human knee in vivo. Because determining knee flexibility requires the application of external loads and the measurement of knee rotations, the new equipment consists of a load application stand and a triaxial goniometer. The triaxial goniometer noninvasively mounts to the leg and directly measures the relative three-degree-of-freedom rotations of the knee. The goniometer incorporates several unique design features that enhance measurement accuracy. The load stand applies pure varus/valgus and external/internal axial moments either individually or in combination through the use of motors controlled by the test subject. Unique to this design are features that enable the application of moments to the knee to minimize shear forces. Other unique design features permit the stand to control hip and knee flexion angles, muscle contraction, and axial loading. To assess the accuracy with which rotations are measured during experiments, three tests were conducted with the equipment. One test evaluated the inherent accuracy of the goniometer, a second test assessed the potential for goniometer slippage during loading, and a third test explored the effect of goniometer mounting on the repeatability of results. A special verification apparatus facilitated evaluation of goniometer inherent accuracy.

A second contribution of the paper is an investigation of the effect of foot constraints (that is, boundary conditions) on flexibility results. To make this investigation, three subjects were tested with the knee at 15° flexion. Results revealed large differences in flexibility between constraining the foot in both external/internal and varus/valgus rotations and permitting the foot to rotate freely in the direction not being loaded. Further, constraint moments as high as 23 Nm were also recorded. These results emphasize that to obtain accurate flexibility results for isolated loads, the foot must be unconstrained by the loading apparatus.

KEY WORDS: goniometer, flexibility, knee, human, varus/valgus moment, axial moment

Epidemiology studies on injuries incurred in Alpine skiing accidents indicate that the ligamentous structures of the knee are the most injury prone components of the musculoskeletal system, constituting approximately 25% of the total number of injuries [*1–4*]. Furthermore, of the four primary ligaments of the knee, the medial collateral ligament (MCL) or the anterior cruciate ligament (ACL) or both are injured ten times more often

[1]Research assistant and professor, respectively, Department of Mechanical Engineering, University of California, Davis, CA 95616.

than either the lateral collateral ligament (LCL) or the posterior cruciate ligament (PCL) [*1,3*]. Focusing on the two ligaments injured most often, two distinct types of injury occur. The first is isolated injury to the ACL and the second is injury to the MCL sometimes with accompanying injury to the ACL. Of interest in this research is the second type of injury which will be designated as an MCL/ACL injury. Through various methods of postaccident analysis, the type of fall most commonly responsible for the second type of injury has been identified as a forward-twisting type fall where the injured leg is externally rotated by means of the leverage of the ski [*1,5*]. During this type of fall, both an external axial moment and a valgus moment would be transmitted by the knee thus implicating these loads acting in combination as a cause of MCL/ACL knee injuries [*1,5,6*].

Previous research on ligament function confirms the role that external axial and valgus moments play in causing MCL/ACL injuries. Ligament sectioning studies have shown that the MCL supports primarily valgus moments [*7–9*] and both internal and external axial moments [*7,10*]. With the MCL intact, the ACL supports anterior tibial forces [*11–13*], hyperextensive moments [*14*], and possibly internal axial moments [*15–17*]. Although the ACL does not support either valgus or external axial moments with the MCL intact, the ACL supports these loads once the MCL is damaged and the knee is flexed [*18*].

Recognizing that axial and varus/valgus moments are the cause of many knee injuries, it is useful to study how the knee displaces under the action of these two loads to understand

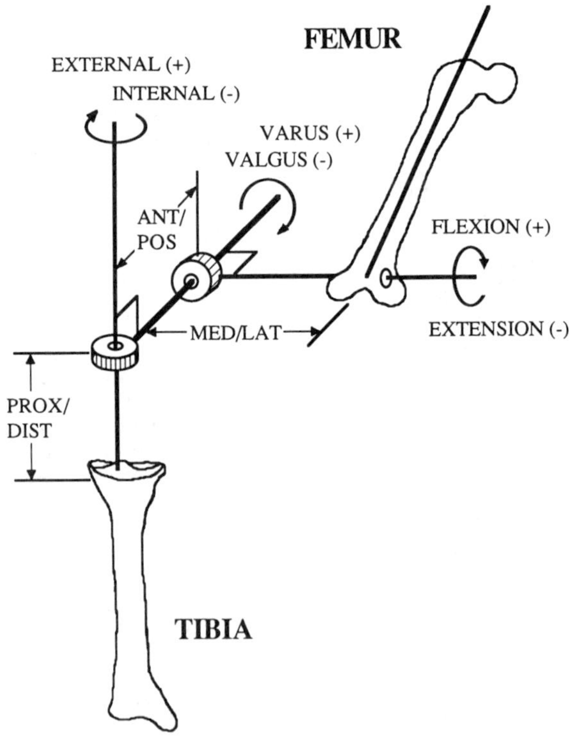

FIG. 1—*The joint coordinate system and an anterior view of the right femur and tibia. The external/internal and flexion/extension rotational axes are fixed to the tibia and femur, respectively, while the varus/valgus rotational axis is fixed to neither bone. Rather the varus/valgus rotational axis floats between and is perpendicular to the remaining two axes.*

better the mechanisms that lead to knee injury. Many previous research efforts have measured rotational displacements both in vitro and in vivo for either load applied singly. These studies have been valuable in identifying variables that affect knee moment-rotation relations. These variables include axial loading (that is, joint compression) [*10,11,19,20*], knee flexion angle [*7,9,21–25*], hip flexion angle [*26*], and muscle contraction [*27–30*]. Lacking from any previous study, however, is a quantitative assessment of how application of the two moments in combination affects knee moment-rotation relations.

Beyond the variables affecting knee moment-rotation relations noted above, an additional variable that must be considered is loading rate. The viscoelastic property of ligament tissue is well known [*31*]. Because knee injuries in skiing undoubtedly occur during situations in which the loading rate is such that this property becomes a factor, there is a need to study how loading rate affects joint displacements. However, epidemiology studies have documented that beginning skiers are the group at greatest risk as far as knee injuries are concerned [*32,33*]. Presumably because of the slower skiing speeds, injury often occurs under loading rates that may be considered quasi-static. Accordingly, studies conducted at these loading rates are the more immediate concern.

With combined varus/valgus and axial moments thought to cause MCL/ACL knee injuries in skiing and no previous study having assessed how these loads applied in combination affect knee rotations, the general objective of this research was to apply these two moments, both individually and in combination, to the knees of human test subjects in vivo and measure the resulting knee rotations. To meet this general objective, three experimental apparatus were developed: an electrogoniometer to measure triaxial rotations between the tibia and femur, a verification apparatus to assess inherent goniometer error, and a load application stand to apply either single or combination moments in vivo. This paper describes the experimental apparatus and presents results of tests undertaken both to assess apparatus performance and to examine the effect of boundary conditions on flexibility results. Results of tests undertaken to quantify flexibility under both single and combination moments are described in a second article.

Methods

Goniometer

Grood and Suntay [*34*] presented the most appropriate coordinate system on which to base our goniometer design. The coordinate system is modeled as a four-bar kinematic chain (Fig. 1) with the linkages interconnected by cylindrical joints, which translate along and rotate around a specific axis. Two of the axes are fixed; one each to the tibia and the femur with the external(+)/internal(−) axis aligning with the long axis of the tibia and the flexion(+)/extension(−) axis traversing through both femoral condyles. The third or varus(+)/valgus(−) axis is fixed to neither bone but rather is the common perpendicular to the other axes. This axis "floats" in relation to both the external(+)/internal(−) and flexion(+)/extension(−) axes depending on tibia-femur displacement. Any relative translation occurs along the rotational axes described above. The benefits of this coordinate system are twofold. The first is that the medically recognized terms commonly used to define joint motion can describe knee rotations and translations within the system. The second is that the joint displacements are obtained independent of the order in which the rotations occur.

Figures 2 and 3 show the goniometer used for the present research. Three miniature potentiometers (Spectrol, 20K, 0.3° resolution), calibrated for linearity and range of motion, measure the relative joint rotations. Because the potentiometers are not collinear with the joint axes of rotation, linkages were necessary to decouple translations between the tibial and femoral attachment clamps. A specially designed dual-parallelogram linkage, inserted

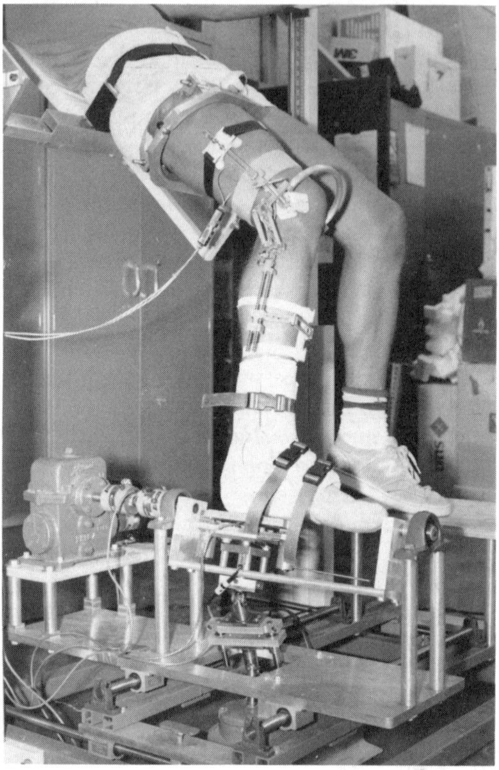

FIG. 2—*The triaxial goniometer attached to a test subject. Note the dual-parallelogram linkage and the four-point goniometer attachment to the leg. The test subject is in 60° knee flexion with the knee under combination internal axial and valgus moments. The linkage that incorporates universal joints to maintain the orientation of the axial moment loading axis with the tibia is also pictured.*

between the goniometer's flexion/extension and varus/valgus rotational axes, specifically decouples medial/lateral and anterior/posterior translations. The linkage consists of four parallel bars pinned to two mutually perpendicular yokes on both the linkage's distal and proximal ends. To decouple distal/proximal translation and transmit the rotations from the tibial attachment clamp to the dual-parallelogram linkage, two parallel hardened-steel rods each slide through two miniature linear ball bearings. This goniometer design uniquely describes the tibial-femoral orientation without having to specify the order in which rotations occur. The total weight of the goniometer is 0.5 kg.

Of critical importance in obtaining accurate results is the method of externally attaching the goniometer to the bony references. Rigidity of fixation is necessary if the goniometer is to follow bone motion while minimizing skin compliance errors. A total of four clamps provide fixation to the right leg—one on the tibia and three on the femur. The tibial clamp follows the design of Hull and Johnson [*35*] and is a C-shaped orthoplast mold contoured to the medial crest. It is kept in place by two Velcro bands, which wrap around the shank. By tightening the bands, the mold snugly clamps around the tibia, thereby preventing medial/lateral and distal/proximal motion of the clamp. An aluminum plate mounted flush with the clamp maintains clamp rigidity as the straps are tightened.

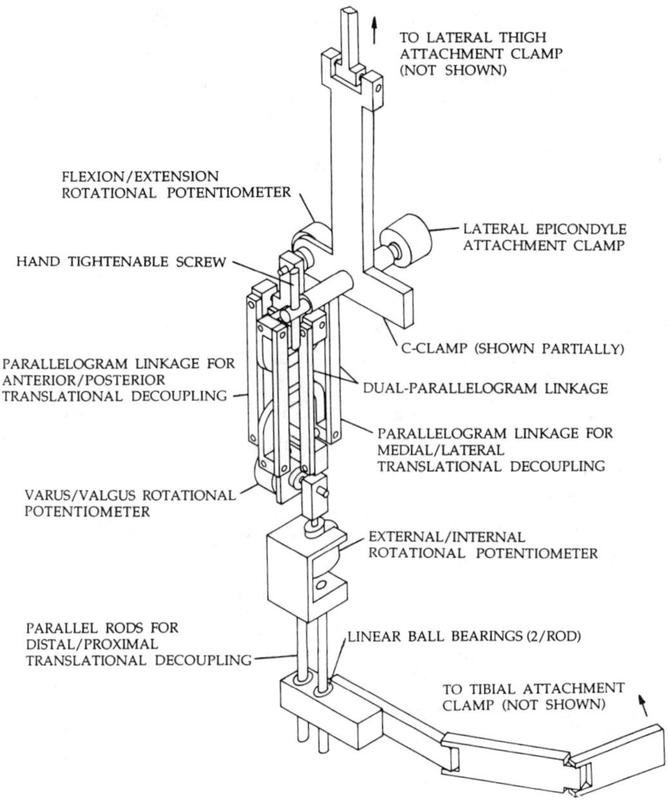

FIG. 3—*Diagram of the triaxial goniometer. Three potentiometers measure rotations independent of sequence according to the coordinate system of Grood and Suntay* [34]. *Because the rotation axes of the goniometer do not lie along those of the adopted coordinate system for the joint, various linkages are necessary to decouple translations from potentiometer rotations. The dual parallelogram linkage provides for medial/lateral and anterior/posterior translations while the parallel rods sliding in linear bearings give proximal/distal decoupling.*

Femoral fixation is at the medial epicondyle, the lateral epicondyle, and the lateral thigh. The medial femoral clamp is a contoured rubber cup fitted to the unique shape of the medial epicondyle. A foam rubber pad placed inside the cup distributes the clamping force on the skin surface, thus improving test subject comfort. The lateral epicondyle clamp is an orthoplast cup and attaches to the end of a spherical bearing to ensure that it conforms to the bony prominences of the lateral epicondyle. An aluminum C-clamp then circles the knee, and a tightenable screw pushes the medial and lateral clamps against the epicondyles. The fourth clamp attaches to the lateral side of the thigh and provides rotary stability of the C-clamp by pressing an orthoplast U-shaped mold against the thigh by way of a Velcro® band.

Because the goniometer axes are aligned with the bone clamps, the alignment of the goniometer axes with the knee is dictated by the bony landmarks to which the clamps attach. The flexion/extension axis of the goniometer is fixed with respect to the femoral clamp and is parallel to a line passing through the center of both attachment clamps. Because the femoral attachment clamps are placed over the center of each condyle, the goniometer measures flexion/extension as rotations about an axis that passes through the centers of the medial and lateral epicondyles. The external/internal axial rotation axis of the goniometer is fixed with respect to the tibial clamp. Because the clamp fits over the medial surface in the middle third of the tibia, the axis lies in the plane of the medial surface. The orientation of the axis in this plane follows the orientation of the anterior and medial borders because the clamp is contoured to fit around these borders.

Verification Apparatus

To assess rotational accuracy, and rotational and translational decoupling, a goniometer verification apparatus was constructed. The apparatus consists of a Plexiglas® support stand (Fig. 4) to which the remainder of the verification hardware attaches. Two aluminum rods, representing the tibia and the femur, provide fixation points for the distal and proximal ends of the goniometer. For ease of attachment to the apparatus, the goniometer's fixation clamps, normally used for mounting the goniometer to the soft tissues around the knee, are removed. Rotations and translations of the apparatus are through manual movement of the lower aluminum rod.

To provide the six goniometer motions, the apparatus uses three instrumented modules. Two of the three modules incorporate a single miniature rotary potentiometer (Spectrol,

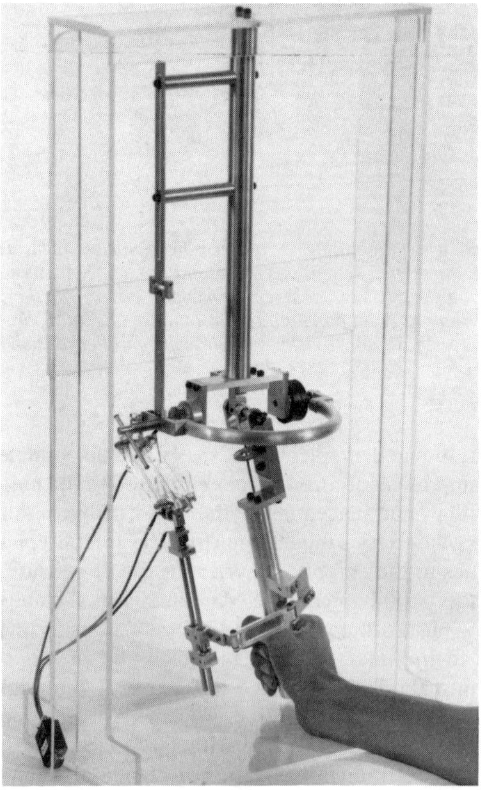

FIG. 4—*The goniometer verification apparatus with varus/valgus module and goniometer. The tibial and femoral attachment clamps were removed for verification. Three different modules offer six-degree-of-freedom displacements, thereby enabling both direct rotational and cross-coupling errors to be assessed.*

20K, 0.3° resolution) to measure a single rotation around a fixed axis. One module is for external/internal rotation while the other is for both flexion/extension and varus/valgus rotations. By rotating the latter module 90°, a single piece of hardware provides for two goniometer rotations. Because the rotation modules must support the weight of both the lower aluminum rod and the distal end of the goniometer, miniature bearings support the load while the potentiometer outputs the resulting rotation. Because of the complexity in including all three rotations into one module, assessment of goniometer rotations in combination was not possible. The translational module, however, provides for translations in all three directions. Three linear potentiometers (ETI Systems, 10K, infinite resolution), each with 1.0 in. (2.54 cm) of linear travel are arranged mutually perpendicular to each other such that a single translation does not affect the other two. The translation module design incorporates Delrin bushings, which slide on parallel rods and prevent the potentiometers from supporting any loads. This module is useful in assessing the degree to which a translation affects the rotational outputs. All potentiometers were calibrated for linearity and range of motion.

Instrumented Load Stand

The load stand (Fig. 5) consists of a tubular steel frame, which completely supports the load-application hardware and test subject. Two worm gear reducer-gearmotor combinations

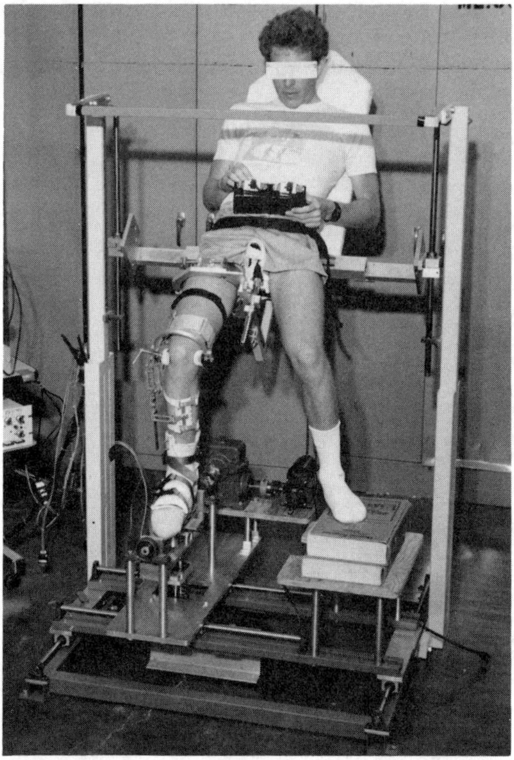

FIG. 5—*The load stand, configured for application of combination moments, with test subject in 60° knee flexion. The motor controller that the test subject is holding permits the test subject to control both magnitude and direction of the applied load.*

(Dayton) provide the necessary torque levels while silicon-controlled rectifier (SCR) controllers (Dayton), modified for direction control, vary load direction and speed. Because the gear motors experience load changes throughout a complete loading cycle, the SCR controllers provide the additional benefit of maintaining a constant output shaft speed independent of the load. Furthermore, the controllers are hand-held, thus enabling the test subject to control loading levels during the experiment. Maximum output rotation rate for each gear reducer is approximately 2 rpm.

The test subject is supported by a bicycle seat, a hip belt, and a padded backrest. The bicycle seat and backrest support the test subject's weight such that any axial force on the tibia can be controlled. Furthermore, a Velcro belt, which crosses over the anterior-superior iliac spines, prevents the hip from rotating relative to the backrest. The entire test subject support apparatus rotates back around an axis that passes through the greater trochanters of each femur. Absolute back angle can then be varied from 0 to 90° with respect to vertical in increments of 22.5°. The purpose of varying the orientation of the torso is to maintain constant hip flexion angle as knee flexion is varied.

In addition to rotating back, the entire support apparatus can translate vertically on hardened steel shafts and linear ball bearings. Such a feature serves two purposes. The first is that by raising and lowering shaft clamps located beneath the bearings, different test subject heights can be accommodated. Furthermore, by fine tuning the seat height, the test subject can then apply different levels of axial force on the tibia. The second purpose is that lowering the test subject's torso also varies knee flexion angle. To vary knee flexion angle, the entire loading carriage also translates anteriorly/posteriorly (Fig. 6). The combination of these two hardware motions allows knee flexion angle to range from 0 to 90°. As a safety feature, a locking mechanism prevents inadvertent movement of the loading

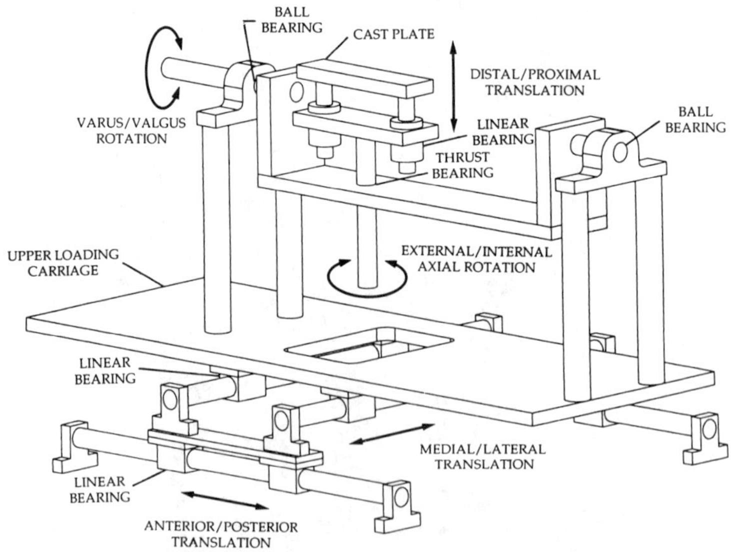

FIG. 6—*The degrees of freedom offered by the load stand. To ensure the absence of coupled loads at the knee, the load stand allows the foot five degrees of freedom, three translations and two rotations (axial and varus/valgus). The foot is constrained from flexing relative to the tibia by a cast (not shown). This constraint is necessary to maintain the knee flexion angle.*

carriage when the test subject is climbing onto the stand. Once the test subject is seated, the carriage is unlocked.

To apply pure moments while minimizing unwanted coupled loads, the foot is connected to the load stand through a system of shafts, which permits five degrees of freedom, three translations, and two rotations (see Fig. 6). The foot is held in a fiberglass cast, which, in turn, is bolted to a cast plate that translates proximally/distally by means of two rods traveling in linear bearings. These linear bearings are housed in a plate that rotates internally/externally by means of the axial moment spindle supported by a thrust bearing. The plate that contains the thrust bearing is supported at either end by two ball bearings, thus offering varus/valgus rotation. Called the upper loading carriage, this whole assembly is then supported by linear bearings translating medially/laterally along shafts, and this, in turn, is supported by linear bearings translating anteriorly/posteriorly along shafts. The anterior/posterior translational degree of freedom has sufficient travel to permit adjustment of knee flexion angle as noted above.

The load stand applies a pure varus/valgus moment as though the entire leg is a cantilever beam. The elevation of the loading axis is approximately at the base of the foot, and the orientation is fixed, being directed anteriorly/posteriorly. Because without muscle contraction the hip is a spherical joint with no moment support capability, the cantilever beam boundary condition is provided by a circular thigh support (see Fig. 2). This support consists of curved and padded clamps that tighten around the thigh to reduce abduction/adduction. Despite these clamps, some degree of abduction/adduction of the thigh occurs as does varus/valgus angulation of the tibia. Accordingly, the foot both rotates and translates medially/laterally. Because the varus/valgus axis remains fixed through the base of the foot, the varus/valgus gear reducer-gearmotor assembly is attached to the upper loading carriage so that it translates with the foot as well.

To apply an axial moment that follows the joint coordinate system, the axial moment axis must track the long axis of the tibia as the stand simultaneously applies a varus/valgus moment. To accomplish this, the axial moment gear reducer-gearmotor assembly is fixed to the upper loading carriage so that this assembly translates with the carriage as varus/valgus loading is applied. The axial moment gear reducer-gearmotor assembly does not rotate with the foot as the tibia assumes some degree of varus/valgus angulation, however, so that a specially designed linkage incorporating universal joints provides a flexible axis to maintain the parallel alignment of the axial moment axis with the tibial long axis.

To prevent the tibia from flexing out of line with the applied moment, thereby maintaining application of moments with the axes of the joint coordinate system, a removable fiberglass cast supported the ankle while fixing it at 90°. The cast required two halves, which were clamped together around the ankle with buckles and straps. Because the test subjects had different foot sizes, an orthopedist formed casts around two persons—one with a small foot and the other with a large one. These two casts enabled the subsequent testing of all subjects through the use of custom-fitted rubber orthotics. Furthermore, each cast had two lengths through the use of a cast extension—a tall one with a height of 41 cm and a short one with a height of 24 cm. The tall cast was necessary to apply varus/valgus moments to the test subject and not cause discomfort. Because the tall cast possibly caused skin shear to the tibial clamp under axial moments, the shorter cast was used for axial moment and combined loading experiments. Assuming no varus/valgus angulation of the tibia, an added benefit of fixing the ankle at 90° is that any axial force the test subject applies will be along the axis of the tibia and, hence, a pure force component (see Fig. 1 of joint coordinate system). This is in contrast to weight bearing, which induces multiple forces at the knee such as when someone gets into a squatting position.

Three strain gage transducers measured the two applied moments and the axial force.

The torsional transducers each consist of a steel shaft mounted with strain gages for measuring the moments. In the case of the axial moment transducer, bearings mounted on either side of the axial moment spindle isolate the shaft from both axial forces and varus/valgus moments. The varus/valgus moment transducer directly connects the gear reducer to the loading shaft. An accuracy check revealed average absolute errors of 0.3 and 0.4 Nm for the axial moment and varus/valgus moment transducers, respectively. The axial load transducer is more sophisticated in design and is located directly below the fiberglass cast. This transducer relies on mechanical decoupling to prevent cross-sensitivity between the desired axial force measurement and the two applied moments. For a pure axial force, average absolute error was 1.0 N. A first-order, least squares fit for the calibration results was calculated for each transducer and included in the data acquisition program for direct conversion of voltage to moments.

Data Acquisition

The data acquisition equipment for the goniometer, verification apparatus, and instrumented load stand includes a Hewlett-Packard Vectra microcomputer and a MetraByte DASH16(12 bit) data acquisition card. The system sampled the three potentiometer and three strain gage channels at 10 Hz using MetraByte's burst data acquisition mode. Because loading was quasistatic, a 10-Hz sampling rate was adequate. Signal conditioning modules (Validyne) amplified the strain gage signals to a level appropriate for the data acquisition system. The data were then digitally filtered using a first-order, low-pass filter.

Tests

A number of sources of variability are inherent in flexibility measurements of the knee using live subjects. These sources fall into one of four categories: (1) inherent to the goniometer, (2) alignment of the goniometer with respect to bony prominences, (3) changing joint properties, and (4) methods of load application. Two sources fall into the goniometer alignment category. One source is the change in goniometer alignment that might occur between cycles in the same trial due to soft tissue movement. As discussed earlier, careful consideration was given to the design of clamps to minimize clamp shifting due to soft tissue motion. But unless the two ends of the goniometer are surgically fixed to the bone, the potential for movement exists. The other source is differences in alignment of the goniometer between trials. Variability is possible if the various clamps are not positioned on the bones identically each time the goniometer is attached. The variability inherent to the goniometer was evaluated using the load verification apparatus. To assess the variability among cycles, among trials, and among methods of load application, three separate tests were conducted.

To assess the variability among cycles in a trial, the first test involved individually applying several cycles of axial and varus/valgus moments at both 15 and 60° knee flexion. Because the purpose behind this test was to determine if the orientation of the goniometer changes over consecutive load cycles, the knee was first preconditioned to reduce this source of variability. As noted above, any change in goniometer orientation would then manifest as differences between individual flexibility curves. Because all tests started with either external axial or varus moments, a second purpose of the cycling tests was to assess the differences in starting with either internal axial or valgus moments. The cycling test involved one subject.

To assess variability among trials, the second test involved first mounting the goniometer and axially cycling the test subject's leg externally and internally through ±20 Nm. The goniometer was then removed from the test subject and remounted with the axial load test cycle repeated. Any differences in the orientation of the goniometer relative to the bony landmarks to which the clamps attach would appear as differences in the flexibility curves. Testing involved one subject.

To quantify any variability either between trials or between cycles, the data over the two load cycles were subjected to a two-sided paired *t* test. Pairs were formed by computing the difference between absolute rotations at equivalent loads for both the loading and unloading portions of the cycle over the full cycle. The criterion for determining whether the rotations were significantly different was a level of significance of 0.05.

The final test sought to assess the effect of boundary conditions on the flexibility results of three test subjects. In the present research, boundary conditions refer to the method of constraining the foot in the load stand during application of moments. Note that "constrained" is with both motors connected whereas "unconstrained" is with only one motor connected, thereby allowing freedom of foot rotation in the remaining motion. Because of the gear-reducer drive, foot movement is prevented if the motor is connected. Because one objective of the present research was to prevent multiple loads from being transmitted to the knee, this study sought to assess if constraining the foot induces large coupled loads, hence altering the flexibility results over the results obtained in the pure moment tests. Therefore, testing included individually cycling both axial and varus/valgus moments to three test subjects at 15° knee flexion with both motors connected and with one motor connected. If the boundary conditions affected the results, then differences in the flexibility curves would be evident between the two sets of boundary conditions.

The protocol for obtaining the flexibility results in the preliminary tests called for three healthy male test subjects with no history of problems to their right knee. (See Table 2*a* for test subject data.) The height of the bicycle seat was adjusted for each test subject such that the leg was suspended from the hip in the gravity field. When the leg was suspended, the angle naturally assumed by the knee was about 15° flexion measured from full extension. Note that hip flexion angle throughout all tests was kept at 0° and the muscles were quiescent. Except for the boundary condition comparison tests, the foot was unconstrained. Before recording data, the test subject operated the hand-held motor controllers to adjust both the limits of loading and the time to complete a full load cycle. This served both to familiarize the subject with the equipment operation and to precondition the knee. Limits of loading were ± 60 Nm for varus/valgus moments and ± 20 Nm for external/internal axial moments with a maximum time span of 60 s per complete load cycle. Time spans for the cycling tests, however, were 30 s per load cycle. Data were collected for two trials of each type of test. Goniometer offsets were taken both before and after each trial with the test subject relaxed and the foot unloaded.

To check that the muscles were quiescent during the tests in which data were recorded, each subject was checked for his ability to maintain relaxation in six major muscles crossing the knee. To perform this check, surface electromyograms were recorded from both heads of the gastrocnemius, the medial and lateral vastii, and the medial and lateral hamstrings during preliminary tests where the foot was unconstrained. Only slight activity was evident in a single but different muscle for each of the three subjects. Activity occurred only in the region near maximum loading and was 3 to 4% for two subjects and 8 to 10% for one subject of that activity level corresponding to maximum voluntary contraction.

Results

Goniometer Error Assessment

The verification apparatus permitted assessment of goniometer rotational accuracy and translational and rotational coupling errors. Because of rotational coupling, all of the goniometer rotations required error correction. The goniometer data were corrected by subtracting from the primary rotation a linear function of primary rotation versus coupled error. Table 1 presents the average and maximum errors obtained after correction from each of the rotational modules and the maximum coupling errors obtained from the translational module. Because of the complexities involved in determining an absolute error that encompasses all combinations of goniometer rotation and translation, only the errors for single apparatus input rotations and translations have been tabulated.

Table 1*a* presents the direct sensitivities for each of the three goniometer rotations. Even though the goniometer can displace more than the values listed, the "limits of rotation" represent the range of rotation over which the knee was expected to displace during flexibility experiments. Note that during all rotation verification tests, only single input rotations were permitted while the remaining rotations and translations were fixed. The "average absolute error" is the absolute value of all errors averaged over a complete rotation cycle. The "maximum positive error" and the "maximum negative error" are then the extremes of error for the input rotations. From the table, flexion/extension has the least error while varus/valgus and external/internal rotations have more.

Table 1*b* tabulates the goniometer rotational coupling errors for each of the three input rotations. Rotational coupling error reflects the amount of coupled motion that the goniometer undergoes for single rotation inputs. As with direct rotation errors, the table gives both average and maximum errors observed for the limits of rotation listed in Table 1*a*. Here, flexion/extension presented the least amount of coupled rotation while external/internal rotation yielded the largest rotational coupling. For instance, ±25° external/internal input rotation resulted in a maximum apparent output rotation of ±1.5° for flexion/extension. Because, during flexibility experiments, knowing flexion angles within ±3° is acceptable, the maximum coupled flexion/extension rotation is within the tolerance.

Finally, Table 1*c* is the coupling of goniometer outputs to ±5 mm translation in three directions. The purpose of conducting the translation tests was to assess the ability of the dual-parallelogram linkage to decouple translations in three mutually orthogonal directions. The table shows that with two exceptions changes in goniometer outputs because of ±5 mm translations are within the ±0.15° uncertainty caused by the 0.3° resolution of the potentiometers.

TABLE 1*a*—*Goniometer direct rotation errors for a single input rotation.*

Input Rotation	Limits of Input Rotation		Average Absolute Error	Maximum Positive Error	Maximum Negative Error
	Minimum	Maximum			
Flex./Extension	-0°	+60°	±0.2°	+0.5°	-0.1°
Varus/Valgus	-10°	+10°	±0.5°	+0.7°	-0.7°
Ext./Internal	-25°	+25°	±0.5°	+0.3°	-0.9°

TABLE 1*b*—*Goniometer rotational coupling for a single input rotation.*

Input Rotation	Ave. Apparent Output Rotation		Max. Apparent Output Rotation	
	Varus/Valgus	Ext./Internal	Varus/Valgus	Ext./Internal
Flex./Extension	±0.1°	±0.2°	±0.3°	±0.4°
	Flex./Extension	Ext./Internal	Flex./Extension	Ext./Internal
Varus/Valgus	±0.2°	±0.2°	±0.4°	±0.3°
	Flex./Extension	Varus/Valgus	Flex./Extension	Varus/Valgus
Ext./Internal	±0.5°	±0.3°	±1.5°	±0.5°

TABLE 1*c*—*Goniometer translational coupling for a single ±5-mm input translation.*

Input Translation	Maximum Apparent Output Rotation		
	Flex./Extension	Varus/Valgus	Ext./Internal
Medial/Lateral	±0.1°	±0.1°	±0.2°
Anterior/Posterior	±0.3°	±0.1°	±0.1°
Distal/Proximal	±0.1°	±0.1°	±0.1°

Repeatability in Flexibility Results

An example plot showing internal/external axial rotation for consecutive cycles of internal/external axial moment loads with the knee at both 15 and 60° flexion is shown in Fig. 7. The results of the paired *t* tests indicated that the null hypothesis could not be accepted at 15° flexion but could be accepted at 60° flexion. Thus, the average difference between the two curves at 15° flexion is significantly different from 0°. The difference is small, however; the results for 15° flexion are repeatable to within 0.40°. The small difference at 15° flexion and the lack of any significant difference at 60° flexion indicate that the orientation of the goniometer relative to the bony prominences did not change permanently as a result of soft tissue movement during a load cycle.

An example plot showing the repeatability in flexibility between trials where the goniometer was remounted is given in Fig. 8. As for the repeatability between cycles at 15° knee flexion, the null hypothesis could not be accepted. In the case of the data in Fig. 8, the two curves are repeatable to within 1.0°. Inasmuch as this difference is less than 5% of full scale rotations, it may be concluded that the goniometer can, in fact, be oriented similarly each time it is mounted on a particular subject.

Boundary Conditions

Table 2 tabulates and Figs. 9 and 10 illustrate the results for the boundary condition tests with both motors connected versus one motor connected. Table 2*a* and *b* tabulate both the primary and coupled rotations for applied varus/valgus and external/internal axial moments, respectively. The tables also include the coupled reaction moments that the varus/valgus and axial moment transducers recorded. Figures 9 and 10 show example plots of both primary and coupled rotations, respectively, for constrained versus unconstrained boundary conditions. Note that the primary and coupled rotations as well as the coupled moments are determined at ± 60 Nm of applied varus/valgus or ± 20 Nm of applied external/internal axial moments. The rotations at these loading limits are defined as terminal rotations (TR). Both

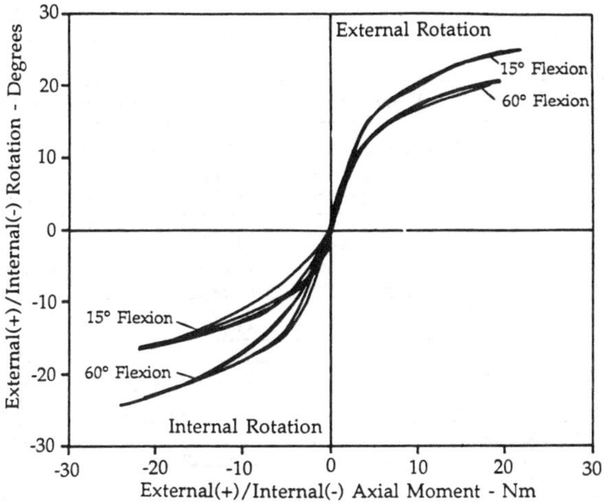

FIG. 7—*The results indicating repeatability in flexibility between successive cycles. The knee was preconditioned before the tests. Results of a paired t-test indicate average differences for external/internal axial rotations of less than 0.40°. Cycle-to-cycle repeatability for varus/valgus rotations was also determined with average differences of less than 0.30°. Results shown are for Test Subject 2.*

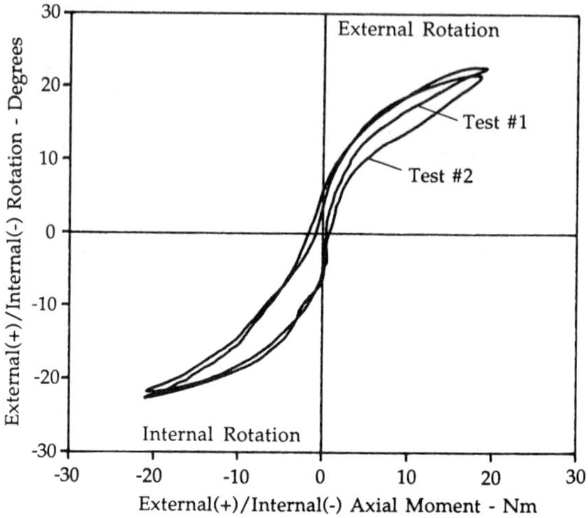

FIG. 8—*The results of goniometer placement tests for a pure axial moment with the test subject in 15° knee flexion. Based on the results of a paired t-test, the average differences between successive mountings of the goniometer are less than 1.0°. Results shown are for Test Subject 1.*

TABLE 2*a*—*The effect of applied varus/valgus moment on primary and coupled rotations at 0° knee flexion.*

		Applied Varus Moment			Applied Valgus Moment		
Test Subject #	Load Case	Primary Varus TR (°) *	Coupled Ext./Int. Rotation (°)	Coupled Ext./Int. Moment (Nm)	Primary Valgus TD (°) *	Coupled Ext./Int. Rotation (°)	Coupled Ext./Int. Moment (Nm)
1	Unconstrained	4.5	1.3	• •	-4.3	-4.4	• •
Age: 24 years	Constrained	6.5	-1.4	-2.6	-2.0	4.9	2.6
Height: 1.83 m	*% Difference*	*44.4*	*-207.7*	• •	*-53.5*	*-211.4*	• •
Weight: 779 N							
2	Unconstrained	9.0	-4.0	• •	-3.7	-0.7	• •
Age: 41 years	Constrained	5.9	-2.4	-10.0	-5.5	10.1	-0.1
Height: 1.75 m	*% Difference*	*-34.4*	*-40.0*	• •	*48.6*	*-1542.9*	• •
Weight: 734 N							
3	Unconstrained	7.6	-5.7	• •	-6.4	1.7	• •
Age: 24 years	Constrained	9.6	-4.8	-10.0	-6.5	13.7	1.4
Height: 1.73 m	*% Difference*	*26.3*	*-15.8*	• •	*1.6*	*705.9*	• •
Weight: 645 N							

TABLE 2*b*—*The effect of applied external/internal axial moment on primary and coupled rotations at 0° knee flexion.*

		Applied External Axial Moment			Applied Internal Axial Moment		
Test Subject #	Load Case	Primary External TR (°) *	Coupled Varus/Valgus Rotation (°)	Coupled Varus/Valgus Moment (Nm)	Primary Internal TR (°) *	Coupled Varus/Valgus Rotation (°)	Coupled Varus/Valgus Moment (Nm)
1	Unconstrained	26.8	7.0	• •	-16.6	-2.7	• •
	Constrained	23.7	4.5	-18.0	-19.5	-1.0	0.5
	% Difference	*-11.6*	*-35.7*	• •	*17.5*	*-63.0*	• •
2	Unconstrained	25.3	2.3	• •	-15.6	-0.8	• •
	Constrained	33.2	2.0	-16.0	-17.4	-0.2	12.3
	% Difference	*31.2*	*-13.0*	• •	*11.5*	*-75.0*	• •
3	Unconstrained	25.6	• •	• •	-25.2	• •	• •
	Constrained	35.0	1.3	-13.0	-31.0	-2.9	23.0
	% Difference	*36.7*	• •	• •	*23.0*	• •	• •

* TR - Terminal Rotation - determined at ±20 Nm external/internal axial and ±60 Nm varus/valgus moments

** Data values either not available or not practical to calculate

Rotation and Moment Sign Conventions: Varus(+)/Valgus(-) and External(+)/Internal(-)

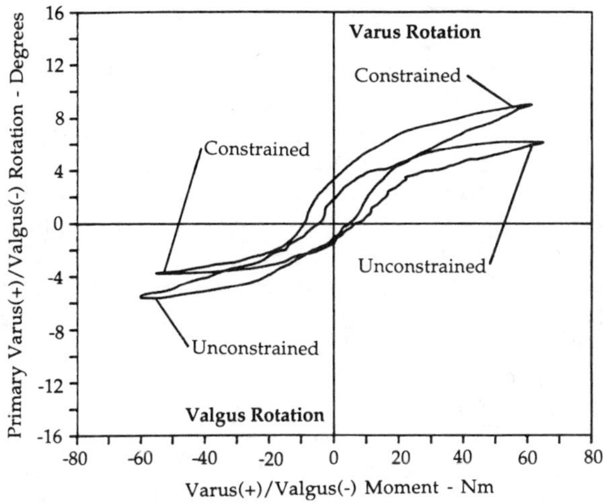

FIG. 9—*The effect of boundary conditions on primary varus/valgus rotations for an applied varus/valgus moment. Differences in flexibility between constrained and unconstrained loading were large indicating that the method of constraining the foot during loading affects the flexibility results. To apply pure varus/valgus moments, the foot must be unconstrained. Results shown are for test Subject 2 in 15° knee flexion.*

the tables and the figures reveal that large differences exist between constrained and unconstrained flexibilities.

In comparing primary varus/valgus rotations for constrained versus unconstrained flexibility, no overall increasing or decreasing trends between the two boundary conditions were observed in either load direction. Nonetheless, absolute differences in TR as great as 3.1°

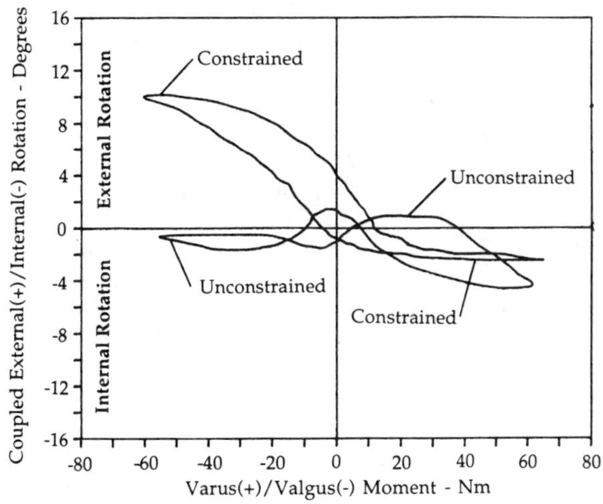

FIG. 10—*The effect of boundary conditions on the coupled external/internal rotations for an applied varus/valgus moment. The directions of the coupled external/internal rotations under constrained boundary conditions were typical for all test subjects; an applied varus moment led to a coupled internal rotation and an applied valgus moment led to a coupled external rotation. For unconstrained boundary conditions, however, the directions of the coupled rotations were not consistent. Results shown are for test Subject 2 in 15° flexion.*

were obtained. Similarly, in external/internal rotation for an axial moment, the relative differences in TR were also large with a maximum absolute difference of 9.4° observed. With the exception of external rotation for test Subject 1, the general trend is for the constrained loading condition to increase external/internal rotation over external/internal rotation in the unconstrained case. Clearly, the method of applying moments can have a large effect on the primary flexibility results.

In addition to the primary rotations, Table 2*a* and *b* also tabulate the coupled rotations for each of the three test subjects. For varus/valgus loading and constrained external/internal rotation, a repeatable and consistent pattern prevailed for all three test subjects: an applied varus moment led to a small coupled internal rotation and an applied valgus moment led to a relatively larger coupled external rotation. With unconstrained loading, however, no consistent and repeatable pattern of coupled external/internal rotation was observed among the three test subjects. Furthermore, the maximum coupled external/internal rotation in the unconstrained case did not, for the most part, occur at the maximum applied varus/valgus moment. On the other hand, for axial loading, a repeatable and consistent pattern prevailed for all test subjects under both constrained and unconstrained varus/valgus rotation: an applied external axial moment led to a coupled varus rotation and an applied internal axial moment led to a coupled valgus rotation. Here, the maximum rotation occurred at the maximum applied moment. In general, the coupled varus/valgus rotations were smaller with the constrained boundary condition. In the table, note that a reversal in coupled rotations occurred between varus/valgus and axial moments: valgus moments led to coupled external rotations, but external axial moments led to coupled varus rotations.

Tables 2*a* and *b* also present the coupled reaction moments applied by the foot to the load stand. For applied varus/valgus moments, the coupled reaction moments are indicative of the coupled external/internal reaction moments because the axial moment transducer remains aligned with the tibia during testing. According to Table 2*a*, these coupled external/internal axial moments are consistent in load direction, with the sign of the reaction moment being generally the same as the coupled rotation. The coupled reaction axial moment ranged in magnitude from 1.4 to 10 Nm. The results for the reaction coupled moments under applied external/internal axial moments must be observed with caution. This is because, under this loading at 15° knee flexion, the thigh rotates axially thereby causing the varus/valgus moment transducer to become disoriented with the knee's varus/valgus rotational axis as defined by the joint coordinate system. Hence, in this situation, the coupled reaction moments that the varus/valgus transducer measures are not varus/valgus moments. Nonetheless, it is still useful to observe the magnitudes of the moments that this transducer recorded. From Table 2*b*, these moments were large compared to the ±20-Nm applied axial moment with one test subject generating a coupled reaction moment of 23.0 Nm. Clearly for both varus/valgus and axial applied moments, the coupled reaction moments can be large compared to the magnitude of the applied moments.

Discussion

Goniometer

Two types of relative motion goniometers have emerged for measuring joint motion in three or more degrees of freedom: the spatial-linkage goniometer [*36–41*] and the triaxial goniometer [*30,42–46*]. Each of these two designs has benefits and drawbacks. Although spatial mechanisms are capable of measuring six degrees of freedom using a kinematic chain, extensive data reduction is necessary. Triaxial goniometers, on the other hand, do not provide relative joint translations, but they require less data reduction because they are capable of measuring rotations directly according to a clinically useful coordinate system

[*44*]. Because knowing joint translations was not required for the present research, the triaxial goniometer was the better choice.

Although the triaxial goniometer is a useful tool in the field of biomechanics research, several design considerations must be addressed before accurate and repeatable results can be expected. The first is that because noninvasive goniometers require external attachment to bony prominences, the method of attachment must address the potential for relative motion between the goniometer and the bones. While impossible to eliminate completely the potential for goniometer movement using noninvasive techniques, numerous researchers have measured joint motion while attaching goniometers to the skin surrounding bony references [*10,30,38,42*]. The present design addressed the attachment problem through the use of a four-point leg attachment (one on the tibia and three on the femur) and a tightenable C-clamp. With the femur generally regarded as the more difficult of the two bones to provide attachment, the C-clamp provided clamping pressure on both epicondyles up to the tolerance level of this subject. The thigh fixture then aided in preventing any rotation of the C-clamp.

The effectiveness of the clamping system is evident to some degree from the cycle-to-cycle repeatability results. The high repeatability of less than 0.4° establishes that the clamping system maintained the orientation of the goniometer from cycle to cycle. Note that the high repeatability does not imply that orientation was maintained within a cycle, however. It is possible that the goniometer orientation shifted during a cycle and that any shift was consistent during successive cycles. As noted earlier, without attaching the goniometer directly to the bone, it is difficult to assess any magnitude of error that might be introduced from such shifting.

A second consideration is that a goniometer must permit translations to occur between the attachment points without letting these translations affect the rotational measurements. Because designs that align goniometer measurement axes with those of the adopted coordinate system imbedded in the knee are impractical and because the axes of the coordinate system shift with knee motion [*21*], most researchers permitted translations to occur by incorporating a parallelogram linkage in their goniometers [*7,22,26,30,35,42,45*]. Typically these parallelogram linkages only transmitted one rotational measurement. McKechnie and Cousins [*43*], however, claimed to overcome goniometer axes misalignment and coordinate system axes shift through the use of a parallel chain mechanism. Consisting of two parallelogram linkages placed in series, this mechanism decouples both medial/lateral and anterior/posterior translations while transmitting three rotations to the potentiometers. The range of motion over which the goniometer decouples translations is unknown, however, because the authors did not present these data. To ensure that the range of motion capabilities was appropriate for the needs of the present research while achieving decoupling from the same two translations as McKechnie and Cousins [*43*], the present goniometer incorporated a dual-parallelogram linkage. Here, the parallelogram linkages were placed in parallel, thereby enabling decoupling over the wide range of motion required by the present research. This feature was critical considering the large loads applied to the knee and the large rotations measured. The accuracy assessment tests using the goniometer verification apparatus verified the ability of this linkage to perform effectively its intended function over the necessary range of motion.

The final consideration is that the rotations be measured directly. To accomplish this task, the goniometer must measure rotations according to a joint coordinate system such as that of Grood and Suntay [*34*]. Chao [*44*] presented one such triaxial goniometer, but the linkages that permit translations to occur resulted in significant "cross talk." Other previously designed three-degree-of-freedom goniometers by Lamoreux [*42*], Markolf et al [*7*], Kuo et al [*45*], and Louie and Mote [*30*] included two parallelogram linkages in separate (that is, parallel) chains to decouple translations but did not measure rotations according to the coordinate system of Grood and Suntay [*34*]. This is because having the parallelogram linkages in two separate chains required that two of the rotational axes be fixed to one bony attachment point while the remaining axis be fixed to the other. But the joint coordinate system that Grood and Suntay [*34*] described requires that only one rotational axis be fixed to each bony segment while the third axis floats between the two. With the present dual-parallelogram consisting of one linkage, one axis is permitted to float while the other two are fixed, thereby allowing the present goniometer to satisfy the requirements of the joint coordinate system.

Verification Apparatus

Sources of error inherent to the goniometer consist of direct measurement errors and coupling errors. Both sources are due to manufacturing imperfections, which may cause (1) the axes of the axial rotation and flexion/extension potentiometers to be disoriented with respect to the rotational axes dictated by the bone clamps and (2) the potentiometer axes not to be perfectly oriented mutually according to the adopted coordinate system. The presence of the translational decoupling linkages and the fixtures to which the bone clamps are attached complicates the goniometer construction to the point where manufacturing imperfections sufficient to affect measurement accuracy are possible. Thus, some quantification of inherent measurement errors was deemed appropriate.

To quantify accurately the inherent error of a goniometer, the input motions must be known to a higher degree of precision than the accuracy capability of the goniometer. Thus, the input motions must also be measured, but the measurement problem is more stringent than the goniometer. A variety of methods have been used to measure inputs and include photogrammetric techniques [*47,48*], discrete calibration points [*39,40*], and another goniometer [*44*], which was the method used here.

In using another goniometer to provide input motions, imprecision can result from two sources. The first is imprecision in direct measurements. With the verification apparatus used here, wirewound rotational linear potentiometers were used. To quantify imprecision in direct measurement, each of the potentiometers in the rotation input modules was calibrated directly. Because of the wirewound construction, imprecision in direct measurements was due solely to the inherent uncertainty, which is $\pm 0.15°$.

The second source is imprecision in the orientation of the goniometer axes with the reference axes and is the more difficult to quantify. Because of the construction of the verification apparatus, imprecision in orientation may be due to one of two causes. One cause is that the fixtures that attach the goniometer to the simulated femur and tibia of the verification apparatus fail to orient the internal/external axial rotation and flexion/extension axes of the goniometer with those of the simulated bones. Also because different modules were used for the rotation inputs, it is possible for the potentiometer axes of the verification apparatus to be disoriented with respect to the axes of the simulated bones when the modules are installed.

To combat the latter cause of disorientation, the design of the rotation modules was simple, resulting in less chance for error stackup than if all modules were combined into one. Further, the manufacturing tolerances were tight. Consequently, although the disorientation between the potentiometer axes and simulated bones was not quantified, the degree of disorientation would not be expected to be of practical concern.

The other cause of disorientation surrounds the fixtures that attach the goniometer to the bones. To combat this cause, the same fixtures without bone clamps used in the experiments were attached to machined surfaces on the simulated bones of the apparatus, thus ensuring that the fixtures provide the same orientation of the goniometer with respect to the simulated bones as that ideally provided by the bone clamps on a leg. Because it is possible that the fixtures did not precisely orient the axes of the goniometer with those of the simulated bones, this disorientation may have been the cause of part of the "inherent" coupling errors in the goniometer. Consequently, the propriety of the term *inherent* might be called into question because these errors could very well be mitigated if the goniometer axes were oriented with respect to those of the verification apparatus. Note, however, that any disorientation in the fixtures would also be present in fixing the goniometer to the real bones if the clamps were, in fact, referenced to the bones as intended. Accordingly, the coupling errors quantified herein are appropriate measurement errors.

Load Stand

Previous studies of in-vivo knee flexibility/stiffness included the development of an apparatus that both supports the test subject and applies the appropriate loads. For the most part, the load stands were only capable of applying either axial moments [*26,30,35*] or varus/valgus moments [*22,29,49*] but not in combination. Only Youm and Bass [*50*] developed a stand with the capability to apply medial/lateral and anterior/posterior forces as well as combination axial and varus/valgus moments. Despite this body of work, in an effort to realize certain design criteria specific to the needs of our research, the present load stand did not follow any of these previous designs.

One primary design criterion was the ability of the load stand to develop pure moment loads at the knee. To meet this criterion, both the method of load application and the necessary degrees of freedom were important considerations. In regards to the method of load application, the method used by several researchers to generate a varus/valgus moment was to force the base of the foot medially/laterally while fixing the lower thigh to the load stand [*22,29,49,50*]. Forcing the foot sideways, however, induces a simultaneous medial/lateral shear force at the knee. To provide a pure moment at the knee without this accompanying shear force, the present load stand applied a pure varus/valgus moment at the foot.

The second important consideration concerned the necessary degrees of freedom. Since pure moments only were desired at the joint, the development of constraint loads had to be avoided. If the movement of the foot were limited to only the degrees of freedom corresponding to the moment loads, then constraint loads would develop due to two causes. One cause is that the loading axis and the natural rotational axis (i.e. functional axis) of the joint although parallel were not collinear. The second cause results from coupled translations and rotations that the knee undergoes when a moment load is applied [*47*]. If the knee is prevented from undergoing these coupled motions, then constraint loads will be developed. Constraint loads from either cause lead to coupled joint rotations and translations thus making it difficult to distinguish between natural joint coupling from a pure moment and joint coupling from multiple loads. Thus, to ensure that pure moments only were actually transmitted by the joint, the load stand had to offer sufficient degrees of freedom so that during loading constraint loads did not develop.

To avoid developing constraint loads at the foot that would introduce loads at the knee other than the desired moments, the load stand offered five degrees of freedom of the foot. The only degree of freedom not permitted in the load stand mechanisms was rotation of the foot about the medial/lateral axis. With the ankle angle fixed by the cast, any rotation of the foot about this axis would result in an undesirable change in the flexion angle of the knee. Because it is desirable for knee flexion angle to be fixed during flexibility experiments, this degree of freedom was not designed into the load stand.

A second design criterion was that the loading axes correspond to those in the coordinate system of Grood and Suntay [*34*]. Because the axial moment axis is fixed to the tibia, the loading axis must follow the tibia orientation. As described earlier, this was achieved for the axial moment by a special linkage that maintained the moment about the long axis of the tibia despite varus/valgus angulation of this bone. The varus/valgus axis, on the other hand, is fixed to neither the thigh nor the femur but is mutually perpendicular to the axial rotation and flexion/extension axes. Thus, if either the tibia rotates in flexion/extension or the femur rotates axially, then the varus/valgus loading axis must track these rotations. Rotation of the tibia in flexion/extension is inhibited by the apparatus, as noted above, but axial rotation of the femur cannot be prevented in axial moment loading with the knee either at or near full extension. This is because, although the varus/valgus moment axis is free to translate, it is not free to rotate with respect to the load stand. Consequently, one limitation of the load stand is that it cannot apply combination moments according to the adopted coordinate system with the knee either at or near full extension. But for flexion angles greater than about 30°, however, the circular thigh support provides a boundary condition such that femoral rotation is minimal and the application of combination moments according to the adopted coordinate system is possible. To permit combination loads for fully extended knees, absolute femur rotation must be known and some means must be provided such that the moment loading axis remains perpendicular to the flexion axis.

The final design criterion was that the load stand be able to control four variables known to affect knee flexibility. Control of two of the variables, hip and knee flexion angles, was accomplished through adjustments in the load stand that positioned the subject. Rather than being directly controlled by the load stand, muscle contraction is a variable that may be controlled by the subject using the procedures outlined by Louie and Mote [*30*]. The remaining variable is axial loading, which may be controlled by either adding weights to the thigh or having the subject bear weight. Either method could conceivably introduce inaccuracy into flexibility measurements. Adding weights to the thigh could cause the goniometer orientation to change due to soft tissue movement, whereas weight bearing might be accompanied by muscle contraction. Preliminary studies would be required to assess which of the methods is preferable.

Another inaccuracy in flexibility measurements during axial loading surrounds the development of loads other than axial force when the tibia assumes a degree of varus/valgus angulation with respect to the load stand. With the medial/lateral translational degree of freedom, no medial/lateral component of the axial force as a result of varus/valgus angulation can be equilibrated at the foot. Thus, the reaction force vector at the foot must always be vertical. Assuming no abduction/adduction of the thigh, this results in a large axial force component and a small varus/valgus moment at the knee. If abduction/adduction of the thigh also occurs, then a medial/lateral component of force also develops. Consequently, because loads other than axial force develop at the knee, the effects of the axial force on knee flexibility cannot be isolated especially during varus/valgus flexibility tests.

Boundary Conditions

The boundary conditions clearly had an effect on the primary and coupled rotations for both varus/valgus and axial moments. Because these differences may be large, the effect of boundary conditions must be considered to obtain accurate flexibility results of the human knee. Recognizing that a large number of knee flexibility/stiffness studies obtained flexibility results with the foot constrained to rotate around a single axis, it is unknown how the coupled reaction loads that the knee generates affected these results. Furthermore, the assessment of any flexibility results presented is complicated by the fact that multiple loads were actually applied. In the interest of obtaining accurate results for isolated loads, the application of moments must be conducted with the foot unconstrained.

Conclusions

Ligamentous knee injuries continue to be a problem in alpine skiing. To better identify both why the problem continues to exist and possible methods for preventing future ligamentous injuries, flexibility information of the human knee under individual and combined moments is needed. To obtain this information, a load stand was developed to control four variables that affect knee strength and a three-degree-of-freedom goniometer was developed to measure the rotations of the knee. Both apparatus offer several advances over those used in previously conducted research. In particular, goniometer advancements include the following: (1) a potentiometer orientation that directly measures the three-degree-of-freedom rotations of the joint according to the clinically relevant coordinate system of Grood and Suntay [*34*]; (2) a specially designed dual-parallelogram linkage, which both decouples the three-degree-of-freedom translations from rotational measurements and allows a wide range of goniometer motion; (3) a tightenable C-clamp and a thigh attachment, which control femoral clamp movement; and (4) a verification apparatus, which quantifies inherent goniometer error. With the present goniometer only able to measure rotations, the measurement of joint translations is not possible. Although the study of translations under shear forces is important from a clinical diagnostic perspective, shear forces were kept to a minimum in the present research, thus obviating the need for a goniometer that measures translations.

For the present load stand, advancements include (1) application of both axial and varus/valgus moments either individually or in combination through the use of permanent magnet gearmotors and SCR controllers, (2) development of pure moments at the knee by allowing five degrees of freedom at the foot, (3) application of moments according to an adopted coordinate system that is clinically relevant, and (4) control of hip flexion angle with varying knee flexion angles. One limitation of the present load stand is its inability to maintain applicability of the joint coordinate system with the knee at less than 30° flexion angles under combined loading.

To evaluate the sources of variability in measuring knee rotations with the goniometer, three performance tests were conducted. Using a specially designed verification apparatus, which enabled inputs of known displacements in all six degrees of freedom, one test determined the inherent accuracy of the goniometer. This test quantified both direct and coupling errors. Combining the average errors for the two types revealed errors of ± 0.7 and $\pm 0.8°$ for varus/valgus and external/internal rotations, respectively. Assessed in the second test was the potential for the goniometer orientation to change permanently from one loading cycle to the next. With less than 0.4° average difference in external/internal rotation and less than 0.3° average difference in varus/valgus rotation between succeeding cycles, this test revealed that the orientation was maintained. The third test explored the effect of goniometer mounting on the repeatability of results. Remounting of the goniometer indicated repeatability to within 1.0° in external/internal rotation between successive mountings. Consequently, the goniometer may be consistently oriented from mounting to mounting.

The boundary condition study showed that boundary conditions have a large effect on both the primary and coupled rotations. To eliminate the large coupled moments that were observed during tests with both motors connected, flexibility tests for single loads must be conducted with only the motor applying the moment constraining the leg. This condition is necessary if pure moments are to be applied.

Acknowledgment

We are grateful to Tyrolia Corporation of Vienna, Austria, and, in particular, Dr. Klaus Hoelzl for the financial support of this research.

References

[1] Johnson, R. J., Pope, M. H., Weisman, G., White, B. F., and Ettlinger, C., "Knee Injury in Skiing—A Multifaceted Approach," *American Journal of Sports Medicine*, Vol. 7, No. 6, 1979, pp. 321–327.

[2] Young, L. R., "Skier Fall Modes and Injury Patterns," in *Ski Trauma and Skiing Safety IV*, W. Hauser, J. Karlsson, and M. Magi, Eds., TUV-Bayern, Munich, 1982, pp. 217–226.

[3] Figueras, J. M., Llobet, M., Bulo, J. M., Morgenstern, R., and Merino, J. A., "The Evaluation of Knee Injuries in Ski Accidents," in *Skiing Trauma and Skiing Safety: Fifth International Symposium, ASTM STP 860*, R. J. Johnson and C. D. Mote, Jr., Eds., American Society for Testing and Materials, Philadelphia, 1985, pp. 141–148.

[4] Shealy, J. E., "Overall Analysis of NSAA/ASTM Data on Skiing Injuries for 1978–1981," in *Skiing Trauma and Safety: Fifth International Symposium, ASTM STP 860*, R. J. Johnson and C. D. Mote, Jr., Eds., American Society for Testing and Materials, Philadelphia, 1985, pp. 302–313.

[5] Shino, K., Horibe, S., Nagano, J., and Ono, K., "Injury of the Anterior Cruciate Ligament of the Knee in Downhill Skiing: Its Pathomechanism and Treatment," in *Skiing Trauma and Safety: Sixth International Symposium, ASTM STP 938*, C. D. Mote, Jr. and R. J. Johnson, Eds., American Society for Testing and Materials, Philadelphia, 1987, pp. 68–86.

[6] Howe, J. and Johnson, R. J., "Knee Injuries in Skiing," *Orthopedic Clinics of North America*, Vol. 16, No. 2, 1985, pp. 303–314.

[7] Markolf, K. L., Mensch, J. S., and Amstutz, H. C., "Stiffness and Laxity of the Knee—Contributions of the Supporting Structures. A Quantitative In-Vitro Study," *Journal of Bone and Joint Surgery*, Vol. 58A, No. 5, 1976, pp. 583–593.

[8] Nagel, D. A., Seering, W., and Piziali, R. L., "Contribution of the Various Knee Ligaments to Transmission of Forces Typical of Skiing," in *Ski Trauma and Skiing Safety III*, R. J. Johnson, M. K. Lamont, W. Hauser, and J. Karlsson, Eds., TUV-Bayern, Munich, 1982, pp. 103–109.

[9] Nielsen, S., Rasmussen, O., Ovesen, J., and Andersen, K., "Rotary Instability of Cadaver Knees After Transection of Collateral Ligaments and Capsule," *Archives of Orthopedic and Traumatic Surgery*, Vol. 103, No. 3, 1984, pp. 165–169.

[10] Shoemaker, S. C. and Markolf, K. L., "Effects of Joint Load on the Stiffness and Laxity of Ligament-Deficient Knees: An In-Vitro Study of the Anterior Cruciate and Medial Collateral Ligaments," *Journal of Bone and Joint Surgery*, Vol. 67A, No. 1, 1985, pp. 136–146.

[11] Hsieh, J. and Walker, P. S., "Stabilizing Mechanisms of the Loaded and Unloaded Knee Joint," *Journal of Bone and Joint Surgery*, Vol. 58A, No. 1, 1976, pp. 87–93.

[12] Butler, D. L., Noyes, F., and Grood, E. S., "Ligamentous Restraints to Anterior-Posterior Drawer in the Human Knee," *Journal of Bone and Joint Surgery*, Vol. 62-A, No. 2, 1980, pp. 259–270.

[13] Sullivan D., Levy, I. M., Sheskier, S., Torzilli, P. A., and Warren, R. F., "Medial Restraints to Anterior-Posterior Motion of the Knee," *Journal of Bone and Joint Surgery*, Vol. 66-A, No. 6, 1984, pp. 930–936.

[14] Brantigen, O. C. and Voshell, A. F., "The Mechanics of the Ligaments and Menisci of the Knee Joint," *Journal of Bone and Joint Surgery*, Vol. 23, No. 1, pp. 44–66.

[15] Piziali, R. L., Rastegar, J., Nagel, D. A., and Schurman, D. J., "The Contribution of the Cruciate Ligaments to the Load-Displacement Characteristics of the Human Knee Joint," *Journal of Biomechanical Engineering*, Vol. 102, No. 11, 1980, pp. 277–283.

[16] Lipke, J. M., Janecki, C. J., Nelson, C. L., McLeod, P., Thompson, C., et al., "The Role of Incompetence of the Anterior Cruciate and Lateral Ligaments in Anterolateral and Anteromedial Instability," *Journal of Bone and Joint Surgery*, Vol. 63-A, No. 6, 1981, pp. 954–960.

[17] Nielsen, S., Ovesen, J., and Rasmussen, O., "The Anterior Cruciate Ligament of the Knee: An Experimental Study of Its Importance in Rotary Knee Instability," *Archives of Orthopedic and Traumatic Surgery*, Vol. 103, No. 3, 1984, pp. 170–174.

[18] Kennedy, J. and Fowler, P. J., "Medial and Anterior Instability of the Knee. An Anatomical and Clinical Study Using Stress Machines," *Journal of Bone and Joint Surgery*, Vol. 53A, No. 7, 1971, pp. 1257–1270.

[19] Wang, C. and Walker, P. S., "Rotary Laxity of the Human Knee Joint," *Journal of Bone and Joint Surgery*, Vol. 56A, No. 1, 1974, pp. 161–170.

[20] Markolf, K. L., Bargar, W. L., Shoemaker, S. C., and Amstutz, H. C., "The Role of Joint Load in Knee Stability," *Journal of Bone and Joint Surgery*, Vol. 63A, No. 4, 1981, pp. 570–585.

[21] Crowinshield, R., Pope, M. H., and Johnson, R. J., "An Analytical Model of the Knee," *Journal of Biomechanics*, Vol. 9, 1976, pp. 397–405.

[22] Markolf, K. L., Graff-Radford, A., and Amstutz, H. C., "In Vivo Knee Stability—A Quantitative

Assessment Using an Instrumented Clinical Testing Apparatus," *Journal of Bone and Joint Surgery*, Vol. 60A, No. 5, 1978, pp. 664–674.

[23] Markolf, K. L., Kochhan, A., and Amstutz, H. C., "Measurement of Knee Stiffness and Laxity in Patients with Documented Absence of the Anterior Cruciate Ligament," *Journal of Bone and Joint Surgery*, Vol. 66-A, No. 2, 1984, pp. 242–253.

[24] Gollehon, D. L., Torzilli, P. A., and Warren, R. F., "The Role of the Posteriolateral and Cruciate Ligaments in the Stability of the Human Knee," *Journal of Bone and Joint Surgery*, Vol. 69A, No. 2, 1987, pp. 233–242.

[25] Grood, E. S., Stowers, S. F., and Noyes, F. R., "Limits of Movement in the Human Knee," *Journal of Bone and Joint Surgery*, Vol. 70-A, No. 1, 1988, pp. 88–97.

[26] Shoemaker, S. C. and Markolf, K. L., "In Vivo Rotary Knee Stability," *Journal of Bone and Joint Surgery*, Vol. 64A, No. 2, 1982, pp. 208–216.

[27] Goldfuss, A. J., Morehouse, C. A., and Le Veau, B. F., "Effect of Muscular Tension on Knee Stability," *Medicine and Science in Sports*, Vol. 5, No. 4, 1973, pp. 267–271.

[28] Pope, M. H., Johnson, R. J., Brown, D. W., and Tighe, C., "The Role of Musculature in Injuries to the Medial Collateral Ligament, *Journal of Bone and Joint Surgery*, Vol. 61A, No. 3, 1979, pp. 398–402.

[29] Olmstead, T. G., Wevers, H. W., Bryant, J. T., and Gouw, G. J., "Effect of Muscular Activity on Varus/Valgus Laxity and Stiffness of the Knee," *Journal of Biomechanics*, Vol. 19, No. 8, 1986, pp. 565–577.

[30] Louie, J. K. and Mote, C. D., Jr., "Contribution of the Musculature to Rotary Laxity and Torsional Stiffness at the Knee," *Journal of Biomechanics*, Vol. 20, No. 3, 1987, pp. 281–300.

[31] Noyes, F. R., DeLucas, J. L., and Torvik, P. J., "Biomechanics of Anterior Cruciate Ligament Failure: An Analysis of Strain Rate Sensitivity and Mechanisms of Failure in Primates," *Journal of Bone and Joint Surgery*, Vol. 56-A, 1974, pp. 236–253.

[32] Campbell, R. J., Ettlinger, C. H., Johnson, R. J., and Pope, M. H., "High Risk Injury Groups in Downhill Skiing," in *Skiing Trauma and Skiing Safety III*, R. J. Johnson, W. Hauser, J. Karlsson, and M. K. Lamont, Eds., TUV-Edition, Munich, 1982, pp. 126–134.

[33] Ekelund, A., Holtmoen, A., and Lystad, H., "Skiing Injuries in Alpine Recreational Skiers," in *Skiing Trauma and Safety: Seventh International Symposium, ASTM STP 1022*, R. J. Johnson, C. D. Mote, Jr., and M.-H. Binet, Eds., American Society for Testing and Materials, Philadelphia, 1989, pp. 41–50.

[34] Grood, E. S. and Suntay, W. J., "A Joint Coordinate System for the Clinical Description of Three-Dimensional Motions: Application to the Knee," *Journal of Biomechanical Engineering*, Vol. 105, No. 5, 1983, pp. 136–144.

[35] Hull, M. L. and Johnson, C., "Axial Rotation of the Lower Limb Under Torsional Loading: I. Static and Dynamic Measurements," in *Skiing Trauma and Safety: Seventh International Symposium, ASTM STP 1022*, R. J. Johnson, C. D. Mote, Jr., and M.-H. Binet, Eds., American Society for Testing and Materials, Philadelphia, 1989, pp. 277–290.

[36] Kinzel, G. L., Hall, A. S., Jr., and Hillberry, B. M., "Measurement of the Total Motion Between Two Body Segments—Analytical Development," *Journal of Biomechanics*, Vol. 5, No. 1, 1972, pp. 93–105.

[37] Kinzel, G. L., Hillberry, B. M., and Hall, A. S., Jr., "Measurement of the Total Motion Between Two Body Segments—II. Description of Application," *Journal of Biomechanics*, Vol. 5, No. 3, 1972, pp. 283–293.

[38] Townsend, M. A., Izak, M., and Jackson, R. W., "Total Motion Knee Goniometry," *Journal of Biomechanics*, Vol. 10, No. 3, 1977, pp. 183–193.

[39] Sommer, H. J., III and Miller, N. R., "A Technique for the Calibration of Instrumented Spatial Linkage Used for Biomechanical Kinematic Measurements," *Journal of Biomechanics*, Vol. 14, No. 1, 1981, pp. 91–98.

[40] Hefzy, M. S. and Grood, E. S., "Sensitivity of Insertion Locations on Length Patterns of Anterior Cruciate Fibers," *Journal of Biomechanical Engineering*, Vol. 108, No. 2, 1986, pp. 73–82.

[41] Shiavi, R., Limbird, T., Frazer, M., Stivers, K., Strauss, A., and Abramovitz, J., "Helical Motion Analysis of the Knee—I. Methodology for Studying Kinematics During Gait," *Journal of Biomechanics*, Vol. 20, No. 5, 1987, pp. 459–469.

[42] Lamoreux, L. W., "Kinematic Measurements in the Study of Human Walking," *Bulletin of Prosthetics Research*, Vol. BPR 10–15, 1971, pp. 3–84.

[43] McKechnie, R. E. and Cousins, S. J., "A Parallelogram Chain Mechanism for Measuring Human Joint Motion," ASME Publication 76-DET-71, 1976.

[44] Chao, E. Y., "Justification of the Triaxial Goniometer for the Measurement of Joint Rotation," *Journal of Biomechanics*, Vol. 13, No. 12, 1980, pp. 989–1006.

[*45*] Kuo, C. Y., Louie, J. K., and Mote, C. D., Jr., "Control of Torsion and Bending of the Lower Extremity During Skiing," in *Skiing Trauma and Safety: Fifth International Symposium, ASTM STP 860*, R. J. Johnson and C. D. Mote, Jr., Eds., American Society for Testing and Materials, Philadelphia, 1985, pp. 91–109.
[*46*] Isacson, J., Gransberg, L., and Knutsson, E., "Three-Dimensional Electrogoniometric Gait Recording," *Journal of Biomechanics*, Vol. 19, No. 8, 1986, pp. 627–635.
[*47*] Blankevoort, L., Huiskes, R., and de Lange, A., "The Envelope of Passive Knee Joint Motion," *Journal of Biomechanics*, Vol. 21, No. 9, 1988, pp. 705–720.
[*48*] Suntay, W. J., Grood, E. S., Hefzy, M. S., Butler, D. L., and Noyes, F. R., "Error Analysis of a System for Measuring Three-Dimensional Joint Motion," *Journal of Biomechanical Engineering*, Vol. 105, No. 5, 1983, pp. 127–135.
[*49*] Bryant, J. T. and Cooke, T. D. V., "Standardized Biomechanical Measurement for Varus/Valgus Stiffness and Rotation in Normal Knees," *Journal of Orthopedic Research*, Vol. 6, No. 6, 1988, pp. 863–870.
[*50*] Youm, Y. and Bass, B. G., "Quantification of Knee Laxity," *SOMA*, Vol. 1, No. 4, 1987, pp. 18–23.

Oliver S. Mills[1] *and Maury L. Hull*[1]

Flexibility of the Human Knee as a Result of Varus/Valgus and Axial Moments in Vivo: Experiments and Results

REFERENCE: Mills, O. S. and Hull, M. L., "**Flexibility of the Human Knee as a Result of Varus/Valgus and Axial Moments in Vivo: Experiments and Results,**" *Skiing Trauma and Safety: Eighth International Symposium, ASTM STP 1104*, C. D. Mote, Jr. and Robert J. Johnson, Eds., American Society for Testing and Materials, Philadelphia, 1991, pp. 35–56.

ABSTRACT: Knee ligamentous injuries persist in the sport of Alpine skiing. To better understand the load mechanisms that lead to injury, pure varus/valgus and pure axial moments were applied both singly and in combination to the right knees of six human test subjects. The corresponding relative knee rotations in three degrees of freedom were measured. Knee flexion angles for each test subject were 15 and 60° for the individual moments and 60° for the combination moments. For both knee flexion angles, hip flexion angle was 0°. Leg muscles were quiescent and axial force was minimal during all tests. Tables of data include sample statistics for each of four flexibility parameters in each loading direction.

Data were analyzed statistically to test for significant differences in flexibility parameters between the test conditions. In flexing the knee from 15 to 60°, the resulting knee rotations under single moments depended on flexion angle with varus, valgus, and internal rotations increasing significantly. Also, rotations were different depending on load direction; varus rotation was significantly different and greater than valgus rotation at both flexion angles. Also external rotation was significantly different and greater than internal at 15° flexion but not 60° flexion. Coupled rotations under single moments were also observed. Applying pure varus/valgus moments resulted in coupled external/internal rotations that were inconsistent and hence not significant. Applying pure axial moments resulted in consistent and hence significant varus/valgus rotations; an external axial moment induced varus rotation and an internal axial moment induced valgus rotation. For combination moments, varus/valgus rotations decreased significantly from those rotations at similar load levels in the single moment studies. Also, a varus moment significantly increased external rotation and a valgus moment significantly decreased internal rotation. These differences indicate significant interaction between corresponding load combinations. These results suggest that load interaction is a potentially important phenomenon in knee injury mechanics.

KEY WORDS: skiing, knee injuries, axial moments, varus/valgus moments, combination moments, rotation

Ligamentous knee injuries remain a persistent problem in Alpine skiing. Epidemiology studies have identified two types of ligamentous knee injuries that primarily occur, the first is isolated injury to the anterior cruciate ligament (ACL) and the second is injury to the medial collateral ligament (MCL) with or without injury to the ACL. Focusing on the second type of injury, designated an MCL/ACL injury, these studies have also identified external axial and valgus moments acting in combination as the dominant loading causing this type

[1]Research assistant and professor, respectively, Department of Mechanical Engineering, University of California, Davis, CA 95616.

of injury [*1–3*]. Previous research on ligament function confirms the potential of these loads to cause MCL injury (for example, Ref *4*) and accompanying ACL injury [*5*].

To understand better injury mechanics when axial and varus/valgus moments are transmitted by the knee, it is useful to study the relation between these loads and the knee rotations which lead to injury. Previously conducted research has examined knee rotations under single varus/valgus moments both in vitro [*4,6–11*] and in vivo [*12–15*]. Other studies have measured rotations as a result of axial moments both in vitro [*4,6–11,16–20*] and in vivo [*13,21–23*] as well. Although this body of previous research is extensive, it does not include any research that studied knee rotations under combination axial and varus/valgus moments.

With combined varus/valgus and axial moments thought to cause the MCL/ACL knee injuries in skiing, and no previous research having studied how the knee rotates under the simultaneous application of these two loads, the general objective of this research was to apply these two moments, both individually and in combination, to the knees of human test subjects in vivo and measure the resulting knee rotations. The equipment to apply the loads quasistatically and measure the triaxial rotations according to a defined coordinate system was presented in another article [*24*] along with an evaluation of equipment performance. This equipment allowed four variables known to affect knee flexibility to be controlled. Identified by the previous research on knee load rotation cited above, the four variables are muscle contraction, axial loading/weight bearing, knee flexion angle, and hip flexion angle. Recognizing these capabilities, the specific objectives of the research reported by the present article were as follows:

(1) to determine the effect of flexion angle on flexibility for pure varus/valgus and axial moments and
(2) to determine the extent to which combined moments affect knee flexibility when compared to single moments.

To provide data on flexibility with the knee in its most lax state, all flexibility tests were conducted with both muscle contraction and axial loading kept to a minimum and hip flexion angle maintained at 0°.

Methods

Equipment and Procedure

To appreciate the testing protocol, the goniometer and load application stand will be briefly described. The goniometer measured the relative three degree-of-freedom rotations of the knee according to the coordinate system of Grood and Suntay [*25*] and attached to the leg at the tibia, the lateral and medial epicondyles, and the thigh. The goniometer provided direct measurement of rotations while the three degree-of-freedom translations were decoupled via a specially designed linkage. An accuracy assessment of the goniometer under individual varus/valgus and external/internal rotations revealed a maximum absolute error of $+0.7°/-0.7°$ and $+0.3°/-0.9°$, respectively. See Mills and Hull [*24*] for further details of the goniometer design and the assessment of its accuracy.

The load application stand supported the test subject so as to enable control of the variables known to affect knee flexibility, while at the same time applying pure varus/valgus and pure axial moments either individually or in combination to the right knee. By definition, pure moments are those that minimally create unwanted shear forces at the knee and are desirable in isolating which loads contribute to total joint angulation. Both moments were applied to the foot through a fiberglass cast which rigidly maintained ankle flexion angle such that the foot was 90° to the shank. To insure that only moment loads were developed at the knee, the cast was connected to the load stand by means of mechanisms which offered five degrees of freedom, three translations, and axial and varus/valgus rotations. Also, other mechanisms maintained the moment loading axes consistent with those in the coordinate system of Grood and Suntay [25]. Operated by a hand-held controller which permitted the test subject to control both loading magnitude and direction, gearmotors provided the necessary torques. Although the gearmotor rotation rate was adjustable to some degree, the range of adjustment restricted the loading rate to quasi-static. To minimize abduction/adduction of the thigh during varus/valgus loading, a clamp secured the upper thigh to the load stand. An accuracy check of the load-stand transducers revealed average absolute errors of 0.3 and 0.4 Nm for axial and varus/valgus moments, respectively. A bicycle seat and backrest supported the test subject. With the inclination of the backrest adjustable as were both the height and inclination of the seat, hip and knee flexion angles could be preset and the axial force (that is, weight) controlled. Refer to Mills and Hull [24] for elaboration of the load application stand.

The testing protocol called for six male test subjects with no prior history of ligamentous injury to their right knees. Table 1 lists the anthropometric data for each subject. Testing consisted of four single moment and two combined moment tests in which loads were applied to the right knees of each individual. The single moment tests included axial and varus/valgus moments each applied at 15 and 60° flexion. The 0° flexion reference was determined as the position assumed by the joint when the subject was seated, the leg was horizontal with the heel simply supported, and the muscles were relaxed. The two combination loading tests included combinations of varus/valgus and axial moments at 60° flexion. Note that combination tests were not possible at 15° knee flexion because femur rotation at the hip altered the orientation of the knee with respect to the coordinate system about which the loading was to follow. Before the tests in which data were recorded, the knee was preconditioned during preliminary loading trials undertaken to familiarize test subjects with the equipment operation.

With the objective of the present study to minimize active muscle contraction, a preliminary study was conducted to assess muscle contraction levels during complete load cycles. Six muscles were chosen for their potential contribution to overall joint flexibility and included vastus medialis and lateralis, medial and lateral heads of the gastrocnemius, biceps femoris, and semitendinosus. During the pure loading tests at 15° knee flexion, muscle activity was monitored on all of the six test subjects using surface electrodes (Motion Control) placed according to Delagi et al. [26]. With the test subjects instructed to be relaxed, no measurable activity was observed in one of the subjects, a small level of activity was observed in a single but different muscle for three of the subjects, and a small level of activity was

TABLE 1—*Test subject anthropometric data.*

Subject	Sex	Age, years	Height, m	Weight, N	PTW,[a] cm
1	M	24	1.83	779	8.9
2	M	41	1.75	734	8.9
3	M	24	1.73	645	8.6
4	M	27	1.73	712	8.5
5	M	26	1.73	712	8.8
6	M	29	1.75	690	9.1
Average		28.5	1.75	712	8.8
Standard deviation		6.4	0.04	45	0.2

[a]PTW = proximal tibial width.

observed in more than one muscle for two subjects. Activity levels were typically about 5% of those corresponding to the levels at maximum voluntary contraction. Also, these activities were observed generally at the extremes of loading. Confident that subjects do not tense muscles appreciably once they are instructed to keep them relaxed, all subsequent flexibility tests were conducted without electromyogram (EMG) monitoring.

Testing on each individual was conducted over two sessions because preliminary studies indicated test subject discomfort from prolonged sitting in the stand if the entire protocol was completed without a break. Hence, the 15° flexion tests were conducted on a different occasion from the 60° flexion tests. With minimal axial force on the knee an objective for the present study, any axial force measured was mainly the weight of the shank since the load-application stand supported the remainder of the test subject's weight. At 60° flexion, however, axial force on the knee was unavoidable because the knee partially supported the weight of the thigh.

The varus/valgus moment tests consisted of cycling between 60 Nm of a varus and a valgus moment over a time span of 60 s. The ±60-Nm moment was chosen because all subjects could tolerate this level. For the present study, varus was loaded first. To transmit the varus/valgus moments to the knee without causing test subject discomfort, a tall (41-cm), removable, fiberglass cast was clamped around both the ankle and the lower leg of the test subject. Before data acquisition, the goniometer offsets were taken with the muscles relaxed, the foot unloaded, and the knee extended. During testing, the foot was allowed to rotate freely either externally or internally which insured that unconstrained varus/valgus moments were transmitted to the knee. The test subject switched load directions through the hand-held controller when 60 Nm of either varus or valgus moment was reached. For the varus/valgus tests as well as the axial moment and combined loading tests, two data runs were obtained to assess repeatability among runs. See Mills and Hull [*24*] for an analysis of repeatability. After a data run, the offsets were rechecked to assess if goniometer slippage occurred. If slippage was evident, then the data run was repeated.

The axial moment tests were conducted similarly to the varus/valgus moment tests except that in the axial moment tests, the leg was unconstrained in varus/valgus rotation and that a shorter cast (24 cm) transmitted the moments. Preliminary data indicated that the tall cast led to increased skin shear during axial moment tests thereby altering the flexibility curves; hence, the shorter cast was used. Offsets were again taken with the leg unloaded and the knee extended. Because no load frequently corresponded to about 10 to 20° external foot rotation, offsets were taken in this position as opposed to 0° foot rotation. Axial moments were then cycled between ±20 Nm with an external axial moment applied first. Other preliminary tests suggested that some of the test subjects would not be able to withstand moments above ±20 Nm. Therefore, this load level was chosen since it was within the tolerance level of all test subjects. The time span for a complete cycle ranged from 50 to 60 s with the offsets rechecked after each test.

To conduct flexibility tests at 60° flexion, the load application stand was adjusted so that the hip flexion angle was 0° when the knee flexion angle was 60°. Since the knee undergoes combination internal axial and varus rotation with increasing flexion [*11*], the offsets were taken once the subject was positioned in the stand so that all plots start at 0° rotation for no load. The procedure for obtaining flexibility data under both varus/valgus and axial moments followed that as described above.

The protocol for combined loading called for running both gearmotors simultaneously. To obtain results over a complete loading cycle, the motor directions were reversed at the same instant when target load levels were reached. These target load levels were 45 and 15 Nm for varus/valgus and axial moments, respectively. Lower load levels than the ones used in the single load studies were chosen because not all subjects could easily tolerate the levels of the single loading tests. Also, the lower load levels in the combination load tests permitted the use of the short fiberglass cast to transmit the moments. Note that throughout all combination tests, the orientation of the femur was nearly constant thereby maintaining applicability of the joint coordinate system (see Fig. 1). As in the single load studies, goniometer offsets were taken at zero load. The combination load protocol consisted of two load cases. Load Case 1 involved simultaneously cycling both external axial and varus moments and then reversing directions at the target load levels for combination internal axial and valgus moments. Load Case 2 involved first combination external axial and valgus moments and then reversing for internal axial and varus moments. With these two tests, all combinations of the two moments were obtained.

Experimental Parameters

To interpret the nonlinear knee flexibility results consistently and meaningfully, four flexibility parameters were defined; Figs. 1 and 2 graphically illustrate these parameters. The first parameter is "laxity" or the range of rotation that the knee undergoes before the soft tissues surrounding the joint significantly restrict movement. The "slope approach" method, which is new to the present research, involved predetermining a common flexibility which is indicative of when the soft tissues begin to restrict movement. The slopes chosen for each moment were based on observing the flexibility plots from all test subjects and determining the slope at which joint stiffening typically occurred. The slopes used were 2.0°/Nm for axial flexibility and 0.17°/Nm for varus/valgus flexibility. The difference in the slopes is because the knee is considerably more flexible in external/internal rotation than in varus/

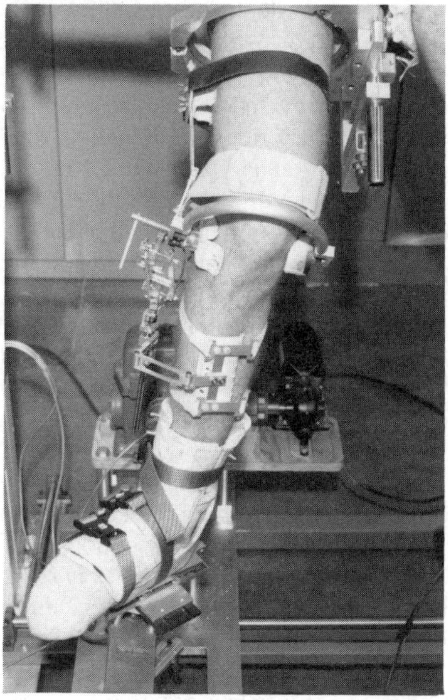

FIG. 1—*Test subject with the knee under combination valgus and external axial moments. Note that rotation of the femur along its long axis is minimal thus maintaining alignment of the varus/valgus moment axis with the varus/valgus axis of rotation in the adopted coordinate system.*

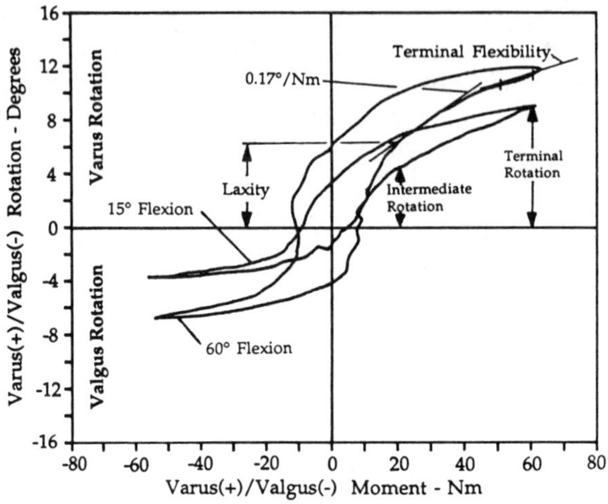

FIG. 2—*The effect of knee flexion angle on varus/valgus rotation for an applied pure varus/valgus moment. Increasing flexion angle from 15 to 60° increased both varus and valgus rotations. Also, varus was more flexible than valgus for both flexion angles. These differences were statistically significant. The parameters used to quantify the varus/valgus flexibility results are illustrated in the figure. Results shown are for Test Subject 2.*

valgus rotation. The joint rotation at which the flexibility curve is first tangent to these slopes for each load direction then becomes the laxity. Laxities were obtained from plotted flexibility curves.

The remaining three parameters provided additional information of joint flexibility for the single-moment tests in both load directions. Intermediate rotation (IR) was the rotation from 0 to 20 Nm for varus/valgus rotation and from 0 to 5 Nm for external/internal rotation. The intermediate rotations were provided in the present study as a means of comparison to rotations repoted by previous researchers. The second parameter, terminal rotation (TR), was the rotation from 0 to 60 Nm in varus/valgus rotation and from 0 to 20 Nm in external/internal rotation. The term was borrowed from Olmstead et al. [*14*] and was modified for the load levels of the present study. Finally, terminal flexibility (TF) was used as an indication of joint flexibility near the knee's limits of rotation and refers to the slope of the flexibility curve between 50 and 60 Nm of varus/valgus moment and between 15 and 20 Nm of axial moment. A linear regression analysis on the data between the aforementioned load values was performed to calculate the slope.

In combined loading, because of the lower moment levels applied, new IR and TR values were required for both the varus/valgus and external/internal rotations. For varus/valgus rotation, IRs remained at 20 Nm, but TRs were reduced to 40 Nm. Because of the generally unquantifiable shape of the varus/valgus flexibility curves in combination loading, no laxity values were tabulated for varus/valgus rotations. For external/internal rotation, IRs remained at 5 Nm (IR1) with a new IR obtained at 10 Nm (IR2). As with varus/valgus, the TRs for external/internal rotation were reduced to 15 Nm. The IR2 at 10 Nm in external/internal rotation and the TR at 40 Nm in varus/valgus rotation were required because it was not possible to reach simultaneously the target levels of both 15-Nm axial and 45-Nm varus/valgus moments with all test subjects. Note that terminal flexibilities were not calculated for the combined loading results.

Results

Varus/Valgus Moments

Figure 2 is an example of a varus/valgus flexibility plot for 15 and 60° flexion angles. Note that the figure graphically represents all four parameters. Figure 2 clearly shows that for both flexion angles, rotations underwent large amounts of hysteresis for complete load cycles. The figure also illustrates that, at 60° flexion, both varus and valgus rotations were greater than the rotations obtained at 15° flexion. Further, the figure illustrates that varus rotations were generally greater than valgus rotations.

The results of the quantitative analysis of the four varus/valgus parameters are summarized in Tables 2*a*, *b*, and *c*. Table 2*a* gives the sample statistics for all four parameters in addition to the statistics for the maximum coupled rotations. Tables 2*b* and *c* give the sample statistics for the differences in parameter values between 15 and 60° flexion and between varus rotation and valgus rotation, respectively. To determine whether statistically significant differences existed, a paired *t*-test was performed. Thus, to assess significance, also given in these tables are values of the *t*-statistic. The value of the *t*-statistic for a level of significance $p = 0.05$ is 2.57 for five degrees of freedom. Those values superscripted by the * symbol indicate statistically significant differences at a level less than 0.05.

The results in Tables 2*b* and *c* indicate that the observations made from Fig. 2 were significant. In particular, the mean differences in both laxity and TR between 60 and 15° flexion were significantly different from and greater than zero for both varus and valgus rotations (Table 2*b*). Consequently, the knee became more flexible at 60° knee flexion. Also the knee became more flexible in varus than valgus regardless of flexion angle. At 15° flexion, neither the mean difference in laxity nor the mean difference in IR was significantly different from zero but the mean difference in TR was significantly different from zero at the 0.10 level (Table 2*c*). At 60° flexion, the mean difference in all parameter values except TF was significantly different from zero at $p < 0.05$.

The final two columns of Table 2*a* give the sample statistics for the maximum coupled external and internal rotations observed in plots such as those shown in Fig. 3 for a pure varus/valgus moment. As is evident from the figure, the maximum coupled rotation did not occur at the maximum applied moment. In fact, for several test subjects, such as the example shown, the maximum coupled rotation was observed near zero applied moment in unloading. Accordingly, because of the difficulty in assigning a primary load direction to a maximum coupled rotation, these two columns only give an indication of the coupled rotation the joint underwent and not the moment direction in which the maximum coupled rotation occurred.

Axial Moments

Figure 4 is an example of an external/internal rotation flexibility plot for both 15 and 60° flexion angles over one complete load cycle. Included on the plot are the graphical representations of all the parameters computed. The flexibility curve illustrates that hysteresis was minimal. Further, Fig. 4 also shows that in flexing from 15 to 60°, internal TR increased and external TR decreased. A final observation apparent in Fig. 4 is that at 15° flexion, external rotation was greater than internal rotation whereas the opposite was true for 60° flexion.

Analogous to Tables 2*a*, *b*, and *c*, Tables 3*a*, *b*, and *c* are a set of tables that summarize the quantitative analysis of the four parameters for internal and external axial rotations. Referring to Tables 3*b* and *c* indicates which of the observations made from Fig. 4 are statistically significant. In flexing the knee from 15 to 60°, the knee became more flexible in internal rotation with mean differences between all three rotation parameters being

Table 2a. Average and Standard Deviation of Varus/Valgus Flexibility Parameters under Single Varus/Valgus Moments Applied to 6 Subjects at 15° and 60° Knee Flexion

	Varus/Valgus Rotations and Flexibility from an Applied Varus Moment				Varus/Valgus Rotations and Flexibility from an Applied Valgus Moment				Total Varus/Valgus Rotation		Maximum Coupled External/Internal Rotation	
Knee Flexion Angle	Laxity	IR	TR	TF [°/Nm]	Laxity	IR	TR	TF [°/Nm]	Laxity	TR		
15°	4.3°± 2.8°	4.5°± 2.5°	8.1°± 3.5°	0.056 ± 0.038	-3.1°± 1.1°	-3.4°± 1.3°	-5.1°± 1.3°	0.014 ± 0.010	7.4°± 2.3°	13.2°± 3.4°	4.0°± 2.0°	-4.8°± 2.2°
60°	9.0°± 4.3°	8.1°± 3.6°	11.8°± 2.9°	0.031 ± 0.033	-5.1°± 1.9°	-4.8°± 1.9°	-7.7°± 1.7°	0.062 ± 0.024	14.1°± 5.8°	19.5°± 4.2°	5.1°± 2.6°	-5.8°± 1.7°

Sign Conventions - Varus (+); Valgus (-); External (+); Internal (-)

Table 2b. Statistical Comparison of Varus/Valgus Flexibility Parameter Differences between 60° and 15° Knee Flexions at the Same Applied Moment

	For an Applied Varus Moment				For an Applied Valgus Moment				Total Varus/Valgus Rotation	
	Laxity	IR	TR	TF [°/Nm]	Laxity	IR	TR	TF [°/Nm]	Laxity	TR
Difference (60° - 15°)	4.7°± 2.6°	3.5°± 1.8°	3.7°± 2.5°	-0.026 ± 0.037	1.9°± 1.8°	1.4°± 2.0°	2.6°± 0.9°	-0.048 ± 0.031	6.6°± 4.0°	6.3°± 2.8°
t Statistic - Paired	4.40*	4.78*	3.66*	1.70	2.67*	1.73	7.06*	3.83*	4.09*	5.63*

Table 2c. Statistical Comparison of Varus/Valgus Flexibility Parameter Differences between Varus and Valgus Applied Moments at the Same Knee Flexion Angle

	For 15° Knee Flexion				For 60° Knee Flexion			
	Laxity	IR	TR	TF [°/Nm]	Laxity	IR	TR	TF [°/Nm]
Difference (Varus - Valgus)	1.2°± 3.6°	1.2°± 3.4°	3.0°± 4.0°	0.042 ± 0.039	4.0°± 3.3°	3.3°± 2.8°	4.1°± 2.4°	-0.031 ± 0.043
t Statistic - Paired	0.80	0.82	1.81	2.62*	2.97*	2.81*	4.16*	1.81

IR - Intermediate Rotation at 20 Nm; TR - Terminal Rotation at 60 Nm; TF - Terminal Flexibility between 50 Nm and 60 Nm

* Indicates significance at $p < 0.05$. Critical value of the t statistic for 5 D.O.F. is 2.57.

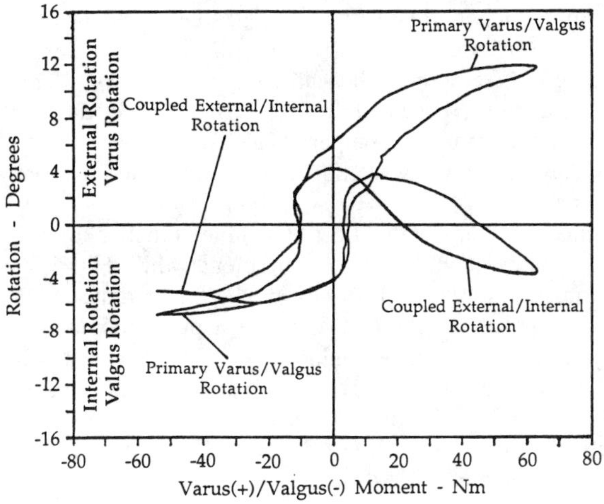

FIG. 3—*Primary varus/valgus rotation and coupled internal/external axial rotation as a result of an applied varus/valgus moment. Because no consistent coupled rotations were observed among the test subjects at both 15 and 60° flexion, mean values of rotation parameters were not significantly different from zero. Results shown are for Test Subject 2 in 60° knee flexion.*

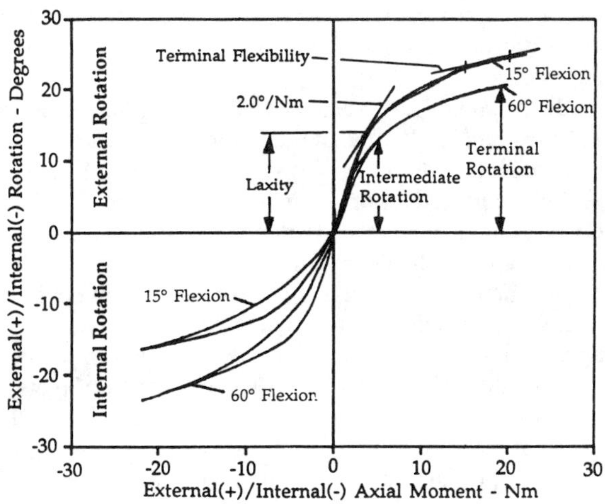

FIG. 4—*The effect of knee flexion angle on internal/external rotation for an applied pure internal/external axial moment. Increasing flexion angle from 15 to 60° increased internal rotation but decreased external rotation. At 15° flexion, external rotation was greater than internal rotation, whereas at 60° flexion, the reverse was evident. Not all these differences apparent in the figure were significant, however. Neither was the decrease in external rotation with flexion significant nor was the difference between external and internal rotations at 60° flexion. The parameters used to quantify the internal/external flexibility results are illustrated in the figure. Results shown are for Test Subject 2.*

significantly different from and greater than zero (Table 3*b*). However, the decrease in TR evident from the figure in external rotation when the knee was flexed from 15 to 60° was not significantly different from zero when all subjects were considered. Mean differences in all parameters except terminal flexibility were significantly different from and greater than zero when external rotation was compared against internal rotation at 15° flexion (Table 3*c*). In contrast, mean differences were not significantly different from zero for any of the parameters at 60° flexion.

Two final columns in Table 3 tabulate the sample statistics for the maximum coupled varus and valgus rotations at ±20-Nm axial moments while Fig. 5 illustrates an example plot of both the primary and coupled rotations. The figure indicates that an external axial moment led to a coupled varus rotation and that a pure internal axial moment led to a coupled valgus rotation. Furthermore, unlike the coupled axial rotations for varus/valgus moment loads, the maximum absolute coupled varus or valgus rotation occurred at the maximum absolute applied axial moment. Because these observations were consistent for all the test subjects, the mean values for both coupled rotations at both flexion angles were significantly different from zero at $p < 0.05$.

Combination Varus/Valgus and Axial Moments

Because of the increased complexity compared to the single loading cases, interpreting the combined loading data required additional information to convey the experimental results. With both loads applied simultaneously, a useful plot is the load-load diagram. On this diagram, axial moment is plotted as a function of varus/valgus moment to assess if the combined loading test approximately followed a straight line between the two load reversal points. With consistency of loading among the test subjects an objective, all combined loading runs had the load-load diagram plotted. Figure 6 plots a superimposed load-load diagram for both Load Cases 1 and 2. Note that neither curve follows a straight line nor returns along the same path. Two test runs were taken from each individual for each load case; flexibility parameters were obtained from the rotation results corresponding to the more linear load-load diagram.

Figures 7 and 8 show example varus/valgus and external/internal flexibility plots respectively for both Load Cases 1 and 2. Plotted in the figures are primary rotation versus primary moment for both external/internal and varus/valgus rotations. As is apparent from Fig. 7, the varus/valgus flexibility curves did not resemble those obtained for single moments. For instance, in Load Case 1, an unloading varus moment led to a maximum varus rotation near zero moment while the valgus half of the curve appeared similar to that obtained in the single loading tests. This increasing rotation with decreasing moment in varus was observed for five of the six test subjects. On the other hand, for all test subjects and Load Case 2, both varus and valgus rotations were near zero at ±40 Nm with the general shape of the flexibility curve unpredictable. Unlike the varus/valgus flexibility plots, Fig. 8 shows that the external/internal flexibility plot more closely resembled the shape of the flexibility curves obtained from single axial moments.

To assess quantitatively how the combined loads affected knee rotations compared to those rotations resulting from single loads, Table 4*a* presents sample statistics for varus/valgus rotation parameters for both single and combined loads, whereas Table 4*b* gives the sample statistics for differences between combined and single moments. Table 4*b* also gives the value of the corresponding *t*-statistic (paired), thus enabling evaluation of mean differences being significantly different from zero. For significance at the $p = 0.05$ level, the critical value of the *t*-statistic is 2.57. Companion tables for internal/external axial rotations are Tables 5*a* and *b*.

Table 3a. Average and Standard Deviation of External/Internal Flexibility Parameters under Single External/Internal Axial Moments Applied to 6 Subjects at 15° and 60° Knee Flexion

	External/Internal Rotations and Flexibility from an Applied External Axial Moment				External/Internal Rotations and Flexibility from an Applied Internal Axial Moment				Total External/ Internal Rotation		Maximum Coupled Varus/Valgus Rotation **	
Knee Flexion Angle	Laxity	IR	TR	TF [°/Nm]	Laxity	IR	TR	TF [°/Nm]	Laxity	TR		
15°	12.8°± 6.0°	16.9°± 5.0°	25.6°± 2.8°	0.423 ± 0.199	-4.1°± 3.5°	-8.8°± 2.9°	-17.6°± 3.8°	0.331 ± 0.127	16.9°± 8.4°	43.2°± 5.0°	4.7°± 1.8°	-4.0°± 2.3°
60°	8.5°± 4.5°	13.8°± 3.9°	24.3°± 2.4°	0.475 ± 0.290	-7.4°± 3.9°	-13.0°± 3.0°	-22.4°± 3.2°	0.360 ± 0.188	15.9°± 3.0°	46.7°± 2.9°	3.0°± 2.3°	-3.6°± 1.9°

Sign Conventions - Varus (+); Valgus (-); External (+); Internal (-)

Table 3b. Statistical Comparison of External/Internal Flexibility Parameter Differences between 60° and 15° Knee Flexions at the Same Applied Moment

	For an Applied External Axial Moment				For an Applied Internal Axial Moment				Total External/ Internal Rotation	
	Laxity	IR	TR	TF [°/Nm]	Laxity	IR	TR	TF [°/Nm]	Laxity	TR
Difference (60° - 15°)	-4.3°± 7.2°	-3.1°± 5.2°	-1.3°± 3.4°	0.051 ± 0.291	3.3°± 2.4°	4.2°± 2.5°	4.8°± 3.1°	-0.029 ± 0.182	-1.0°± 8.6°	3.5°± 3.8°
t Statistic - Paired	1.47	1.45	0.95	0.43	3.46*	4.08*	3.80*	0.40	0.27	2.25

Table 3c. Statistical Comparison of External/Internal Flexibility Parameter Differences between External Axial and Internal Axial Applied Moments at the Same Knee Flexion Angle

	For 15° Knee Flexion				For 60° Knee Flexion			
	Laxity	IR	TR	TF [°/Nm]	Laxity	IR	TR	TF [°/Nm]
Difference (Ext. - Int.)	8.7°± 5.0°	8.1°± 4.8°	8.1°± 4.5°	0.093 ± 0.153	1.1°± 7.9°	0.8°± 5.4°	2.0°± 4.8°	0.115 ± 0.454
t Statistic - Paired	4.25*	4.08*	4.43*	1.48	0.34	0.37	0.99	0.62

IR - Intermediate Rotation at 5 Nm; TR - Terminal Rotation at 20 Nm; TF - Terminal Flexibility between 15 Nm and 20 Nm

* Indicates significance at $p < 0.05$. Critical value of the t statistic for 5 D.O.F. is 2.57.

** Data for 15° are for 5 subjects

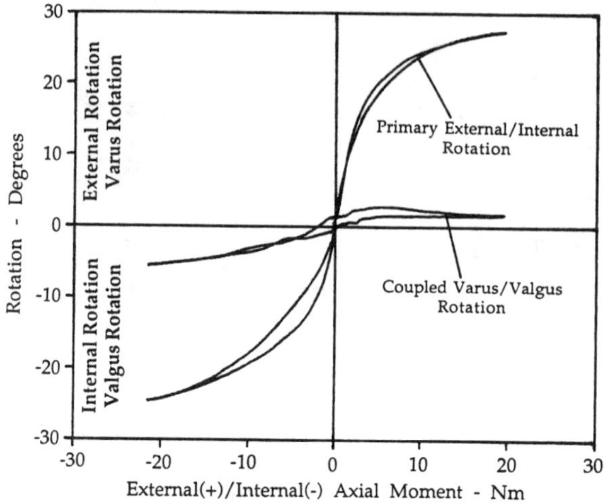

FIG. 5—*Primary internal/external axial rotation and coupled varus/valgus rotation as a result of an applied internal/external axial moment. Because a pure external axial moment consistently led to a coupled varus rotation and a pure internal axial moment consistently led to a coupled valgus rotation, mean rotations were significantly different from zero at both 15 and 60° flexion. Results shown are for Test Subject 3 in 60° knee flexion.*

Before discussing the results in the tables, it is worth elaborating on several aspects of the data presented. Referring first to Table 4*a*, note that it includes columns pertaining to maximum absolute varus and valgus rotations. Because these rotations did not necessarily occur at the maximum absolute varus/valgus moment, the average TR values are different from the average Max values in some cases. Also notice that neither laxity nor terminal flexibility was evaluated for varus/valgus rotations. Referring to Fig. 7, the shape of the

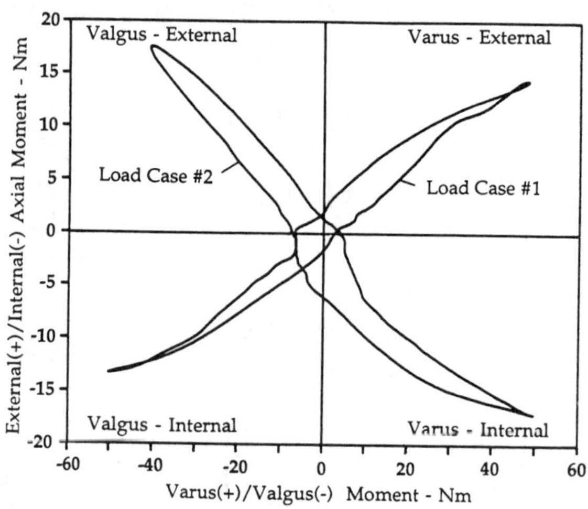

FIG. 6—*Load-versus-load diagram for combination varus/valgus and external/internal axial moments. This plot illustrates the loading path for both Load Case 1 and Load Case 2. Load Case 1 is external axial/varus and internal axial/valgus, while Load Case 2 is external axial/valgus and internal axial/varus. Results shown are for Test Subject 2 in 60° knee flexion.*

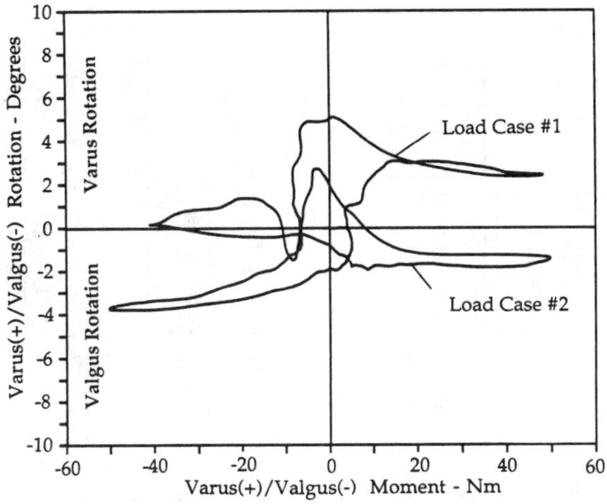

FIG. 7—*Varus/valgus rotation versus varus/valgus moment under combination varus/valgus and internal/external axial moments. The flexibility curve for Load Case 1 illustrates that varus rotation increased during unloading with the maximum rotation near zero moment. In contrast, the magnitudes of both varus and valgus rotations for Load Case 2 were near zero. Both varus and valgus rotations under combination moments were significantly different and less than the rotations under pure varus/valgus moments. Consequently, interaction between all moment combinations was significant. Results shown are for Test Subject 2 in 60° knee flexion.*

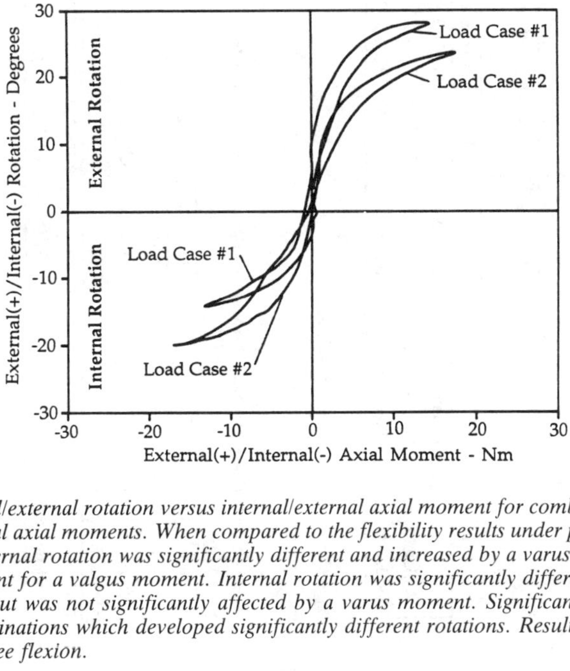

FIG. 8—*Internal/external rotation versus internal/external axial moment for combination varus/valgus and internal/external axial moments. When compared to the flexibility results under pure internal/external axial moments, external rotation was significantly different and increased by a varus moment but was not significantly different for a valgus moment. Internal rotation was significantly different and decreased by a valgus moment but was not significantly affected by a varus moment. Significant interactions existed between load combinations which developed significantly different rotations. Results shown are for Test Subject 2 in 60° knee flexion.*

Table 4a. Average and Standard Deviation of Varus/Valgus Flexibility Parameters under Combination Moments Applied to 6 Subjects at 60° Knee Flexion

	Varus/Valgus Rotations from an Applied Varus Moment				Varus/Valgus Rotations from an Applied Valgus Moment			Total Maximum Rotation
	IR	TR	Max. Rot.		IR	TR	Max. Rot.	
Single Moment	8.2°± 3.6°	10.7°± 3.2°	10.7°± 3.2°	Single Moment	-4.7°± 2.0°	-6.7°± 1.8°	-6.7°± 1.8°	17.4°± 4.8°
With External Axial Moment (LC #1)	4.4°± 1.2°	5.5°± 2.0°	7.0°± 2.1°	With Internal Axial Moment (LC #1)	-3.9°± 1.4°	-4.6°± 1.5°	-4.6°± 1.4°	11.6°± 2.7°
With Internal Axial Moment (LC #2)	0.2°± 1.1°	1.3°± 1.6°	3.5°± 0.9°	With External Axial Moment (LC #2)	0.4°± 0.9°	0.9°± 1.3°	-1.7°± 0.8°	5.2°± 0.5°

Sign Conventions - Varus (+); Valgus (-)

Table 4b. Statistical Comparison of Varus/Valgus Flexibility Parameter Differences between Combination and Single Moments at the Same Applied Moment

	For an Applied Varus Moment				For an Applied Valgus Moment			Total Maximum Rotation
	IR	TR	Max. Rot.		IR	TR	Max. Rot.	
Difference (w/External - Single)	-3.7°± 4.0°	-5.2°± 3.6°	-3.7°± 3.1°	Difference (w/Internal - Single)	-0.8°± 1.1°	-2.1°± 1.1°	-2.1°± 1.1°	-5.8° ± 3.3°
t Statistic - Paired	2.26	3.56*	2.91*	t Statistic - Paired	1.69	4.64*	4.75*	4.23
Difference (w/Internal - Single)	-7.9°± 3.9°	-9.4°± 3.5°	-7.2°± 3.1°	Difference (w/External - Single)	-5.1°± 2.3°	-7.5°± 2.6°	-5.0°± 1.9°	-12.2° ± 4.7°
t Statistic - Paired	5.01*	6.53*	5.68*	t Statistic - Paired	5.47*	7.19*	6.61*	6.30

IR - Intermediate Rotation at 20 Nm; TR - Terminal Rotation at 40 Nm

LC #1 - Load Case #1 (Varus/External - Valgus/Internal); LC #2 - Load Case #2 (Varus/Internal - Valgus/External)

* Indicates significance at $p < 0.05$. Critical value of the t statistic for 5 D.O.F. is 2.57.

Table 5a. Average and Standard Deviation of External/Internal Flexibility Parameters under Combination Moments Applied to 6 Subjects at 60° Knee Flexion

	External/Internal Rotations from an Applied External Axial Moment					External/Internal Rotations from an Applied Internal Axial Moment				Total External/ Internal Rotation	
	Laxity	IR1	IR2	TR #		Laxity	IR1	IR2	TR ##	Laxity	IR2
Single Moment	8.5°± 4.5°	14.3°± 3.9°	19.0°± 3.5°	22.2°± 2.7°	Single Moment	-7.4°± 3.9°	-11.8°± 3.4°	-16.6°± 3.6°	-19.7°± 3.9°	15.9°± 3.0°	35.6°± 4.8°
With Varus Moment (LC #1)	17.1°± 5.5°	19.6°± 4.2°	25.5°± 3.8°	**	With Valgus Moment (LC #1)	-7.8°± 1.9°	-9.1°± 2.2°	-13.4°± 2.9°	-15.8°± 4.8°	24.9°± 6.2°	39.0°± 5.3°
With Valgus Moment (LC #2)	9.6°± 3.0°	13.0°± 3.0°	18.2°± 2.7°	21.6°± 2.6°	With Varus Moment (LC #2)	-9.5°± 4.6°	-11.9°± 3.3°	-16.4°± 4.1°	-18.0°± 3.4°	19.1°± 7.3°	34.7°± 6.7°

Sign Conventions - External (+); Internal (-)

Table 5b. Statistical Comparison of External/Internal Flexibility Parameter Differences between Combination and Single Moments at the Same Applied Moment

	For an Applied External Axial Moment					For an Applied Internal Axial Moment				Total External/ Internal Rotation	
	Laxity	IR1	IR2	TR #		Laxity	IR1	IR2	TR ##	Laxity	IR2
Difference (w/Varus - Single)	8.6°± 5.4°	-5.3°± 3.4°	6.5°± 4.4°	**	Difference (w/Valgus - Single)	0.4°± 4.5°	-2.7°± 2.4°	-3.1°± 2.7°	-3.9°± 2.3°	9.0°± 4.8°	3.4°± 4.9°
t Statistic - Paired	3.92*	3.82*	3.59*	**	t Statistic - Paired	0.23	2.75*	2.79*	2.90*	4.57*	1.69
Difference (w/Valgus - Single)	1.1°± 5.4°	-1.3°± 4.4°	-0.8°± 4.2°	0.5°± 4.5°	Difference (w/Varus - Single)	2.1°± 3.2°	0.1°± 3.6°	-0.1°± 4.4°	-1.7°± 4.6°	-3.2°± 6.8°	-0.9°± 6.5
t Statistic - Paired	0.49	0.70	0.45	0.21	t Statistic - Paired	1.60	0.03	0.06	0.84	1.15	0.34

IR - Intermediate Rotation at 20 Nm; TR - Terminal Rotation at 40 Nm

LC #1 - Load Case #1 (Varus/External - Valgus/Internal); LC #2 - Load Case #2 (Varus/Internal - Valgus/External)

* Indicates significance at $p < 0.05$. Critical value of the t statistic for 5 D.O.F. is 2.57.

** Statistics not practical to calculate because of only one subject

Data for "With Valgus (LC #2)" are for 4 subjects

Data for "With Valgus (LC #1)" are for 3 subjects and data for "With Varus (LC #2)" are for 5 subjects

varus/valgus flexibility curves made computing these parameters impractical. In regard to Table 5, TR values for external rotation in Load Case 1 could not be computed because the corresponding moment level of 15 Nm was not reached for the majority of the subjects.

Table 4*b* indicates that the combined loading significantly affected both varus and valgus rotations compared to the single load case. The mean difference in varus rotations with combined varus and external axial moments was significantly different from and less than zero at the 0.05 level for the TR and Max rotations. Although the mean difference in IR was not significantly different from zero at the 0.05 level, it was significant at the 0.10 level. Also, the mean difference in all three parameters with a combined varus and internal axial moment was significantly different from and less than zero. Similarly, the mean differences in parameters quantifying valgus flexibility were significantly different from and less than zero for both axial moments. Consequently, the effect of an axial moment in either direction was to decrease generally varus/valgus flexibility relative to the flexibility registered for a pure varus/valgus moment.

In contrast to varus/valgus flexibility in which mean differences were significantly different from zero for both internal and external axial moments, mean differences in internal/external axial flexibility were significant only for selected combinations of varus/valgus moments. Table 5*b* indicates that external flexibility was changed significantly with the addition of a varus moment but not a valgus moment. Furthermore, the effect of the varus moment was to cause external flexibility to increase. Mean differences in flexibility parameters (except laxity) in internal rotation with a valgus moment were significantly different from zero and decreased relative to the flexibility for a pure internal axial moment. However, mean differences with a varus moment were not significantly different from zero.

Discussion

With the primary objective of this study being to determine the extent to which combined moments affect the knee moment-rotation relation when compared to single moments, it was necessary to design an experimental apparatus to both apply loads and measure the triaxial rotations, conduct experiments under both single and combined loads, and then quantitate the data to allow for meaningful comparison. Of the four parameters used to quantitate results, both laxity and terminal flexibility were computed using specialized procedures. In the case of laxity, the specialized procedure was new. The motivation behind the new procedure was to yield a value that would be consistent with the definition of the term. The definition of laxity used herein is the movement that the knee undergoes before the structures surrounding the joint offer "substantial" resistance to the movement. To reflect this definition, the slope-approach method of the present research computed laxity as the rotation up to a predetermined slope beyond which the knee became less flexible. This method of computing laxity is independent of the initial stiffness, the terminal stiffness, or any arbitrary load levels on which others have based laxity computations [*4,7,12,19, 21–23*].

While the slope approach method is compatible with the definition of laxity given above, some degree of subjectivity was necessary to implement the procedure. To judge when the resistance to movement became "substantial," the load-rotation records of all subjects were examined and the slope values were then selected. The object of the examination was to determine a slope value that would correspond to the region in the flexibility plots where the slope decreased for all subjects. The slope values used achieved this objective in the judgement of the investigators who made the examination.

As with laxity, different procedures have been used to quantify terminal flexibility/stiffness, but the procedure used was selected to improve the accuracy of this parameter. One procedure has been to calculate stiffness analytically from curve fits [*4,12,27,28*]. These curve fits, however, approximated the whole load-rotation relation thus possibly losing accuracy in the specific region near the load reversal point. Another procedure was to "eye" the slope at the load reversal point [*14*]. Again the accuracy of this procedure was limited due to the inherent variability. To improve the accuracy, the present procedure computed terminal flexibility similar to Bryant and Cooke [*15*] by a linear regression on the loading part of the curve between predetermined load levels. Further, load levels were selected so as to confine this computation to a narrow region of rotation near the load reversal point.

Inaccuracies in the transducers used to measure physical quantities and the inability to control variables precisely which might affect measured quantities introduced sources of variability into quantitative results. In our previous paper [*24*], we discussed in detail the transducer inaccuracies as well as how the load application stand was designed to control known sources of variability (that is, knee and hip flexion angles, coupled loads, muscle activity, axial force, and loading rate). That discussion wil not be repeated here. Rather, the discussion will focus on those sources particular to these tests and not elaborated previously.

One source of variability that was not completely eliminated was muscle activity. Although the load apparatus was adjusted to support the tests subjects' weight, and the subjects were instructed to keep muscles relaxed, the preliminary study showed evidence of relatively low levels (maximum of 5% of maximal voluntary contraction [MVC]) of muscle activity particularly at higher load levels. What effect these low muscle activity levels might have had on the varus/valgus rotation results was investigated by Goldfuss et al. [*29*] who concluded that unconscious muscle activity has no affect on measures of varus/valgus flexibility. Whether this conclusion is also valid for axial flexibility is difficult to assess because of a lack of available data comparing flexibility at low versus no level of muscle activity. However, note that because activity was registered only at high load levels, any effect would be primarily on those parameters computed at these load levels. Thus, the TR and TF parameters would be affected whereas laxity and IR would not.

A second source of variability particularly in the parameters (except total rotations) in axial rotation surrounded the set point for zero rotation. With these parameters being quantified for each direction of rotation, the definition of the setpoint directly influenced parameter values. Because the goal of this research was to quantitate the load rotation of the knee, the setpoint was the position of the joint in the unloaded state. As noted in the **Methods** section, the setpoint was established by monitoring the moment transducers for zero load. Accordingly, any inaccuracy in identifying zero load could be manifest as a shift in the setpoint. With the average absolute accuracy of the axial moment transducer being 0.3 Nm, setpoint differences could have been as large as about 1°. Any difference would then appear to decrease the value of all rotation parameters in one rotation direction by the difference amount and increase those values in the other by the same amount.

A final source of variability in the results at 15° flexion revolved around the control of this angle. The initial angle of the knee in these tests was the angle naturally assumed when the leg was suspended in the gravity field, the muscles were relaxed, and no moment loads were applied. Measured from full extension, this angle was not the same for each subject varying by a maximum ±4° about 15° which was the average angle. Further, monitoring the knee flexion angle throughout the tests using the goniometer showed some variation in this angle. Inasmuch as the load rotation of the knee is sensitive to flexion angle between full extension and about 30° flexion [*11,20*], differences in this angle initially as well as changes in this angle about the initial position would introduce variability into the parameter values.

Because of the variability in the parameters chosen to quantify knee flexibility as a result of both knee joint structural differences and the aforementioned sources, it was necessary to perform hypothesis tests on parameter sample statistics to determine what experimental conditions significantly affected knee flexibility. To enhance the sensitivity of the testing procedure by negating the effects of the large within-sample variation, a paired *t*-test was chosen [*30*]. Without this enhancement (that is, the unpaired *t*-test), neither would the increase in varus rotations in flexing from 15 to 60° be significant (Table 2*b*) nor would the decrease in internal rotation with a combined valgus/internal axial moment be significant (Table 5*b*). Consequently, the paired *t*-test was valuable in identifying differences that might otherwise have gone undetected.

Comparison with Previous Research

Comparisons between the present work and previous research need to be made with caution because the methods used to obtain flexibility/stiffness data were not consistent. The following three considerations potentially contribute to inconsistencies in the results: the differences in the testing apparatus; the state of the knee (that is, in vitro versus in vivo); and the anthropometry, age, and gender of specimens or test subjects. Nonetheless, comparisons with previously done work are important in the assessment of the results obtained in the present research. Note that since no previous research quantified either laxity or TF as in the present work, quantitative comparisons with other work will only involve IR and/or TR. Further, as a result of differences in determining zero rotation references, only total rotations will be compared.

A number of workers conducted experiments which explored the effect of both moment direction and flexion angle on varus/valgus moment-rotation relations in vitro [*4,6–8,10,11*]. Although these studies were conducted at a variety of load levels, they are consistent in reporting that both varus and valgus rotations at 60° flexion were generally increased over those rotations at 15° flexion. This agrees with the results of the present study. Using test apparatus that permitted coupled motions as did the test apparatus here, the studies by Markolf et al. [*7*], Gollehon et al. [*10*], and Grood et al. [*11*] applied load levels of ±20 Nm at flexion angles of 15 to 20°. Thus, results can be compared quantitatively. Average total rotations of 13.5° [*7*], 14.5° [*10*], and 10° [*11*] are similar to the average of 13.2° in Table 2*a*. Two of these studies also applied moments at 60° knee flexion. The total rotation of 17.1° reported by Gollehon et al. [*10*] compares closely with the total rotation of 19.5° in Table 2*a*, whereas the 13.1° of Grood et al. [*11*] is lower.

Several studies applied varus/valgus moments and measured the resulting varus/valgus angles in vivo [*12–15*]. Although all of these studies applied moment levels of ±20 Nm, only the study by Markolf et al. [*13*] applied moments at a flexion angle of 20°, which is comparable to that here, so that comparison will be limited to this study. The average total rotation of 12.3° given by Markolf et al. [*13*] agrees closely with the average 13.2° from Table 2*a*. Thus, the total rotations reported by previous in-vivo and in-vitro studies at a load level and flexion angle similar to that here compare favorably to the results here.

Since much research has been conducted on knee flexibility/stiffness in vitro under axial loading, comparisons with this body of work are also of interest. Among these in-vitro studies are those by Wang and Walker [*16*], Crowninshield et al. [*6*], Hseih and Walker [*1*], Markolf et al. [*4,7*], Lipke et al. [*18*], Nielsen et al. [*8*], Shoemaker and Markolf [*19*], Gollehon et al. [*10*], Blankevoort et al. [*20*], and Good et al. [*11*]. The majority of these studies examined the effect of flexion angle on the total rotation between some predefined load limits. While the load limits varied, the results were consistent in that total rotation increased somewhat as the joint was flexed from 15 to 60°. This is similar to the finding here in which Table 3*a* shows larger total rotations at 60 than 15° flexion. Restricting attention to the two studies by Gollehon et al. [*10*] and Grood et al. [*11*], a meaningful quantitative comparison can be made. Similar to the varus/valgus comparison, the load levels were approximately the same as that for the IR values in Table 3*a*, and as mentioned previously, both investigators used experimental techniques in which joint motion was not constrained. At both 15 and 60° flexion, the average values of 39 and 44° [*10*] and 34 and 40° [*11*], respectively, were larger than the average total IR of 25.7 and 26.8° (15 and 60° flexion) from Table 3*a*. Although subject age and passive muscle tension might be offered as factors to account for this difference, the agreement between in-vitro and in-vivo results in varus/valgus rotations discourages such an accounting.

Comparisons to the results of the in vivo studies are complicated by differences in test variables. The in vivo studies by Shoemaker and Markolf [*21*], Markolf et al. [*13*], Louie and Mote [*22*], and Hull and Johnson [*23*] all used subject samples that were comparable in average age to that here, but no study duplicated the combinations of load level and flexion angles. Further, only the studies by Shoemaker and Markolf [*21*] and Markolf et al. [*13*] were conducted at consistent maximum load levels which were ±10 Nm. At 20° flexion the average total rotations of 41 [*21*] and 29.9° [*13*] were higher than the average total IR of 25.7° at ±5 Nm here which is expected due to the higher load levels. Thus, the results of this study agree qualitatively with what would be expected due to differences in test variables from previous in vivo studies.

The present study observed significant coupled varus rotation with an external axial moment and significant coupled valgus rotation with an internal axial moment. One explanation for this finding is that during external/internal rotation, the motion of the condyles on the tibial plateau, within the constraints of the supporting ligaments, is such that the condyles ride up onto the menisci. This thereby shifts the tibia in either varus or valgus rotation depending on the axial moment direction.

Reports of varus/valgus rotations under axial moment loads from previous in-vitro studies are conflicting. Gollehon et al. [*10*] applied ±4.5-Nm axial moments to 17 specimens but found no "consistent or meaningful coupled rotations in either magnitude or direction in intact knees." Also, Grood et al. [*11*] concurred with this finding. In contrast, Blankevoort et al. [*20*] applied ±3 Nm to 4 knee specimens and found coupled rotations consistent with those reported here.

Combination Varus/Valgus and Axial Moments

The rotations observed for some of the combined loads suggest that rotations are a result of complex interactions between the ligaments and the articular surfaces. Interaction was apparent for both varus/valgus and internal/external axial flexibilities. For varus/valgus flexibility, axial moments in both directions significantly decreased both varus and valgus rotations. If interaction was not a factor so that rotations from single moments were additive, then based on the coupled rotation results from the pure load tests, varus rotations would be expected to increase under the application of a combination varus/external axial moment, whereas valgus rotations would increase under a combination valgus/internal axial moment. Because the changes in rotations were opposite to these expectations, interaction was evident. Also, because neither an external axial moment induced a coupled valgus rotation nor an internal axial moment caused a coupled varus rotation, the significant decrease in both these rotations for combination valgus/external axial and varus/internal axial moments indicates interaction between these loads as well. Thus interaction was prevalent in varus/valgus flexibility for all combinations of loads.

In contrast to the case for varus/valgus flexibility, interaction in internal/external axial rotations was apparent for selected load combinations rather than all load combinations.

Recall that external rotation was significantly changed and increased by a varus moment but not by a valgus moment, whereas internal rotation was significantly changed and decreased for a valgus moment but not changed by a varus moment. Because neither varus nor valgus moments induced predictable coupled internal/external axial rotations, interaction was likely for the two moment combinations in which changes were significant, but not the other two.

Beyond the apparent interaction between load combinations, another observation of interest is the increase in varus rotation that occurred in combination external axial and varus moments during unloading. Depicted in Fig. 7 for load Case 1, this result was observed for five of the six test subjects, and the maximum varus rotation consistently occurred near zero moment. Moreover, in examining the load-load curves for each of the test subjects, no sudden increases in varus moment were observed which would lead to the rotation increases. One observation of note in all of the load-load diagrams was that as the varus moment approached zero, about 5 Nm of an external axial moment was present. Recalling that a single external axial moment led to coupled varus rotation, it is possible that without the presence of a varus/valgus moment, the external axial moment caused a sudden increase in varus rotation. This is plausible considering that most of the coupled varus rotations in the single axial moment studies occurred within 5 Nm of the start of the axial loading tests.

Inasmuch as the motivation behind this research was to gain a more thorough understanding of the mechanics of knee ligamentous injuries incurred in falls which develop combination axial and varus/valgus moments, the final issue meriting discussion is the relevance of the results reported here to injury mechanics. To appreciate this relevance, it must first be recognized that ligament injury (that is, midsubstance tearing) is a strain-related phenomenon. Accordingly, a complete understanding of injury mechanics ultimately requires relating load to strain. To establish such a relation there are two possible approaches. One approach is to relate load first to displacements and then displacements to strain while the other approach is to relate load directly to strain bypassing the displacement measures.

The results of this research have utility regardless of which approach is followed. If the first approach is followed, then the results of this research are directly useful here since they provide the load-displacement relations. If the second approach is followed, then the results are also useful in that they guide experimental protocol. One important aspect of this protocol surrounds the interactions between loads. Although ligament strain probably cannot be inferred directly from joint displacements, displacements nevertheless bear some relation to strain since strain is dictated by the relative motion between the two bones. Accordingly, the interactions between moments in causing rotations reported here will likely occur between moments in causing strains as well so that the study of these interactions should be part of the experimental protocol.

Conclusions

1. Load direction significantly affected knee flexibility for both varus/valgus and axial moments. For terminal varus/valgus rotations at both 15 and 60° flexion angles, varus was significantly different from and greater than valgus rotation. For axial rotations at 15° flexion, terminal external rotation was significantly different from and greater than terminal internal rotation, whereas at 60° flexion, no significant differences were observed.
2. The rotation of the knee under both varus/valgus and external/internal axial moments was also significantly affected by flexion angle. In flexing from 15 to 60°, mean differences in both varus and valgus terminal rotations were significantly different from and greater than zero indicating an increase in flexibility with flexion angle. On the

other hand, in flexing from 15 to 60°, the mean difference in terminal external rotation was not significantly different from zero, whereas that difference in internal rotation was significantly different from and greater than zero.

3. Both varus/valgus and axial moments produced coupled rotations. Of the two loading modes, only axial moments produced consistent coupled rotations; external axial moments resulted in significant varus rotation, and internal axial moments resulted in significant valgus rotation. For both moments, the coupled rotations were large when compared to the laxity values obtained from the single moment tests.
4. Combined loads with the knee at 60° flexion led to rotations that exhibited significant interactions when compared to rotations obtained from the single moment tests at the same load level and flexion angle. For varus/valgus rotations, axial moments in both directions produced rotations in which significant interaction was evident for all load combinations. For axial rotations, interaction was significant for selected load combinations. Especially, the combinations of varus/external and valgus/internal moments interacted, whereas the combinations of valgus/external and varus/internal did not.
5. Because interaction between external axial and valgus moments in valgus rotation was significant, the interaction between combined loads is a potentially important phenomenon in the mechanics of knee ligamentous injury and, in particular, MCL/ACL injury. Future research seeking to relate ligament strain to the injury causing loads should quantitatively evaluate the importance of this phenomenon.

Acknowledgment

We are grateful to the Tyrolia Corporation of Vienna, Austria and in particular Dr. Klaus Hoelzl for financially supporting this research.

References

[1] Johnson, R. J., Pope, M. H., Weisman, G., White, B. F., and Ettlinger, C., "Knee Injury in Skiing—A Multifaceted Approach," *American Journal of Sports Medicine*, Vol. 7, No. 6, 1979, pp. 321–327.

[2] Howe, J. and Johnson, R. J., "Knee Injuries in Skiing," *Orthopedic Clinics of North America*, Vol. 16, No. 2, 1985, pp. 303–314.

[3] Shino, K., Horibe, S., Nagano, J., and Ono, K., "Injury of the Anterior Cruciate Ligament of the Knee in Downhill Skiing: Its Pathomechanism and Treatment," in *Skiing Trauma and Safety: Sixth International Symposium, ASTM STP 938*, C. D. Mote, Jr. and R. J. Johnson, Eds., American Society for Testing and Materials, Philadelphia, 1987, pp. 68–86.

[4] Markolf, K. L., Mensch, J. S., and Amstutz, H. C., "Stiffness and Laxity of the Knee—Contributions of the Supporting Structures. A Quantitative In-Vitro Study," *Journal of Bone and Joint Surgery*, Vol. 58A, No. 5, 1976, pp. 583–593.

[5] Kennedy, J. and Fowler, P. J., "Medial and Anterior Instability of the Knee: An Anatomical and Clinical Study Using Stress Machines," *Journal of Bone and Joint Surgery*, Vol. 53A, No. 7, 1971, pp. 1257–1270.

[6] Crowninshield, R., Pope, M. H., and Johnson, R. J., "An Analytical Model of the Knee," *Journal of Biomechanics*, Vol. 9, 1976, pp. 397–405.

[7] Markolf, K. L., Bargar, W. L., Shoemaker, S. C., and Amstutz, H. C., "The Role of Joint Load in Knee Stability," *Journal of Bone and Joint Surgery*, Vol. 63A, No. 4, 1981, pp. 570–585.

[8] Nielsen, S., Rasmussen, O., Ovesen, J., and Andersen, K., "Rotary Instability of Cadaver Knees after Transection of Collateral Ligaments and Capsule," *Archives of Orthopedics and Trauma Surgery*, Vol. 103, No. 3, 1984, pp. 165–169.

[9] Nielsen, S., Ovesen, J., and Rasmussen, D., "The Anterior Cruciate Ligament of the Knee: An Experimental Study of Its Importance in Rotary Knee Stability," *Archives of Orthopedics and Trauma Surgery*, Vol. 103, No. 3, 1984, pp. 170–174.

[*10*] Gollehon, D. L., Torzilli, P. A., and Warren, R. F., "The Role of the Posteriolateral and Cruciate Ligaments in the Stability of the Human Knee," *Journal of Bone and Joint Surgery*, Vol. 69A, No. 2, 1987, pp. 233–242.

[*11*] Grood, E. S., Stowers, S. F., and Noyes, F. R., "Limits of Movement in the Human Knee," *Journal of Bone Joint Surgery*, Vol. 70-A, No. 1, 1988, pp. 88–97.

[*12*] Markolf, K. L., Graff-Radford, A., and Amstutz, H. C., "In Vivo Knee Stability—A Quantitative Assessment Using an Instrumented Clinical Testing Apparatus," *Journal of Bone and Joint Surgery*, Vol. 60A, No. 5, 1978, pp. 664–674.

[*13*] Markolf, K. L., Kochan, A., and Amstutz, H. C., "Measurement of Knee Stiffness and Laxity in Patients with Documented Absence of the Anterior Cruciate Ligament," *Journal of Bone and Joint Surgery*, Vol. 66-A, No. 2, 1984, pp. 242–253.

[*14*] Olmstead, T. G., Wevers, H. W., Bryant, J. T., and Gouw, G. J., "Effect of Muscular Activity on Varus/Valgus Laxity and Stiffness of the Knee," *Journal of Biomechanics*, Vol. 19, No. 8, 1986, pp. 565–577.

[*15*] Bryant, J. T., and Cooke, T. D. V., "Standardized Biomechanical Measurement for Valgus/Varus Stiffness and Rotation in Normal Knees," *Journal of Orthopedic Research*, Vol. 6, No. 6, 1988, pp. 863–870.

[*16*] Wang, C. and Walker, P. S., "Rotary Laxity of the Human Knee Joint," *Journal of Bone and Joint Surgery*, Vol. 56A, No. 1, 1974, pp. 161–170.

[*17*] Hseih, H. and Walker, P. S., "Stabilizing Mechanisms of the Loaded and Unloaded Knee Joint," *Journal of Bone and Joint Surgery*, Vol. 58A, No. 1, 1976, pp. 87–93.

[*18*] Lipke, J. M., Janecki, C. J., Nelson, C. L., McLeod, P., Thompson, C., et al., "The Role of Incompetence of the Anterior Cruciate and Lateral Ligaments in Anteriolateral and Anteriomedial Instability," *Journal of Bone and Joint Surgery*, Vol. 63-A, No. 6, 1981, pp. 954–960.

[*19*] Shoemaker, S. C. and Markolf, K. L., "Effects of Joint Load on the Stiffness and Laxity of Ligament-Deficient Knees: An In-Vitro Study of the Anterior Cruciate and Medial Collateral Ligaments," *Journal of Bone and Joint Surgery*, Vol. 67A, No. 1, 1985, pp. 136–146.

[*20*] Blankevoort, L., Huiskes, R., and deLange, A., "The Envelope of Passive Knee Motion," *Journal of Biomechanics*, Vol. 21, No. 9, 1988, pp. 705–720.

[*21*] Shoemaker, S. C. and Markolf, K. L., "In Vivo Rotary Knee Stability," *Journal of Bone and Joint Surgery*, Vol. 64A, No. 2, 1987, pp. 208–216.

[*22*] Louie, J. K. and Mote, C. D., Jr., "Contribution of the Musculature to Rotary Laxity and Torsional Stiffness at the Knee," *Journal of Biomechanics*, Vol. 20, No. 3, 1987, pp. 281–300.

[*23*] Hull, M. L. and Johnson, C., "Axial Rotation of the Lower Limb Under Torsional Loading: I. Static and Dynamic Measurements," in *Skiing Trauma and Safety: Seventh International Symposium, ASTM STP 1022*, R. J. Johnson, C. D. Mote, Jr., and M. H. Binet, Eds., American Society of Testing and Materials, 1989, Philadelphia, pp. 277–290.

[*24*] Mills, O. S. and Hull, M. L., "Flexibility of the Human Knee Due to Varus/Valgus and Axial Moments in Vivo: Apparatus Design and Performance Evaluation," in this volume, pp. 11–34.

[*25*] Grood, E. S., and Suntay, W. J., "A Joint Coordinate System for the Clinical Description of Three-Dimensional Motions: Application to the Knee," *Journal of Biomechanical Engineering*, Vol. 105, No. 5, 1983, pp. 136–144.

[*26*] Delagi, E. F., Perotto, A., Azzeti, J., and Morrison, D., *Anatomical Guide for the Electromyographer—The Limbs*, Charles C Thomas, Springfield, IL, 1975.

[*27*] Piziali, R. L., Rastegar, J., and Nagel, D. A., "Measurement of the Nonlinear, Coupled Stiffness Characteristics of the Human Knee," *Journal of Biomechanics*, Vol. 10, No. 1, 1977, pp. 45–51.

[*28*] Seering, W. P., Piziali, R. L., Nagel, D. A., and Schurman, D. J., "The Function of the Primary Ligaments of the Knee in Varus-Valgus and Axial Rotation," *Journal of Biomechanics*, Vol. 13, No. 9, 1980, pp. 785–794.

[*29*] Goldfuss, A. J., Morehouse, C. A., and LeVeau, B. F., "Effect of Muscular Tension on Knee Stability," *Medicine and Science in Sports*, Vol. 5, No. 4, 1973, pp. 267–271.

[*30*] Dougherty, E. R., *Probability and Statistics for the Engineering and Computing Sciences*, Prentice-Hall, Englewood Cliffs, NJ, 1990, pp. 473–478.

Gregory S. Berns,[1] *Maury L. Hull,*[2] *and Hugh A. Patterson*[3]

Design and Performance Evaluation of an Automated System to Determine Knee Flexibility in Vitro

REFERENCE: Berns, G. S., Hull, M. L., and Patterson, H. A., "**Design and Performance Evaluation of an Automated System to Determine Knee Flexibility in Vitro,**" *Skiing Trauma and Safety: Eighth International Symposium, ASTM STP 1104*, C. D. Mote, Jr. and Robert J. Johnson, Eds., American Society for Testing and Materials, Philadelphia, 1991, pp. 57–76.

ABSTRACT: An automated system was designed to study the complete flexibility functions of the knee in vitro. The system allows five degrees of freedom with flexion angle being fixed, although adjustable from 0 to 45°. Loads corresponding to each of the five motions can be applied independently and in any combination. The effect of weight bearing on knee flexibility can also be studied by including axial force as one of the five loads. The relative motions are accurately measured with linear and rotary variable differential transformers (LVDTs and RVDTs), and the loads are measured with strain gage transducers. The system is digitally controlled with a closed feedback loop, allowing for any combination of programmed loads. A control algorithm on an IBM PC/AT monitors the loads on each axis and continuously adjusts stepping motors to follow programmed loads correctly. The machine coordinate system corresponds to clinically accepted definitions of motion yet retains sequence independence for rotations. Results demonstrate the repeatability of using a functional definition of axis placement to align the leg within the machine and the utility of the full flexibility functions of the knee, notably in the determination of significant load interactions and coupled motions.

KEY WORDS: biomechanics, knee, flexibility, automated system, five degrees of freedom

To prevent knee injuries from occurring, a thorough understanding of the load response of the joint must first be obtained. The load response refers to the deformations that occur in either the joint or its structures or both when loads are transmitted through it. Load transmission generally occurs from two types of events. The first is the use of muscles to move either the leg or the body. The second type of load transmission can occur from the application of an external load (for example, a fall in alpine skiing), in which case the inertia of the leg and body resists the load. In either event, when loads are transmitted through the joint, the ligaments and menisci must support these loads. Because these are soft tissues, they will deform, leading to a relative deformation of the femur and the tibia. The amount of deformation divided by the applied load is termed flexibility. The load response of the knee refers to both the magnitude of flexibility and the amount of soft tissue deformation, measured by strain. Because excessive strain leads to injury, by determining the relationship of load to displacement and displacement to strain, the types of loads to which the knee is

[1]Research assistant, Biomedical Engineering Graduate Group, University of California, Davis, CA 95616.
[2]Professor, Department of Mechanical Engineering, University of California, Davis, CA 95616.
[3]Lecturer, Department of Human Anatomy, University of California, Davis, CA 95616.

most susceptible to injury can be deduced. This paper is concerned with measuring the load-to-displacement (flexibility) relationship.

To study knee injuries accurately, one must have the capability of realistically simulating the conditions under which they occur. The knee is sufficiently complex so that any simplification of real-world loading conditions may significantly affect the results. Because injuries typically occur from combinations of loads, an accurate study of injury mechanics should examine as many combinations of loads as is deemed necessary to identify the most injurious ones. Consequently, the experimental apparatus must have the capability of applying any possible combination of loads.

While few studies have examined the effects of load combinations on the knee, much work has been done in determining single-load flexibilities and the contribution of specific structures in the knee to this. Early work on the mechanics of knee injury was aimed at determining the function of individual ligaments [*1*], and many groups have extended the method of ligament cutting to determine function [*2–9*]. The extension of this technique centers around improvements in instrumentation to measure joint displacements and, in some cases, correlating results with clinical reports of injury [*10,11*]. However, any conclusions from experiments of this type necessarily rely on the assumption that ligament functions do not interact with each other, that is, cutting one ligament does not affect the function of the remaining structures. Clearly, this cannot be entirely valid because several structures are intimately related to one another (for example, the two cruciate ligaments). We believe that any study aimed at determining ligament function should be performed in the most realistic manner possible—on intact knees.

While we do not yet fully understand the mechanics of knee injury, we do understand which variables might contribute to injury. We therefore have enough information to design a system capable of studying the effect of these variables on both knee flexibility and soft tissue strain, the parameters associated with injury.

One variable that may significantly affect joint flexibility and hence knee injury is muscle activity. Some studies of flexibility have been performed in vivo [*10,12–14*] to investigate the effect of muscle activity. And, while it has been shown that muscle activity increases joint stiffness [*12–14*], the role of the musculature in preventing injuries is still unclear [*15–17*]. These studies show that, even though voluntary muscle contraction probably does not occur rapidly enough to prevent knee injury, the instantaneous level of muscle activity significantly affects joint stiffness. Therefore, any realistic study of injury mechanisms must account for muscle activation.

Two other variables that may significantly affect joint mechanics are weight bearing and flexion angle. Because weight bearing seats the femoral condyles in the menisci, it is reasonable that joint flexibility would decrease [*5,9*]. Weight bearing, however, may simply be considered as one of the loads applied to the joint and does not necessitate separate consideration. Flexion angle, however, significantly alters the geometry of the joint and should be considered as a separate variable [*3,4,6,18*].

Recent studies have shown that constraints on knee motion imposed by experimental apparatus dramatically affect the biomechanics of the joint and the strain patterns of the ligaments [*19,20*]. Because the knee allows both translations and rotations, any constraints that prevent natural motion will bias the measurements during load application. Therefore, the most accurate study of knee mechanics and injury requires an apparatus that allows six degrees of freedom.

Beyond the variables already mentioned, the rate of loading is another important variable to consider in injury mechanics. Affecting the biomechanics of the knee joint are the material properties of the ligament, particularly their viscoelasticity [*21–24*]. Because the ligaments exhibit this behavior and knee injury may occur during falls in which the loading rate is relatively high, there is a need to study how loading rate affects injury mechanics. However, knee injury during skiing also occurs during slow fall situations. Thus, the need for multiple degree-of-freedom studies under quasistatic loads exists as well. We have therefore decided to concentrate on these latter studies.

One objective of this study was to design a system capable of studying the knee in such a way that the data would represent the most reliable simulation of injury possible. Thus, the primary design criterion was to apply any combination of external loads to intact knee specimens while still allowing the joint to move naturally. Secondary requirements were the need to simulate muscle activity and vary flexion angle. Such a system, which enables a full characterization of joint flexibility, including load couplings and interactions, is necessary to improve the understanding of injury mechanics.

A second objective was to evaluate the performance of the system; specifically, the application of this system to study knee flexibility requires the ability to apply accurately and reliably multiple loads simultaneously. Considering the time constraints of using fresh cadaveric specimens, the system must apply these loads in a reasonable amount of time also. Our evaluation considered such criteria as the repeatability of aligning a specimen within the system, the repeatability of obtaining flexibility measurements, and the time required to apply loads.

Methods and Materials

Coordinate System

Before any measurements of joint flexibility can be made, a coordinate system must be established at the knee. A coordinate system serves a dual purpose as a reference for displacement measurements and as a set of axes for load application. Our system was designed around the coordinate system described by Grood and Suntay [*25*]. The coordinate system has the advantage of corresponding to clinically accepted definitions of joint motion. It also has the desirable property of sequence independence of rotations.

This coordinate system fixes one axis to the tibia and one axis to the femur. The third axis "floats," being unfixed to either bone but intersecting the other two axes at right angles (see Fig. 1). To correspond to the anatomical axes, the fixed tibia axis runs longitudinally. Internal/external rotation occurs about this axis. Either of the two other axes may be fixed to the femur. The femur-fixed axis could be placed running laterally through the femoral condyles, corresponding to flexion/extension. The varus/valgus axis would then float. Alternatively, the varus/valgus axis, which is directed anteriorly/posteriorly, could be attached to the femur at the point of contact with the tibial plateau, in which case the flexion axis floats. Even though flexion angle was fixed in our experiments, we used the former setup for consistency with prior research. In either case, one achieves rotational independence of the three axes while still retaining clinically accepted definitions of motion.

Mechanical and Electrical Components

An apparatus was designed and constructed with the following capabilities:

(1) five degrees of freedom are allowed with flexion/extension being fixed, although adjustable from 0 to 45°;
(2) loads corresponding to each of the remaining five motions can be applied independently and in any combination;
(3) the relative joint motions can be measured in the coordinate system with linear and rotary variable differential transformers (LVDTs and RVDTs);

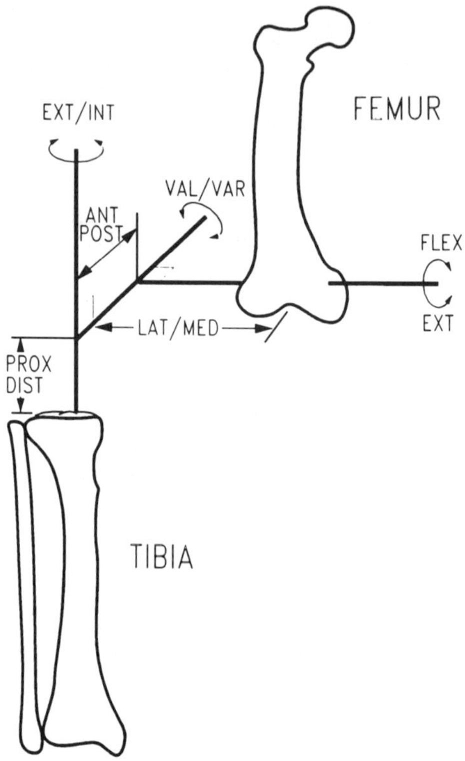

FIG. 1—*Coordinate system incorporated in the apparatus. The internal/external axis is fixed to the tibia, while the flexion/extension axis is fixed to the femur. The varus/valgus axis is fixed to neither bone but "floats," being mutually perpendicular to the other two axes. Rotations in this coordinate system are sequence independent and coincide with clinically accepted definitions of motion.*

(4) the position of the leg can be adjusted to allow for alignment of the coordinate axes with the anatomical axes;
(5) the joint can be subjected to either programmed load or displacement sequences by means of digitally controlled direct current (dc) stepping motors;
(6) elongation of the anterior cruciate ligament (ACL) and medial collateral ligament (MCL) can be recorded with appropriate transducers during load application.

The apparatus (Figs. 2, 3, and 4) consists of two units, the tibia unit and the femur unit, each holding the respective bones. Both units apply specific loads and enable corresponding movements. When mounted in the apparatus, the leg is positioned on its side so that medial/lateral translation is in the vertical direction. Both the tibia and femur are potted in cylindrical tubes with polymethylmethacrylate (PMMA). During potting, the bones are held in place with four pairs of screws tightened to a snug fit against the periosteum. This serves the additional purpose of preventing rotation of the hardened PMMA within the tubes under application of external torques. Each of the bones is coupled to its respective unit through two concentric pairs of cylinders, used to align the specimen. The inner cylinders clamp to the bone tubes and can translate vertically by means of threaded shafts and hand knobs. These shafts couple the bone to a larger cylinder which has shafts attached to the outside and are perpendicular to the inner ones (see Figs. 3 and 4). This allows adjustment in the horizontal direction. Because two of these clamping mechanisms are attached to each bone, the tibia and femur may be translated and rotated independently with respect to the apparatus. When the desired position is achieved, the shafts may be fixed with lock nuts.

Of the six degrees of freedom possible, the tibia unit allows two degrees of freedom: internal/external rotation and proximal/distal translation. Internal/external rotation is achieved by nesting the tibia bone clamps within a third outer cylinder which is free to rotate about its long axis (see Fig. 3). This outer rotation is accomplished by supporting the outer cylinder proximally by three cam followers and distally by a shaft attached to a plate capping the end of the cylinder. The shaft, supported in a pillow block, is driven by a dc stepping motor through a 300:1 gear reduction. This allows for a maximum applied internal/external torque of approximately 200 N/m on the tibia. To provide proximal/distal translation, the entire unit is mounted on linear ball bearings parallel to the tibial axis. The axial force, which

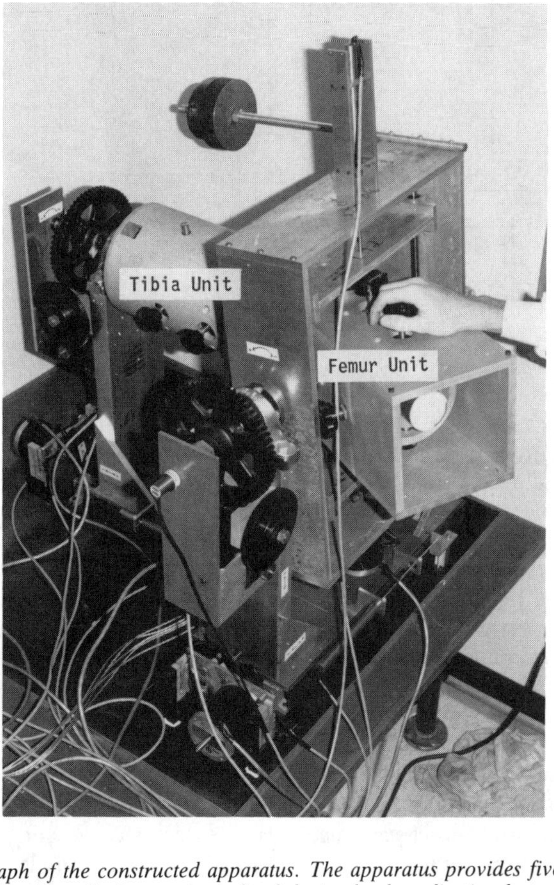

FIG. 2—*Photograph of the constructed apparatus. The apparatus provides five degrees of freedom. The sixth degree of freedom, flexion angle, is fixed during load application but can be adjusted from 0 to 45°. Included in the hardware are the tibia and femur clamps, which form an adjustable alignment system. Each bone may be adjusted independently in six degrees of freedom relative to the mechanical hardware. This allows alignment of the functional axes of the knee with those of the apparatus. Loads corresponding to each of five motions can be applied either singly or in any combination by means of computer-controlled DC stepping motors. Loads are measured by strain gage transducers, and displacements are measured by rotational and linear variable differential transformers.*

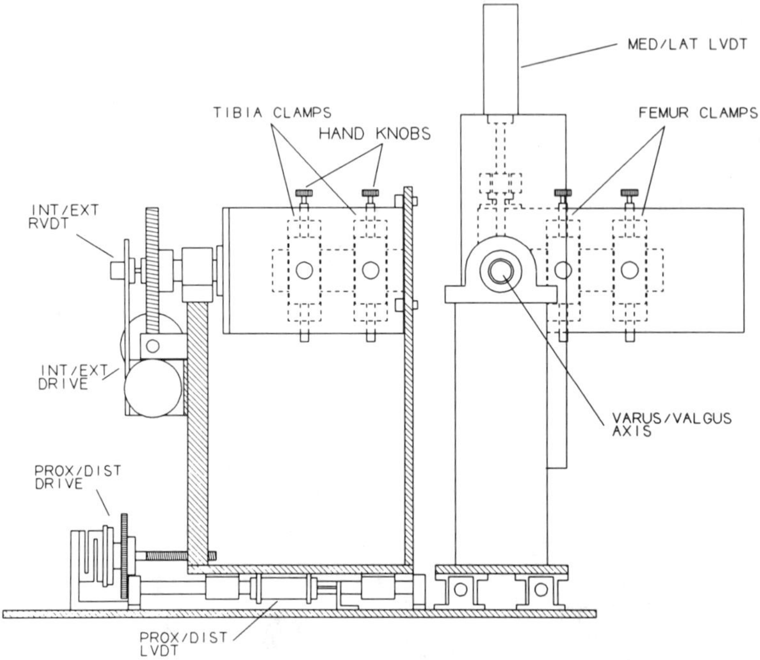

FIG. 3—*Side view of the apparatus. The tibia unit provides two of the degrees of freedom, internal/external axial rotation and proximal/distal translation.*

corresponds to joint compression, is developed through a screw mechanism and a 5:1 gear reduction, allowing for a maximum force of 1000 N.

The femur unit allows four degrees of freedom: varus/valgus and flexion/extension rotations and medial/lateral and anterior/posterior translations. Flexion/extension is achieved by nesting the femur bone clamps within an outer box which is allowed to rotate about an axis perpendicular to its top and bottom faces by means of shafts and ball bearings (see Figs. 3 and 4). The flexion angle may be fixed through a locking arm. The box is also allowed to translate vertically, which corresponds to medial/lateral motion, through linear ball bearings. This translation is driven through a screw mechanism similar to that described above. Varus/valgus rotation is achieved by mounting the whole assembly in a large frame to which shafts are attached and supported by pillow blocks. A stepping motor and gear reduction apply varus/valgus torques up to 200 N/m. Anterior/posterior translation is allowed by mounting the varus/valgus pillow blocks on a carriage supported by linear ball bearings and driven by a screw mechanism with forces up to 1000 N.

Provision for simulating muscle contraction is provided by cables and pulleys. Cables with load-sensing rings can be sutured to the tendons of the major muscle groups crossing the knee (the quadriceps, biceps femoris and semitendinosus, and gastrocnemius). The cables can be routed around pulleys to a screw mechanism that applies tension.

Because each of the motors used has a holding torque of 2.2 N/m, a large gear reduction is necessary to increase the load applied to the knee. This gear reduction is to reduce the displacement of the driving shaft for each step of the motor. Because each increment of the motor results in a 1.8° shaft rotation, the gear train reduces this even further. The net result

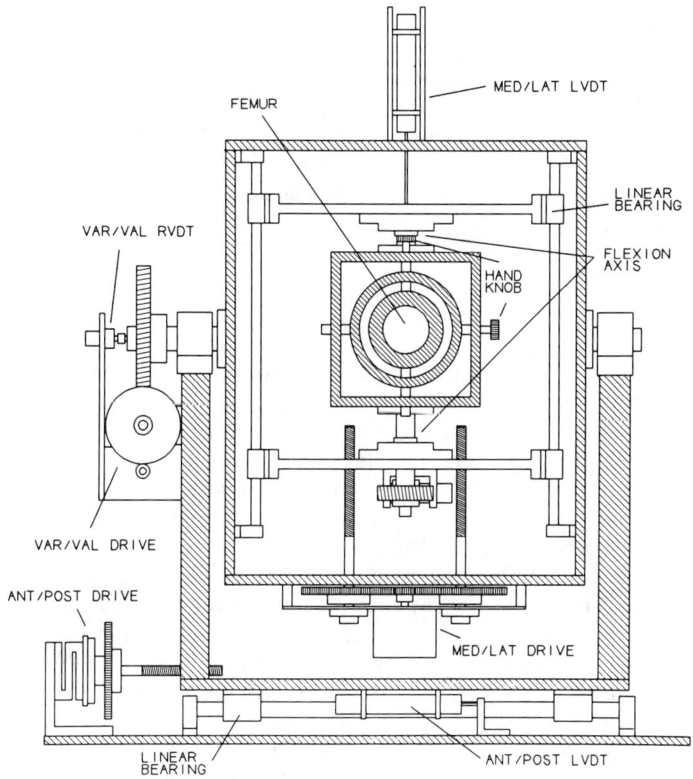

FIG. 4—*Femoral view of the apparatus. The femur unit provides four of the degrees of freedom, flexion/extension and varus/valgus rotations and medial/lateral and anterior/posterior translations.*

is that extremely fine control of load and displacement is possible on each of the five instrumented motions.

We designed a custom motor controller and driver tailored to the specific needs of our system. This device consists of essentially two stages. The controller stage accepts a four-bit address from a computer, three of which specify the motor to be moved; the fourth bit indicates the direction of motion either clockwise (1) or counterclockwise (0). This stage also accepts a trigger pulse from a computer, signifying when to step the motor. The controller takes these inputs and, through a series of logic devices, determines which of the four stepping motor coils should be energized. The driver stage amplifies the outputs from the logic devices through four power transistors corresponding to each of the four coils. The result of this circuit is that each coil is driven with a 12-V square wave.

Measuring loads and displacements requires specific transducers. Each of the three forces is measured through two Z-transducers with conventional strain gages mounted to the motor supports. The two torques are measured directly on the driven shafts through 90° strain gage arrays. Relative bone translations are measured through three LVDTs mounted parallel to each of the linear carriages. Internal/external and varus/valgus rotations are measured through two RVDTs attached to the shafts.

In considering the accuracy of displacement measures, the limiting factor is the apparatus compliance rather than the errors inherent in the various motion transducers. This is because the motion transducers are attached to various points on the apparatus frame away from the cylinders in which the bones are potted. Consequently, any deflection in the frame between the bone cylinders and the motion transducers will appear as an apparent movement of the joint itself. To evaluate the compliance inherent in the apparatus, a length of steel tubing was inserted in place of a leg. The tube measured 6.35 cm (2.5 in.) in diameter with 3.2-mm (0.125-in.) wall thickness, giving a modulus of rigidity of 57 200 N/m^2. All forces were applied to a level of 400 N, while varus/valgus torque was applied to 150 N/m, and internal/external torque was applied to 100 N/m. Displacements that occurred from these loads could then be attributed to compliance in the mechanical structures. The system compliance was then subtracted from subsequent displacement measurements.

System Control

To apply accurately loads of desired magnitude, closed loop control of the stepping motors was necessary. This is because the knee exhibits nonlinear behavior including hysteresis. Consequently, the relationship between applied load and actuator movement cannot be predicted a priori, thus obviating the possibility of open loop control.

The necessity of closed loop control imposes certain hardware and software requirements upon the system. One requirement is the ability to monitor rapidly all the loads being applied. Because loads are transduced through strain gages and monitored by the analog/digital board of the computer, this requirement is readily satisfied. The second requirement is the ability to use this information by means of a control algorithm to control motor movements. Satisfying the second requirement is more complex and necessitates meeting performance criteria concerning the stability and rate of convergence to the desired loads. The control algorithm was developed specifically to meet these criteria.

The control of the system of five stepping motors is partitioned into cycles, in which each cycle consists of three components. The first component samples the load transducers for each of the five motors by a sequential scan and analog-to-digital conversion of the five loads. Each channel is sampled 100 times at 555 Hz to obtain an average voltage for that cycle. Using predetermined calibration factors, the actual load is then computed. The second component of each control cycle consists of a comparison between the actual loads and the target loads. The target loads are read from a file stored on disk with each record containing the five loads corresponding to each motor. This file may contain several hundred records, the contents of which determine the path through load space, which will be discussed shortly. For every load that deviates more than a threshold value (4.0 N for forces, 0.4 N/m for torques) a correction is applied to the corresponding motor, the correction being the third component of each control cycle.

To correct the five motors, three parameters are required for each motor: direction, speed, and distance. Direction is self-explanatory. Speed is controlled by the rate at which pulses are sent to each motor driver. Because dc stepping motors are constant power actuators, there is an inverse relationship between output torque and rotation rate. At greater knee displacements the joint becomes less flexible, which requires more output torque and hence a slower speed from the motor. The amount of necessary motor torque depends not only on joint flexibility, but also on the friction in the system gear drives. Because it is difficult to predict joint flexibility and gear friction, the relationship between joint reaction load and maximum motor speed was determined by trial and error. The best results were obtained by using a second-order polynomial speed function that decreases as load increases. This was determined individually for each of the five motors.

The final parameter for motor control is distance, which is determined by the number of pulses sent to each driver, termed a "hop." It should be emphasized that the hop size varies for each motor between control cycles, and while the following description applies to one motor in one cycle, the actual implementation controls all five motors simultaneously.

To achieve both rapid convergence and stability, the hop size for each control cycle is determined through an adaptive approach. At the beginning of each control cycle, the load on each motor is compared to the load in the previous cycle. If the current load deviation is less than 40% of the previous deviation from the target load, then the hop size is halved. If the current load deviation is greater than 60% of the previous deviation, then the hop size is doubled. An upper limit of 512 pulses, which because of gear reductions corresponds to 3.1° for the rotations and 3.3 mm for the translations, prevents the hop size from doubling indefinitely. If the current load deviation falls between 40 and 60% of the previous deviation, then the hop size remains unchanged. Finally, if the current load has overshot the target load, then the direction is reversed and the hop size is halved. This is summarized in Table 1.

Specimen Alignment

Specimens were aligned in the apparatus according to the functional axes of the knee. The tibia was aligned so that the apparatus axis of internal/external rotation coincided with that of the joint, whereas the femur was aligned in an effort to make the varus/valgus axis of both the joint and apparatus coincide. The alignment protocol called for first aligning the tibia and then the femur. Initially, each specimen was placed in the apparatus by visual approximation. The protocol then required the placement of the tibia axis by minimization of the coupled loads induced by internal/external rotation. This was achieved by successive applications of ±14° rotations in 2° increments. After each rotation the magnitudes and directions of the coupled loads were examined and the leg was repositioned to try to minimize them. Depending on the initial placement, it took from three to twelve iterations of this procedure to obtain a satisfactory placement. A placement was accepted when all three coupled translational forces were less than 20 N. Varus/valgus torque was generally not significant under application of internal/external rotation. The varus/valgus axis was similarly placed in the femur using ±5° varus/valgus rotations. In this case, the prime indicator of misalignment was proximal/distal force. Placement was accepted when this was less than 20 N.

We evaluated the repeatability of the alignment protocol by performing two sets of load-displacement (flexibility) measurements on a single cadaver leg on two separate days. Be-

TABLE 1—*Summary of actions taken on the number of pulses sent to each motor in successive control cycles.*

Condition[a]	Action
$\lvert P_{ij} - T_i\rvert > 0.6\,\lvert P_{i(j-1)} - T_i\rvert$	$\Delta_{ij} = 2.0\Delta_{i(j-1)}$
$\lvert P_{ij} - T_i\rvert < 0.4\,\lvert P_{i(j-1)} - T_i\rvert$	$\Delta_{ij} = 0.5\Delta_{i(j-1)}$
$\lvert P_{ij} - T_i\rvert \geq 0.4\,\lvert P_{i(j-1)} - T_i\rvert$ and $\lvert P_{ij} - T_i\rvert \leq 0.6\,\lvert P_{i(j-1)} - T_i\rvert$	$\Delta_{ij} = \Delta_{i(j-1)}$
$\mathrm{sgn}(P_{ij} - T_i) \neq \mathrm{sgn}(P_{i(j-1)} - T_i)$	reverse direction

[a] P_{ij} = actual load on the ith motor (i = 0,1,2,3,4) in the jth cycle.
T_i = target load for the ith motor.
Δ_{ij} = number of pulses sent to the ith motor in the jth cycle.

tween the two experiments the leg was removed from the apparatus and stored at 4°C overnight. Each experiment was preceded by the complete alignment protocol without any reference to previous positioning. The comparison of these two experiments is described in the **Results** section.

Flexibility Evaluation

To determine joint flexibility functions (that is, load-displacement relations), we programmed a load sequence that first applied varus/valgus, medial/lateral, internal/external, and anterior/posterior loads individually. Table 2 summarizes the maximum loads applied. To investigate the effects of combined loading, each of the six possible load pairs was then applied. Each load pair sequence was determined by a cloverleaf-shaped path in the load-load plane (see Fig. 5). Each of the radii of the cloverleaf was specified by four points. When all six load pairs were applied, the entire sequence including both single and paired loads was repeated with a constant 400 N of joint compression. The entire load sequence consisted of approximately 400 points, which required about 9 h to complete at three different flexion angles.

After system compliance was subtracted, measured displacements were used in a multivariable regression analysis to determine the flexibility functions. We used a polynomial model with single load terms up to fourth order and interaction terms (that is, paired loads) to second order. Equation 1 models the effect of the five loads (x_i) on each of the five displacements (y_i).

$$y_i = a_i + \sum_{j=1}^{5} b_{ij}x_j + \sum_{j=1}^{5}\sum_{k=1}^{5} c_{ijk}x_jx_k + \sum_{j=1}^{5} d_{ij}x_j^3 + \sum_{j=1}^{5} e_{ij}x_j^4 \tag{1}$$

where the a_i, b_{ij}, c_{ijk}, d_{ij}, and e_{ij} are polynomial constants. Note that the constants c_{ijk} for $j \neq k$ correspond to load interaction terms. The statistical significance of each coefficient was evaluated according to the F-test probability obtained from a multivariable analysis of variance (ANOVA). We accepted only those coefficients that were significantly different from zero at the $p < 0.05$ level.

Results

Specimen Alignment

Figures 6 and 7 illustrate the effect of repositioning the leg within the apparatus. Given the initial placement, it was observed that only medial/lateral and anterior/posterior coupled loads were significant under tibial rotation; therefore, these were the only coupled loads minimized in alignment of the tibia. Repositioning the leg reduced these loads by approximately a factor of 8. Similar results were obtained using the varus/valgus axis for the femur.

TABLE 2—*Maximum levels of applied loads.*

Load	Maximum
Varus/valgus	60 N/m
Medial/lateral	200 N
Internal/external	20 N/m
Anterior/posterior	200 N
Compression (proximal)	400 N

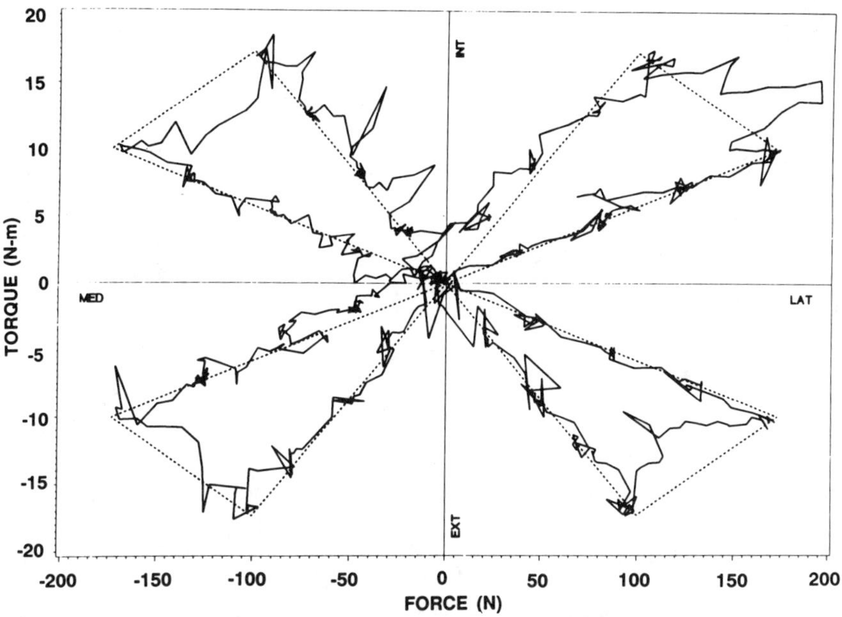

FIG. 5—*Stability and tracking of the control algorithm for combinations of medial/lateral force and internal/external torque. The broken line represents the programmed sequence. Each radial line is defined by four points. Showing no instability, actual loads converge to programmed points. An adaptive control algorithm is used to achieve stability while at the same time giving an acceptable rate of convergence. The time to follow this programmed load sequence is about 25 min.*

The repeatability of the alignment protocol is illustrated in Figs. 8 and 9. Figure 8 shows that internal/external flexibility was relatively unaffected by the realignment. This could indicate either that the alignment procedure is highly repeatable or that internal/external flexibility is insensitive to misalignment. Because previous evidence indicates that tibial rotation is probably not the best indicator for axis misalignment [*26*], the results for other loads were examined as well. The effect on medial/lateral flexibility is illustrated in Fig. 9, which also shows good repeatability between trials.

Using a paired *t*-test on the magnitudes of the flexibility response for Trials 1 and 2 for each of the resultant displacements, we determined the overall repeatability between trials. Table 3 summarizes the differences in displacements given the various applied loads. Translations were repeatable to within 0.83 mm. Varus/valgus angle was repeatable to within 0.49°, and internal/external angle was repeatable to within 1.47° (under medial/lateral force). These values probably represent slightly larger differences than those from realignment alone as a result of confounding of the viscoelastic effects. Given that the specimens were not preconditioned, the paired differences may be due in part to differences between the first and second load cycles.

System Performance

Table 4 summarizes the compliance of the various axes of the machine. All compliances were determined by linear regression over the range of applied loads. All five axes displayed a highly linear relationship of displacement to load ($r^2 > 0.97$). When the system compliance

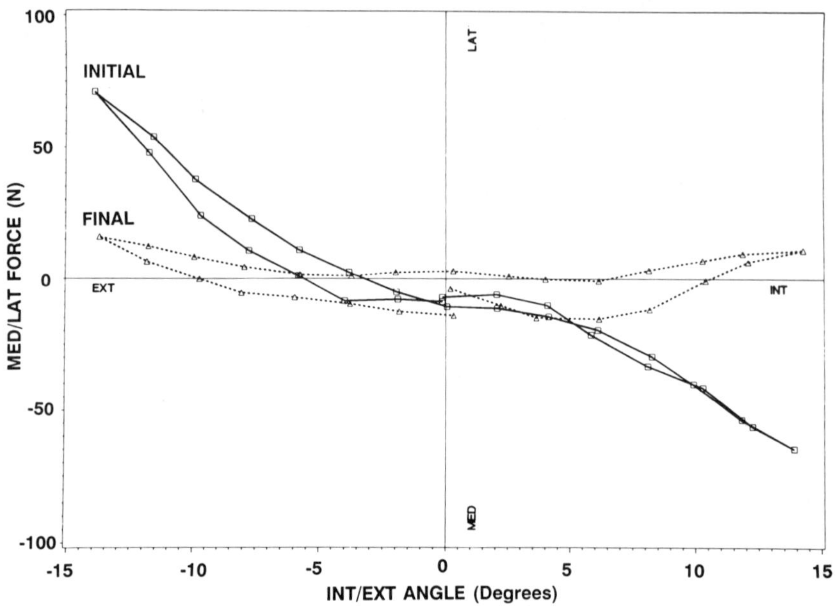

FIG. 6—*Using internal/external rotation and coupled medial/lateral force to reposition the leg within the apparatus. Repositioning is accomplished with the tibia and femur clamps. The final position results in significantly less coupling of medial/lateral force.*

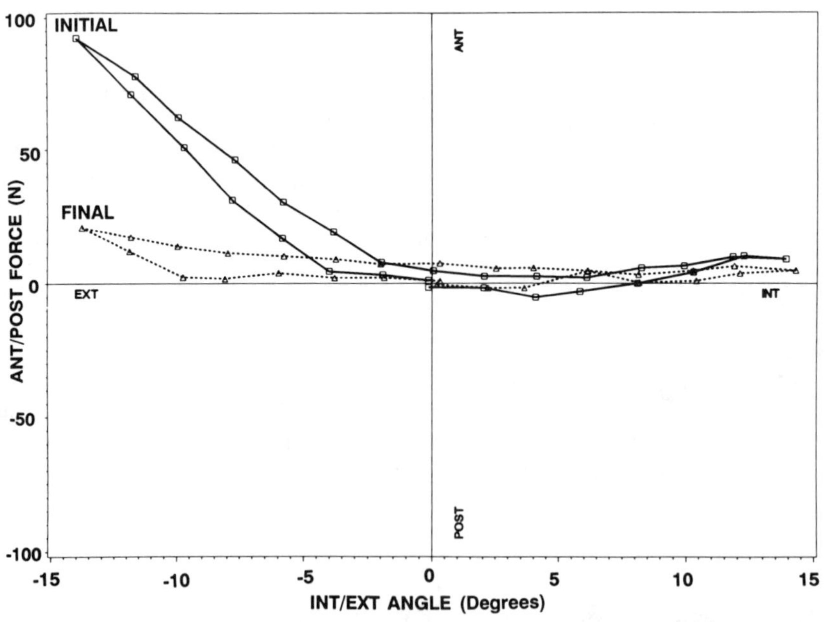

FIG. 7—*Using internal/external rotation and coupled anterior/posterior force to reposition the leg within the apparatus. The final position results in significantly less coupling to anterior/posterior force.*

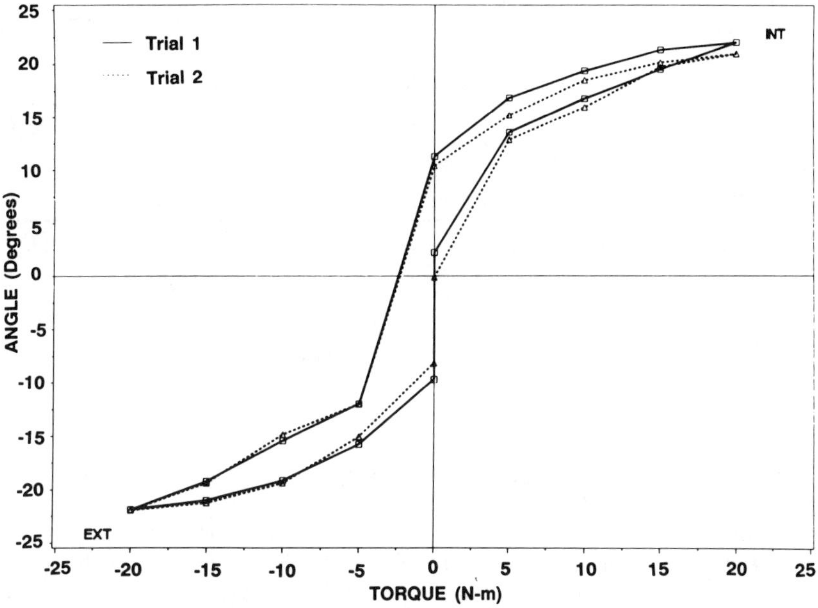

FIG. 8—*The effect of the alignment procedure on internal/external flexibility. The difference between the magnitudes of the two trials is not significantly different from zero* (p > *0.05*).

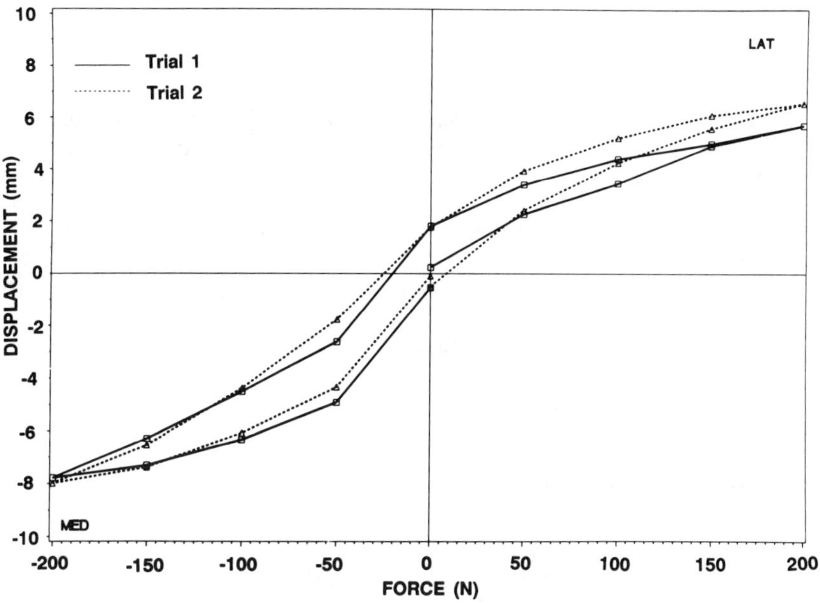

FIG. 9—*The effect of the alignment procedure on medial/lateral flexibility. The difference between the magnitudes of the two trials is not significantly different from zero* (p > *0.05*).

TABLE 3—*Repeatability of measured parameters.*

	Applied Load			
Displacement[a]	Var/Val	Med/Lat	Int/Ext	Ant/Post
Var/val, °	0.49[b]	0.27	0.33	0.42
Med/lat, mm	...[c]	0.35	0.83	...
Int/ext, °	0.84	1.47	...	0.24
Ant/post, mm	...	0.41	...	0.83

[a]Rows represent the difference between Trials 1 and 2 in the magnitude of displacement for each of the applied loads.

[b]Values, when given, are the absolute mean differences in magnitudes between Trials 1 and 2.

[c]Where no value is given, the difference in magnitude was not significantly different from zero ($p > 0.05$).

is subtracted from subsequent displacement measurements, the accuracy is approximately 0.5 mm for translations and 0.25° for rotations.

As stated before, the evaluation criteria for system performance were stability and rate of convergence. The stability of the control algorithm was achieved through an adaptive approach. The remaining criterion is rate of convergence. Convergence rate averaged 15 to 20 s for each programmed load point. This depended upon the difference between successive points.

The stability of the system is illustrated in Fig. 5. This shows a subset of a load sequence containing combinations of medial/lateral force and internal/external torque. The programmed path was given by four points along each radius. The actual path followed by the system did indeed converge on each of the programmed points.

Knee Flexibility

Figure 10 shows an example of a flexibility plot obtained from the application of combinations of varus/valgus and internal/external torques. The flexibility function that yielded the plot in Fig. 10 is given by:

$$\begin{aligned} \text{VVANG} = & -0.198 + 0.174(\text{VV}) + 0.096(\text{IE}) \\ & - 0.00114(\text{VV})^2 + 0.00144(\text{VV})(\text{IE}) \\ & - 0.00019(\text{VV})^3 + 2.8 \times 10^{-7}(\text{VV})^4 \end{aligned} \quad [2]$$

TABLE 4—*Flexibility of machine axes.*

Axis	Flexibility
Varus/valgus	0.013 °/N/m
Medial/lateral	0.003 mm/N
Internal/external	0.003 °/N/m
Proximal/distal	0.008 mm/N
Anterior/posterior	0.023 mm/N

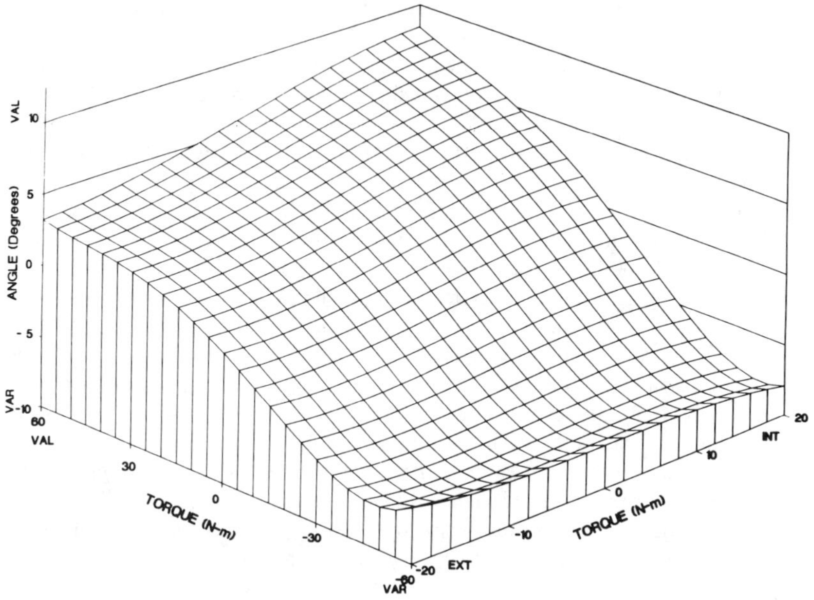

FIG. 10—*Flexibility function for varus/valgus angle as a result of combinations of varus/valgus and internal/external torque. At constant varus/valgus torque, varus/valgus angle changes with internal/external torque, indicating that varus/valgus angle is coupled to axial torque. However, this coupling changes as varus/valgus torque changes, indicating that internal/external and varus/valgus torques interact.*

where

VVANG = varus/valgus angle in degrees (valgus positive),
VV = varus/valgus torque in N/m (valgus positive), and
IE = internal/external torque in N/m (internal positive).

From Eq 2 and Fig. 10, both of which show the effect of the two torques on varus/valgus angle, two important observations emerge. Not surprisingly, varus/valgus torque has a significant effect on varus/valgus angle. Note, however, that internal/external torque also has an effect on varus/valgus angle. Thus, one observation is that internal/external torque couples to varus/valgus rotation. Furthermore, the magnitude of this effect depends on the level of varus/valgus torque. Therefore, the second observation is that internal/external and varus/valgus torques interact with each other. The effect of internal/external torque appears to be maximum when a valgus torque is also applied to the knee.

Discussion

The goals of this study were to design an automated system that applies external loads to the knee while allowing the joint to move naturally with five degrees of freedom and to evaluate its capabilities. Our results indicate that promising new studies may be undertaken with such a system. Because of the paucity of data describing knee and ligament mechanics under both pure and combined loading, we anticipate that this system will enable the collection of significant new data that represent more accurate simulations of knee injury.

But before these experiments can be performed, certain aspects of protocol must be resolved, especially in the area of specimen alignment.

Perhaps the single most important aspect of the experimental protocol is the alignment of the leg within the apparatus. It is notoriously difficult to obtain repeatable results from one specimen to another, and this can be attributed to four sources of variation. The first is individual variation in material properties of the soft tissue structures of the joint. It has been well documented that isolated ligament preparations display variability in material properties from one subject to another [*18,23,24,27*], although the exact contribution to variation in overall joint mechanics may be due to a number of variables, including sex and age [*28*]. The second source of variation relates to differences in bone geometry. Bone geometry manifests in the attachment points for ligaments. Different bone geometries yield different insertion points and hence affect the biomechanics of the knee [*29,30*]. One would expect larger boned individuals to have stiffer and stronger joints, but we are unaware of any studies demonstrating a positive correlation. A third source of variation is soft tissue geometry. Although soft tissue geometry cannot be completely separated from bone geometry, the size and the shape of the ligament itself certainly affect its function [*22*]. Finally, variations in joint measurements can be attributed to experimental errors, specifically the errors introduced by misalignment of a leg within a fixed axis machine. Neglecting systematic errors such as machine compliance, imprecise alignment will inflate the variance of measured quantities. Of these four sources, only the fourth is substantially under control by the researcher.

Historically, the approach to specimen alignment has centered on increasing the accuracy of using bony landmarks [*3,6,13,31,32*]. This has the advantage of using landmarks that are easily palpable in live subjects, but its main drawback is that to obtain good repeatability, landmarks are typically chosen at widely spaced points on the bones. This means that the entire lower limb geometry, from femoral head to distal tibia, determines the coordinate system setup at the knee. Clearly, variations of these distant points can profoundly affect experimental results.

Because of the potential variability introduced into displacement measurements by using bony landmarks to align specimens, we have sought to minimize this variability by aligning specimens in the apparatus according to the functional axes of the knee. Recall that the design of the apparatus is such that the tibia unit allows one rotational degree of freedom (internal/external axial rotation), while the femur unit allows two rotational degrees of freedom (varus/valgus rotation and flexion/extension rotation). Since the apparatus was constructed such that the three axes about which these rotations occur intersect at a common point (the origin of the apparatus coordinate system), the alignment procedure determines the location of the apparatus origin within the knee and the orientation of the knee in the coordinate system of the apparatus. With the tibia unit offering only internal/external axial rotation, the only functional axis that can be used for tibia alignment is the internal/external axial rotation axis. However, with the femur unit offering two rotational degrees of freedom, the choice must be made to align either the functional varus/valgus axis or the functional flexion/extension axis with the corresponding axis of the femur unit. Both functional axes cannot be simultaneously aligned with the apparatus axes because the functional axes do not intersect; the functional axis in flexion/extension is approximately along a line connecting the medial and lateral epicondyles, whereas the functional varus/valgus axis passes through the point of contact of the tibial plateau with either the medial (for varus rotation) or lateral (for varus rotation) femoral condyle. Because the apparatus applies valgus/valgus torques and not flexion/extension torques, errors will be minimized by aligning the functional varus/valgus axis not the functional flexion/extension axis. Note that even though the knee specimen is aligned with the femur unit using the functional varus/valgus axis, the flexion/

extension axis of the apparatus is the axis actually fixed to the femur as demanded by the coordinate system illustrated in Fig. 1.

The approach of using a functional axis definition appears to be sound based on the repeatability tests. Although similar results can undoubtedly be obtained from the accurate use of bony landmarks, the question remains as to which method offers more consistent placement over a range of individuals. Because joint mechanics are determined largely by the internal geometry of the joint rather than by external geometry of the bones, we believe that the functional placement of axes is fundamentally better than using external landmarks. Future experiments should ascertain this.

The system itself performed as necessary, the primary concern being the ability of the control algorithm to converge to programmed points within reasonable time. To achieve stability and rapid convergence, the developmental effort centered on a technique for determining hop size. Two techniques were investigated to determine the optimum hop size for each control cycle. The first technique involved programming hop size as a function of load. This necessitated a predetermined relationship between hop size and load. Because the joint is more flexible around the origin in load space (that is, the laxity region), various functions were investigated that increased the hop size in this region. Around the laxity region, it is desirable to move the motors quickly and in large hops because of the large amount of motion necessary to develop loads. Unfortunately, this invariably led to oscillations (that is, instability) at higher loads. If at higher loads the joint flexibility declines more steeply than originally anticipated, then large hops lead to oscillations about the desired point. If one takes a more conservative approach using small hops, however, then the convergence rate to points in the laxity region is frustratingly slow.

To alleviate the difficulties with the first technique, a second technique was developed in which the hop size is determined through an adaptive approach. Rather than using programmed distance-load functions, an algorithm adjusted the hop size from cycle to cycle based on the difference between actual loads and target loads. The power of the control algorithm lies in its adaptability. In the laxity region, the hop size quickly doubles until the system nears the target load, where it then repeatedly halves until it zeroes in on the target load. In the low flexibility region, the hop size remains small, thus avoiding oscillations.

Although the system converged on individual programmed points, the actual path through load space was generally quite tortuous. This is an important consideration in the interpretation of flexibility functions. Because the system may approach a given point from any direction, which is unpredictable as a result of the possibility of overshoot, a given data point may be obtained from either the loading or unloading side of the hysteresis curve. Because the regression procedure fits a polynomial through all the data points, hysteresis is effectively averaged out.

The utility of the regression functions lies in the identification of significant load couplings and interactions and also in the determination of the relative contributions of different loads to specific displacements. By determining the gradient of each function, a particular load combination to which the dependent variable is most sensitive can be identified. For example, starting at the origin of Fig. 10, the gradient, which indicates the direction of maximum increase, has a slope of 0.174°/N/m in valgus and 0.096°/N/m in internal torque. Since positive values represent valgus angle, these two numbers represent the flexibility of valgus angle in each of these two applied loads. Thus, to maximize valgus angle, one should apply valgus and internal torques in the ratio of 0.174:0.096 (or 1.8:1), respectively. To maximize varus angle, one would simply reverse the direction of torque application but keep the ratio the same.

The motivation for designing an automated system was to be able to quantitate the load response of the knee joint toward the goal of gaining a more thorough understanding of knee injury mechanics. As noted in the beginning of the paper, the load response includes both the flexibility of the joint as well as the actual strain developed in the ligaments. Specifically, the ligaments most commonly injured, the medial collateral and anterior cruciate, are of primary interest. The flexibility results are useful in identifying couplings between loads and displacements, interactions between loads, and the sensitivity of displacements to specific loads. However, the applicability of such results to injury mechanics can only be hypothetical without concomitant data detailing ligament strains. With strain sensors such as those used either by Renstrom et al. [*16*] or Edwards et al. [*31*], it is possible to instrument the two ligaments of interest and to record ligament strain data together with flexibility data using our automated system. This is the next step in our research program, and the results will be reported in subsequent communications.

Conclusions

The primary motivation for the design of the system was the necessity to apply multiple loads while still allowing natural joint motion. This necessity in turn set the criteria of automated control. The development of our system demonstrated that first, the knee can be integrated into an automated control environment in a stable manner. Second, the system can apply programmed load sequences in a reasonable period of time.

The results presented in this paper can be summarized as follows.

1. The use of a functional definition for axis placement was shown to be highly repeatable. This method of specimen alignment may be used as an alternative to bony landmarks.
2. When combinations of loads are applied, significant load couplings and interactions appear that are not evident from single load experiments. An example showing the coupling between varus/valgus and internal/external torque is presented. Internal/external torque also interacts with varus/valgus torque.
3. Using a gradient analysis of the flexibility functions, it is possible to determine the combinations of loads that maximize a particular motion. The example of varus/valgus angle is shown to be maximized when varus/valgus and internal/external torques are applied in a ratio of 1.8:1, respectively.

Acknowledgments

We gratefully acknowledge the financial support of Tyrolia Corporation (Vienna, Austria), the Foundation for Chiropractic Education and Research, and the Department of Mechanical Engineering, University of California, Davis.

References

[*1*] Brantigan, O. C. and Voshell, A. F., "The Mechanics of the Ligaments and Menisci of the Knee Joint," *Journal of Bone and Joint Surgery*, Vol. 23, No. 1, 1941, pp. 44–66.

[*2*] Butler, D. L., Noyes, F. R., and Grood, E. S., "Ligamentous Restraints to Anterior-posterior Drawer in the Human Knee," *Journal of Bone and Joint Surgery*, Vol. 62-A, No. 2, 1980, pp. 259–270.

[*3*] Crowninshield, R., Pope, M. H., and Johnson, R. J., "An Analytical Model of the Knee," *Journal of Biomechanics*, Vol. 9, No. 5, 1976, pp. 397–405.

[*4*] Furman, W., Marshall, J. L., and Girgis, F. G., "The Anterior Cruciate Ligament—A Functional Analysis Based on Postmortem Studies," *Journal of Bone and Joint Surgery*, Vol. 58-A, No. 2, 1976, pp. 179–185.

[*5*] Hseih, H. H. and Walker, P. S., "Stabilizing Mechanisms of the Loaded and Unloaded Knee Joint," *Journal of Bone and Joint Surgery*, Vol. 58-A, No. 1, 1976, pp. 87–93.

[6] Markolf, K. L., Mensch, J. S., and Amstutz, H. C., "Stiffness and Laxity of the Knee—the Contributions of the Supporting Structures," *Journal of Bone and Joint Surgery*, Vol. 58-A, No. 5, 1976, pp. 583–593.

[7] Piziali, R. L., Rastegar, J., Nagel, D. A., and Schurman, D. J., "The Contribution of the Cruciate Ligaments to the Load-Displacement Characteristics of the Human Knee Joint," *Journal of Biomechanical Engineering*, Vol. 102, 1980, pp. 277–283.

[8] Piziali, R. L., Seering, W. P., Nagel, D. A., and Schurman, D. J., "The Function of the Primary Ligaments of the Knee in Anterior-Posterior and Medial-Lateral Motions," *Journal of Biomechanics*, Vol. 13, No. 10, 1980, pp. 777–784.

[9] Wang, C. J. and Walker, P. S., "Rotatory Laxity of the Human Knee Joint," *Journal of Bone and Joint Surgery*, Vol. 56-A, No. 1, 1974, pp. 161–170.

[10] Kennedy, J. C. and Fowler, P. J., "Medial and Anterior Instability of the Knee," *Journal of Bone and Joint Surgery*, Vol. 53-A, No. 7, 1971, pp. 1257–1270.

[11] Kennedy, J. C., Weinberg, H. W., and Wilson, A. S., "The Anatomy and Function of the Anterior Cruciate Ligament," *Journal of Bone and Joint Surgery*, Vol. 56-A, No. 2, 1974, pp. 223–235.

[12] Markolf, K. L., Graff-Radford, A., and Amstutz, H. C., "In Vivo Knee Stability," *Journal of Bone and Joint Surgery*, Vol. 60-A, No. 5, 1978, pp. 664–674.

[13] Olmstead, T. G., Wevers, H. W., Bryant, J. T., and Gouw, G. J., "Effect of Muscular Activity on Valgus/Varus Laxity and Stiffness of the Knee," *Journal of Biomechanics*, Vol. 19, No. 8, 1986, pp. 565–577.

[14] Shoemaker, S. C. and Markolf, K. L., "In Vivo Rotatory Knee Stability," *Journal of Bone and Joint Surgery*, Vol. 64-A, No. 2, 1982, pp. 208–216.

[15] Pope, M. H., Johnson, R. J., Brown, D. W., and Tighe, C., "The Role of the Musculature in Injuries to the Medial Collateral Ligament," *Journal of Bone and Joint Surgery*, Vol. 61-A, No. 3, 1979, pp. 398–402.

[16] Renstrom, P., Arms, S. W., Stanwyck, T. S., Johnson, R. J., and Pope, M. H., "Strain within the Anterior Cruciate Ligament During Hamstrings and Quadriceps Activity," *American Journal of Sports Medicine*, Vol. 14, No. 1, 1986, pp. 83–87.

[17] White, A. A., III and Raphael, I. G., "The Effect of Quadriceps Loads and Knee Position on Strain Measurements of the Tibial Collateral Ligament," *Acta Orthopaedica Scandinavica*, Vol. 43, No. 1, 1972, pp. 176–187.

[18] Butler, D. L. and Stouffer, D. C., "Tension-Torsion Characteristics of the Canine Anterior Cruciate Ligament—Part II: Experimental Observations," *Journal of Biomechanical Engineering*, Vol. 105, No. 2, 1982, pp. 160–165.

[19] Andriacchi, T. P., Mikosz, R. P., Hampton, S. J., and Galante, J. O., "Model Studies of the Stiffness Characteristics of the Human Knee Joint," *Journal of Biomechanics*, Vol. 16, No. 1, 1983, pp. 23–29.

[20] Inoue, M., McGurk-Burleson, E., Hollis, J. M., and Woo, S. L. Y., "Treatment of the Medial Collateral Ligament Injury," *American Journal of Sports Medicine*, Vol. 15, No. 1, 1987, pp. 15–21.

[21] Dunn, M. G. and Silver, F. H., "Viscoelastic Behavior of Human Connective Tissues: Relative Contribution of Viscous and Elastic Components," *Connective Tissue Research*, Vol. 12, 1983, pp. 59–70.

[22] Haut, R. C. and Little, R. W., "Rheological Properties of Canine Anterior Cruciate Ligaments," *Journal of Biomechanics*, Vol. 2, No. 3, 1969, pp. 289–298.

[23] Noyes, F. R., DeLucas, J. L., and Torvik, P. J., "Biomechanics of Anterior Cruciate Ligament Failure: an Analysis of Strain-Rate Sensitivity and Mechanisms of Failure in Primates," *Journal of Bone and Joint Surgery*, Vol. 56-A, No. 2, 1974, pp. 236–253.

[24] Woo, S. L. Y., Gomez, M. A., Seguchi, Y., Endo, C. M., and Akeson, W. H., "Measurement of Mechanical Properties of Ligament Substance from a Bone-Ligament-Bone Preparation," *Journal of Orthopaedic Research*, Vol. 1, No. 1, 1983, pp. 22–29.

[25] Grood, E. S., and Suntay, W. J., "A Joint Coordinate System for the Clinical Description of Three-Dimensional Motions: Application to the Knee," *Journal of Biomechanical Engineering*, Vol. 105, No. 2, 1983, pp. 136–144.

[26] Rastegar, J., Piziali, R. L., Nagel, D. A., and Schurman, D. J., "Effect of Fixed Axes of Rotation on the Varus-Valgus and Torsional Load-Displacement Characteristics of the in-vitro Human Knee," *Journal of Biomechanical Engineering*, Vol. 101, No. 2, 1979, pp. 134–140.

[27] Dorlot, J. M., Ait Ba Sidi, M., Tremblay, G. M., and Drouin, G., "Load Elongation Behavior of the Canine Anterior Cruciate Ligament," *Journal of Biomechanical Engineering*, Vol. 102, No. 3, 1980, pp. 190–193.

[28] Noyes, F. R. and Grood, E. S., "The Strength of the Anterior Cruciate Ligament in Humans and Rhesus Monkeys," *Journal of Bone and Joint Surgery*, Vol. 58-A, No. 8, 1976, pp. 1074–1082.

[29] Hefzy, M. S. and Grood, E. S., "Sensitivity of Insertion Locations on Length Patterns of Anterior Cruciate Ligament Fibers," *Journal of Biomechanical Engineering*, Vol. 108, No. 1, 1986, pp. 73–82.
[30] Sidles, J. A., Larson, R. V., Garbini, J. L., Downey, D. J., and Matsen, F. A., "Ligament Length Relationships in the Moving Knee," *Journal of Orthopaedic Research*, Vol. 6, No. 4, 1988, pp. 593–610.
[31] Edwards, R. G., Lafferty, J. F., and Lange, K. O., "Ligament Strain in the Human Knee Joint," *Journal of Basic Engineering*, Vol. 92, No. 1, 1970, pp. 131–136.
[32] Lewis, J. L., Lew, W. D., and Schmidt, J., "Description and Error Evaluation of an in vitro Knee Joint Testing System," *Journal of Biomechanical Engineering*, Vol. 110, No. 3, 1988, pp. 238–248.

Timothy P. Quinn[1] and C. D. Mote, Jr.[1]

A Six-Degree-of-Freedom Acoustic Transducer for Rotation and Translation Measurements Across the Knee

REFERENCE: Quinn, T. P. and Mote, C. D., Jr., "**A Six-Degree-of-Freedom Acoustic Transducer for Rotation and Translation Measurements Across the Knee,**" *Skiing Trauma and Safety: Eighth International Symposium, ASTM STP 1104*, C. D. Mote, Jr. and Robert J. Johnson, Eds., American Society for Testing and Materials, Philadelphia, 1991, pp. 77–93.

ABSTRACT: An acoustic transducer design to measure the relative translations and rotations across the knee with no mechanical coupling between the tibia and femur is presented. Platforms attached to femoral and tibial tracking fixtures hold acoustic sources and receivers, respectively. The distance from each source to each receiver is measured by the acoustic transit time, and the translations and rotations across the knee joint are computed. For rotations less than 30° around the expected operating position, the resolution of the transducer is 0.3°; for translations less than 1.5 cm around the expected operating position, the resolution is 0.03 cm. Theoretical error analysis using a Monte Carlo method shows that the uncertainty in the measurement depends on the relative position of the sources and receivers. The analysis predicts the worst case resolution of the transducer as 0.09 cm in translation and 0.6° in rotation when the receiver platform is translated 8.0 cm parallel to the source platform. The transducer and fixturing system are demonstrated on a cadaver specimen for applied anterior force and applied internal-external rotation. Errors as a result of (soft tissue) motion of the transducer relative to the bone during *in-vivo* measurements are assessed on the cadaver specimen. For internal-external rotation, the error caused by soft tissue motion is a maximum of 0.5 cm in translation and 1.8° in rotation. For applied anterior force, the error as a result of soft tissue motion is a maximum of 0.16 cm in translation and 2.7° in rotation.

KEY WORDS: acoustic transducer, rotations, displacements, knee, error analysis, soft tissue motion, skiing injury

About 32% of all skiing injuries occur at the knee [*1*]. Past investigators studying skiing injuries [*2–6*] have measured the rotations across the knee as a function of the applied loading in an attempt to understand normal knee motion. To study the kinematics of the knee, it is often necessary to measure the complete, six-degree-of-freedom (DOF) motion across the joint [*2*]. Instrumented spatial linkages [*7–10*] and biplanar photographs or X-rays [*10–12*] have been used for these measurements. Errors in the measurements made with mechanical linkages result from the stick-slip, backlash, and large mass commonly found. Biplanar X-rays are not suitable for repeated in-vivo experiments.

Suntay et al. [*10*] presented theoretical and experimental analyses for the spatial resolution of a six-DOF linkage and for the spatial resolution of a biplanar X-ray technique. The linkage consisted of seven links constructed of aluminum blocks and stainless steel rods connected by rotary potentiometers. They found resolutions of 0.5 mm in translation and

[1]Graduate student and professor and chairman, respectively, Department of Mechanical Engineering, University of California, Berkeley, CA 94720.

0.6° in rotation with both methods. The linkage showed 0.3 mm and 0.2° hystereses for a 20-mm anterior-posterior (A-P) translation and a 72° flexion. The weight of the linkage was not given. Lewis et al. [*9*] gave the spatial resolution for a similar linkage as 0.7 mm for translation and 0.7° for rotation.

Techniques using acoustic sources and receivers have been applied to measurement of the complete motion of other joint systems. Andrews [*13*] described a system of sonic emitters and microphones to find the six-DOF motion of the wrist. Three acoustic sources were placed on each of the two articulating bones, and large linear arrays of spatially fixed microphones were used to digitize the position of the sources. No error analysis was reported; the results of tests conducted on a mechanical joint gave instant centers of rotation repeatable to 1 mm. A similar method was used by Siegler et al. [*14*] and Chen et al. [*15*] to measure motions of the ankle. They reported that the position of the sources could be determined to within 1 mm but gave no error bounds on the computed rotations and translations. Engin et al. used redundant emitters with large, spatially fixed linear arrays of microphones to measure the six-DOF motion of the shoulder [*16–19*], elbow [*20*], and hip [*21,22*]. Four sources were used to describe a spatially fixed reference frame for the fixed articulating bone, and six sources were attached to the moving bone with fixtures. A complex procedure was used to select the three sources on the moving bone that best represent rigid body motion. The resolution of the system in translation was measured to be approximately 1 mm [*16*]. For rotation, the resolution in determining the center of rotation was reported to be 1.5 cm [*18*]; no resolutions for the actual rotations were reported.

Error in measured joint motions in vivo arises from two sources: (1) error caused by the limited spatial resolution of the device and (2) error in tracking the articular bones because of the motion of intervening soft tissue. Few studies have measured the error of soft tissue motion on the tracking of the bone. In tests on cadaver specimens, Daniel et al. [*23*] quantified the difference in measurement of anterior laxity with a knee arthrometer strapped to the outside of the limb and with transducers directly attached to the bone. They reported an error of 0.44 mm because of soft tissue motion. Edixhoven et al. [*24*] measured the three-dimensional motion across the knee of two cadaver specimens using biplanar X-rays during an A-P laxity test to determine the accuracy of measurements made with linear displacement transducers that tracked the tibial tuberosity and the patella. They found that femur fixation through the soft tissue led to errors of 10% in the total A-P laxity measured. A scheme to correct for soft tissue motion is used in the Genucom Knee Analysis System (Faro Medical Technologies, Inc., Montreal, Canada), an instrumented spatial linkage and six-DOF dynamometer. The motion of the femur, which is held between padded posts, is first measured through the soft tissue when a load is applied to the tibia. These data are used to correct for motion of the femur in later tests when only motion of the tibia is measured. After correction, errors caused by soft tissue motion of 1 mm are claimed; no errors are given for rotational motion.

Work has been done to understand theoretically the error in joint motion parameters measured experimentally. Several authors [*25–28*] reported parametric studies on the errors of helical axis estimation based on uncertainties in the marker data. Panjabi et al. [*27*] assumed a normally distributed error in the position of landmark data and calculated the effect on the prediction of the center of rotation. Veldpaus et al. [*29*] described errors in the translation vector and rotation matrix as a function of the spatial distribution of marker data.

To compare joint motion tests of different subjects, a reproducible coordinate system must be established. Chao [*30*] and Grood and Suntay [*31*] presented similar knee joint coordinate systems based on skeletal landmarks using eulerian angles; Lewis et al. [*9*] and

Blankevoort et al. [*11*] commented on the difficulty of finding repeatable joint coordinate systems based on skeletal landmarks.

The purpose of this paper is to present an acoustic transducer to measure the translations and rotations across the knee that uses no mechanical couplings between the tibia and femur, thereby avoiding stick-slip and backlash problems of linkage systems. A coordinate system, based on the finite helical axis of the knee in flexion-extension, is used to represent the motion. (The motion between two rigid bodies measured at two different points in the motion can be described as rotation about a specified finite helical axis and translation along it [*32*].) Theoretical and experimental analyses of the resolution of the instrument are presented. The application of the instrument and fixtures is demonstrated using cadaveric tests with applied anterior force and applied internal-external rotation. The error due to motion of the transducer relative to the bone for *in-vivo* measurements is assessed.

The Six-DOF Acoustic Knee Transducer

Fixtures strapped to the tibia and femur are used to track the bone. Platforms attached to the tibial and femoral tracking fixtures hold acoustic receivers and sources, respectively. The femoral fixture is thermoplastic and extends over the anterior surface of the distal end of the thigh (Fig. 1). Two lobes grip the condyles of the femur and are clamped there with a Plexiglas C-clamp. The receiver platform, mounted at the lateral side of the tibia, is made from light, stiff, graphite composite sandwich plate. The tibial fixture is an Ecko II knee orthosis (Orthomedics, Brea, California) modified by cutting away the hinge. The receiver platform is attached to the frontal part of the orthosis. The source platform weighs 0.15 N, the receiver platform weighs 1.55 N, and, together with the fixturing devices, the total weight of the transducer is 5.5 N.

Four ultrasonic microphones (receivers) with 40-kHz natural frequency are held in a 9- by 9-cm square. The supersonic sources are high-voltage sparks across 0.25-mm gaps. Three sources are rigidly mounted at the corners of a 7.8-cm, equilateral triangular, graphite composite platform.

A schematic of the transducer is shown in Fig. 2. Twelve bit counters, driven by an 8-MHz clock, count the time from the initiation of the source to reception of the shock wave by the receiver. A flash coil, when triggered, applies 400 V across the spark gap; the four counters are reset at each spark. The omnidirectional microphones resonate at 40 kHz because of the impinging shock wave. The voltage output from each microphone is amplified and compared to a threshold. If it exceeds the threshold, the comparator stops the counter. The counter values are then placed sequentially on the bus, and the cycle is repeated for each subsequent source. The microphone (Science Accessories Corp., Southport, Connecticut) responses are independent of the source location for a given radius in its frontal half space. A three-source cycle is completed in 31.3 ms. The period of the shortest possible cycle is calculated from the transit time and the settling time of the microphones. The microphone settling time is about 0.25 ms, and the shock transit time for a 20-cm separation between source and receiver is 0.58 ms allowing a three-source cycle to be completed in 2.5 ms or at a maximum rate of 400/s.

The transit time of the shock wave from each source to each receiver is the distance between them divided by the speed of sound. The distances from the ith source to the jth receiver, c_{ij}, are interpolated in time so that they are predicted simultaneously. The coordinates of each receiver (x_j^r, y_j^r, z_j^r) are determined from the coordinates of the three sources (x_i^s, y_i^s, z_i^s) and the simultaneous distances c_{ij} by solution of the equations

$$(x_j^r - x_i^s)^2 + (y_j^r - y_i^s)^2 + (z_j^r - z_i^s)^2 - c_{ij}^2 = 0, i = 1, 2, 3 \; j = 1, 2, 3, 4 \qquad (1)$$

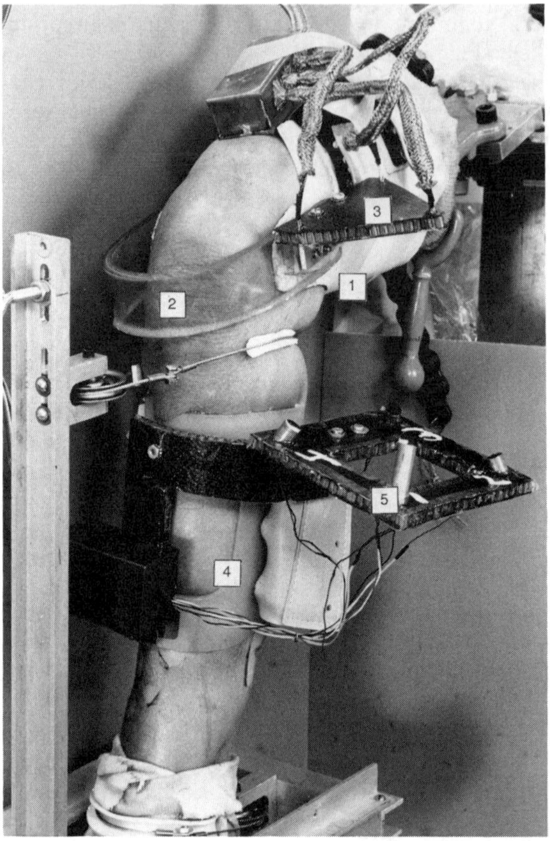

FIG. 1—*The six-DOF acoustic transducer. The femur is tracked by a molded thermoplast fixture clamping the distal thigh with lobes molded over the condyles of the femur* (1). *The lobes are held in place with a Plexiglas C-clamp* (2). *The source platform* (3), *made from graphite composite sandwich plate, is screwed to the clamp. The tibia is tracked with a modified knee brace* (4). *The receiver platform* (5) *is also made from graphite composite sandwich plate. The source and receiver platforms are shown in their initial position.*

Newton's method with damping [*33*] is used to determine the (x_j^r, y_j^r, z_j^r). The analysis is repeated for each receiver following each three-spark cycle. The overall rate at which the translations and rotations are determined is then 32/s.

Because three points on a rigid body are sufficient to determine its position and orientation, there is one redundant receiver. A least squares algorithm is used to determine the relative rotations and translations. The rotation matrix **R** and translation vector **v** of the receiver fixture with respect to the source fixture are computed using an algorithm developed by Veldpaus and Spoor [*34*]. If all receivers lie in the same plane, a coordinate system exists where all receivers have a common coordinate and a degree of redundancy is lost; therefore, one receiver is elevated 2.0 cm from the plane of the other three.

The anatomical reference coordinate system is based on the finite helical axis for a knee flexion between 0 and 90° (termed the large rotation axis system or LRAS) [*32*]. The finite helical axis is computed in each of six trials of applied flexion from 0 to 90°. These six axes are averaged, and the *Y*-coordinate axis is aligned with this averaged helical axis. The location

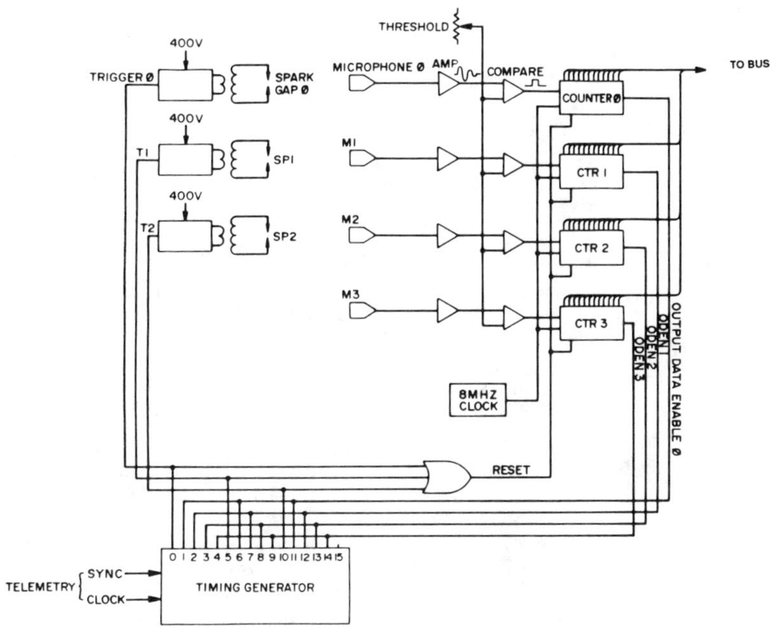

FIG. 2—*Schematic of the six-DOF acoustic transducer.*

of the tibial tubercle is also measured with this system in six trials by positioning a receiving microphone over it; this is the only bony landmark used to identify the coordinate system. The origin of coordinates is at the intersection of the averaged, finite helical axis with the normal plane containing the tibial tubercle (Fig. 3). The direction of the X-axis is defined by the intersections of the plane normal to the helical axis containing the tibial tubercle and the plane parallel to the long axis of the femur containing the helical axis. The Z-axis is the positive normal to the X-Y plane. The "reference coordinate system" (X-Y-Z) is fixed to the femur. A coordinate system that is initially coincident with the reference coordinate system is fixed to an extension of the tibia and is referred to as the "body fixed coordinate system." Euler angles are used to describe the rotation as in the gyroscopic system presented by Chao [*30*]. The order of the rotations are first β about the Y-axis giving a rotated coordinate system $X' - Y' - Z'$ ($Y = Y'$), then α about the X'-axis giving a rotated coordinate system $X'' - Y'' - Z''$ ($X'' = X'$), and finally γ about the body Z-axis ($Z'' =$ body Z). The rigid body rotation matrix is then given by

$$\mathbf{R} = \begin{bmatrix} \cos(\beta)\cos(\gamma) - \sin(\alpha)\sin(\beta)\sin(\gamma) & -\cos(\alpha)\sin(\gamma) & \sin(\alpha)\cos(\beta)\sin(\gamma) + \sin(\beta)\cos(\gamma) \\ \cos(\beta)\sin(\gamma) + \sin(\alpha)\sin(\beta)\cos(\gamma) & \cos(\alpha)\cos(\gamma) & \sin(\beta)\sin(\gamma) - \sin(\alpha)\cos(\beta)\cos(\gamma) \\ -\cos(\alpha)\sin(\beta) & \sin(\alpha) & \cos(\alpha)\cos(\beta) \end{bmatrix} \tag{2}$$

The relative rotations α, β, and γ correspond to varus-valgus, flexion-extension, and internal-external rotations, respectively (Table 1). Positive α, β, and γ correspond to valgus, flexion, and external rotations. The relative translations along the X, Y, and Z axes are δx, δy, and δz corresponding to anterior-posterior, medial-lateral, and proximal-distal translations, respectively. Positive δx, δy, and δz correspond to anterior, lateral, and proximal translations.

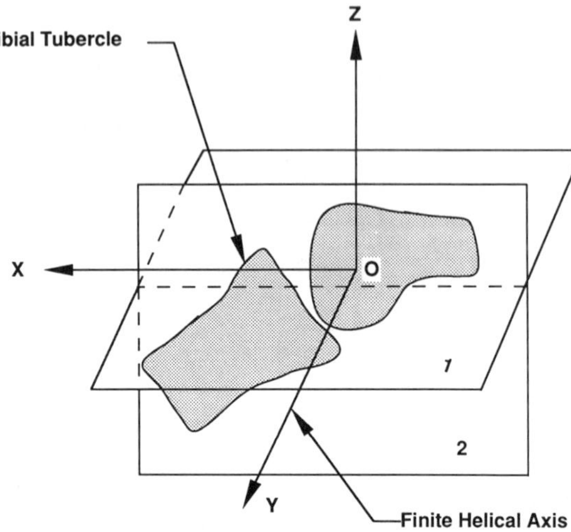

FIG. 3—*Large rotation axis system. Plane 1 contains the finite helical axis and is parallel to the long axis of the femur. Plane 2 is perpendicular to the finite helical axis and contains the tibial tubercle. The origin **O** is the intersection of plane 2 with the finite helical axis. The* Y *axis is the finite helical axis for a rotation from 0 to 90°. The* X *axis is parallel to the intersection of plane 1 with plane 2. The* Z *axis is the positive normal to the* X-Y *plane.*

Because the position and orientation of the LRAS reference frame is not known before measurement of the finite helical axis, a machine tool bed is used to find the locations of the sources in a "temporary coordinate system" scribed on the source platform. The origin and orientation of the LRAS coordinate system is found with respect to this temporary coordinate system, and, finally, the locations of the sources are transformed into the LRAS system. All subsequent data are reduced in the LRAS system.

Each time the source fixture is mounted on a subject, the helical axis and tibial tubercle measurements are required to determine the LRAS. Hart and Mote [*32*] found that the helical axis could be determined to within 4.0°, 2.8 mm, and 0.1 mm in orientation, position, and axial translation, respectively, in tests in which the source and receiver fixtures were removed and remounted.

TABLE 1—*The measured resolutions of the six-DOF acoustic transducer and the range of the applied motion around the initial position (see Fig. 1).*

Motion	Corresponding Motion	Resolution of the Transducer	Range of Applied Motion
α	varus-valgus	0.1°	±6°
β	flexion-extension	0.3°	±30°
γ	internal-external	0.2°	±30°
δx	anterior-posterior	0.02 cm	±1.5 cm
δy	medial-lateral	0.01 cm	±1.5 cm
δz	proximal-distal	0.03 cm	±1.5 cm

Methodology

Transducer Resolution

The precisions of the measurements of the relative motion of the source and receiver platforms for translations less than ±1.5 cm and rotations less than ±30° around the initial position were determined by translating and rotating the receiver platform by specified values relative to the source platform using a machine tool bed. In the initial position shown in Fig. 1, the source platform was 10 cm directly above, and parallel to, the receiver platform. The coordinate system used to present the results has approximately the same origin and orientation as the LRAS.

To assess the dependence of the instrument measurement error on the position of the receiver platform relative to the source platform, a Monte Carlo simulation was performed [*35*]. The positions of the receivers were calculated after undergoing simulated rigid body motion according to

$$\mathbf{p}_{2j} = \mathbf{R}\,\mathbf{p}_{1j} + \mathbf{v},\ j = 1, 2, 3, 4 \tag{3}$$

where $\mathbf{p}_{1j}$ and $\mathbf{p}_{2j}$ are the initial and the final positions of the receiver. The distances from the sources to the receivers, c_{ij}, were then calculated using Eq 1. Normally distributed, zero mean, random errors with standard deviation σ were used to perturb the calculated distances. Perturbed rotations and translations were computed using the perturbed c_{ij}. Standard deviations of the rotations and translations from the initial position to the final position were calculated for 10 000 trials. The nondimensional errors in the translations are defined by

$$\varepsilon_x = \frac{\sigma_x}{\sigma},\ \varepsilon_y = \frac{\sigma_y}{\sigma},\ \varepsilon_z = \frac{\sigma_z}{\sigma} \tag{4a}$$

where σ_x, σ_y, and σ_z are the standard deviations in δx, δy, and δz. The nondimensional errors in the rotations are defined by

$$\varepsilon_\alpha = \frac{\sigma_\alpha d}{\sigma},\ \varepsilon_\beta = \frac{\sigma_\beta d}{\sigma},\ \varepsilon_\gamma = \frac{\sigma_\gamma d}{\sigma} \tag{4b}$$

where d (= 7.78 cm) is the mean length between the three sources and σ_α, σ_β, and σ_γ are the standard deviations in the angle measurements in radians.

The errors in each translation and rotation component were calculated for simulated rigid body translations and rotations from the initial position shown in Fig. 1. The same coordinate system and initial position were used in the cadaver experiment described below.

Applied Force and Rotation Tests

Tests were conducted to demonstrate the use of the transducer and to assess the error caused by motion between the tracking fixtures and the bone.

A human cadaver leg was severed 7 cm distal to the trochanter of the femur, and the femur was exposed an additional 7 cm distally (see Figs. 1 and 4). The cadaver leg was stored at −30°C and thawed to room temperature before the experiment. The proximal end of the femur was then fixed to the table using a standard pipe clamp. The knee flexion angle was 66°.

In the first series of tests, a bracing fixture was used to apply a single force in the anterior direction through the knee joint center for flexion-extension. Two cables passed around the

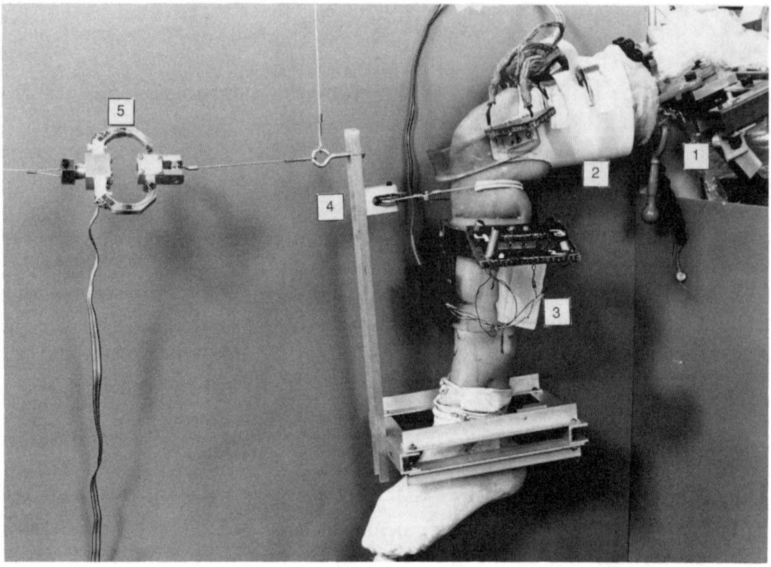

FIG. 4—*The femur of the cadaver specimen was clamped to the table with a standard pipe vise* (1). *In the fixtured case, the femur and tibia were tracked with the femoral fixture* (2) *and tibial fixture used in vivo* (3). *In the screwed case, the source platform was clamped to the chair, and the receiver platform was screwed to the tibia (not pictured). The bracing fixture* (4) *allowed an anterior force to be applied through the center of rotation for flexion-extension. The force was applied to the bracing fixture through a cable, and a force transducer* (5) *monitored the tension in the cable.*

leg: one just distal to the knee joint line and the second just proximal to the malleoli (see Fig. 4). The two cables were padded with molded orthoplast. The fixture did not constrain varus-valgus or internal-external rotations of the tibia. The force was applied to the bracing fixture by a cable that passed around a pulley at a 24° angle to the long axis of the femur. Because the distance between the pulley and the bracing fixture was large (125 cm), medial-lateral and proximal-distal translations of the tibia were minimally constrained. Tension was applied to the cable by manually pulling it down around the pulley. The tension was measured with a force transducer in line with the cable having a resolution of 1.6 N. The displacement of the cable was measured with a linear variable differential transformer (LVDT) and plotted versus the tension to monitor the progress of the test. The three rotations and three translations across the knee were measured with the acoustic transducer. The tension in the cable and the motion at the knee were recorded on laboratory computers during the tests.

To measure the motion of the fixtures relative to the bone, the tests were first performed with the acoustic transducer clamped to the leg as described above for live subjects. This is termed the *fixtured case*. The tests were then repeated with the receiver platform screwed to the tibia and the source fixture clamped to the table along with the femur. This is termed the *screwed case*. The relative motion between the tibia and the femur was measured. Differences between the two test measurements were assumed to be tracking errors between the fixtures and skeleton. Care was taken to ensure that the source platform remained in the same position and orientation so that the two cases could be compared in the same coordinate system. Five tests of three loading cycles each were performed for each of the two cases.

In the second series of tests, the foot was attached to a six-degree-of-freedom dynamometer mounted on a pedestal bearing with the axis of rotation of the bearing aligned with the long axis of the tibia. An internal-external rotation of the foot was applied by the experimenter. A strongly three-dimensional loading at the knee occurred (see Ref *2*). Five tests consisting of three loading cycles were performed for the screwed case and also for the fixtured case.

The applied anterior force was the input for the first series of tests, and torsion about the Z-axis at the foot (M_z) was the measure of the input for the internal-external rotation tests. The relative translations and rotations were defined to be zero at the initiation of each anterior force test. Because it is difficult to start internal-external rotation at the same reference position, the relative rotations and translations for that series of tests were measured from the γ midway between its extreme values. This choice for the zero reference of the relative translations and rotations gave approximately symmetric data about the M_z = 0 axis. The results of the 15 loading cycles for the screwed and fixtured cases were averaged, and a standard deviation was computed for each point along the loading axis. For the anterior force series, the data from the portion of the loading cycle from null anterior force to the maximum anterior force were used in the averaging, and, for the internal-external rotation tests, the data from maximum external to maximum internal rotation were used. The statistical differences between the fixtured and screwed cases were measured with a two-tailed, unpooled variance, t test. The hypothesis that the means of the two populations were the same was rejected if the significance level was less than 0.05.

Transducer Resolution and Accuracy: Results and Discussion

The recorded results during movement of the source and receiver platforms relative to one another using a machine tool bed are shown in Fig. 5. The mean measured responses in the translations and rotations other than in the applied translation or rotation were less than ± 0.001 cm for the translations and $\pm 0.01°$ for the rotations. The transducer exhibits no hysteresis. The root mean square (rms) relative errors for translations less than 1.5 cm and rotations less than 30° around the initial position are 0.03 cm in translation and 0.3° in rotation (see Table 1).

The principal source of measurement error in the relative positions of the two platforms is the movement of the spark location at the source. Because the two electrodes of the source protrude about 0.13 cm and the spark initiates anywhere along the gap, the location of the spark varies by 0.13 cm. From the measurements, the uncertainty of the spark location is partially compensated for through the least squares reduction of the redundant measurements.

The Monte Carlo error analysis predicts how the resolution of the transducer depends on the position of the platforms relative to the initial position shown in Fig. 1. The errors in the components of translation and rotation are found to be linear in σ. The predicted errors in the translations and rotations for simulated rotations around the coordinate axes are shown in Fig. 6. The range of α rotation is limited to $\pm 10°$ based on physiological limits in varus-valgus rotation. The error ε_α is insensitive to the values of α or β. Its maximum increase from the initial error in the range of rotations studied is 14% at $\gamma = 20°$. The values ε_β, ε_γ, and ε_z are insensitive to rotations from the initial position with maximum increases of 7% at $\alpha = -10°$, 8% at $\gamma = 20°$, and 9% at $\gamma = 20°$, respectively. The value ε_x is nearly linear in γ, reaching a maximum increase in the interval studied of 20%; ε_x is insensitive to rotations α and β. The value ε_y is most sensitive to rotation β with a maximum increase of 12% at $\beta = -20°$.

The predicted errors for translations from the initial position along the coordinate axes are shown in Fig. 7. ε_α, ε_β, and ε_z are sensitive to translations from the initial position in the X and Y directions with maximum increases of 80% at $\delta y = 8.0$ cm, 88% at $\delta x = -8.0$ cm, and 215% at $\delta x = 8.0$ cm, respectively. The values ε_γ, ε_x, and ε_y vary slowly with the

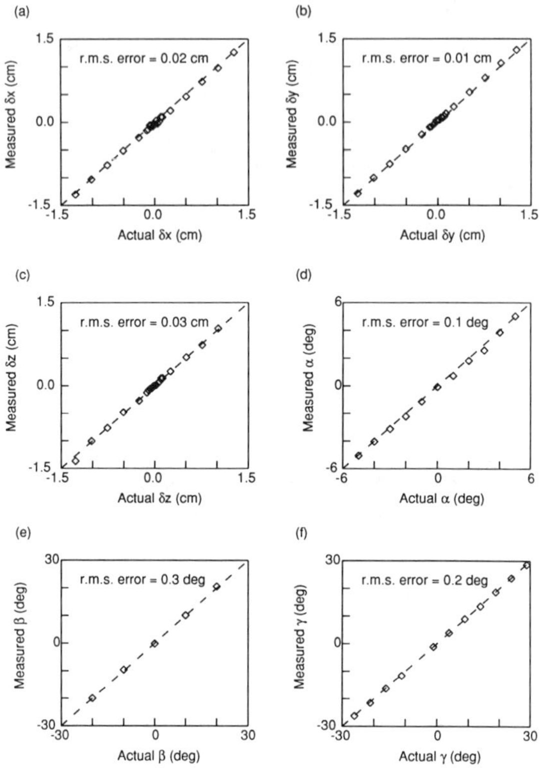

FIG. 5—*The resolution of the six-DOF acoustic transducer. The receiver platform is moved relative to the source platform.*

translations with maximum increases of 30% at $\delta z = -6.0$ cm, 75% at $\delta y = -8.0$ cm, and 61% at $\delta x = 8.0$ cm, respectively.

The predicted errors increase as the distance between the source and receiver platforms increases. In the measurement of the errors in translation presented in Fig. 5, the error of the transducer is measured near the initial position shown in Fig. 1 and represents an average error around the initial position. The theoretical error calculations predict how the error depends on the position of the receiver platform as the platform moves away from the initial position. Therefore, for the worst case at the extreme of motion in the x direction, the resolution in measurement of δz decreases to 0.09 cm (a decrease of 215%). If the actual resolutions in rotation presented in Fig. 5 are the resolutions of the transducer at the initial position, the worst case resolution for β is 0.6° at $\delta x = -8.0$ cm.

Anterior Force and Internal-External Rotation Tests: Results and Discussion

The results from the anterior force tests for the screwed case and fixtured case are shown in Fig. 8. The rotation α is small (less than 2°) for the screwed tests, with smaller angle α measured in the fixtured tests. The maximum difference is 1.9° at 87.4 N (for the fixtured tests $\alpha = 1.9°$, standard deviation [sd] 0.3; for the screwed tests $\alpha = -0.1°$, sd 0.2; Table 2). The response β is also less than 2° over the range of motion. The greatest difference in

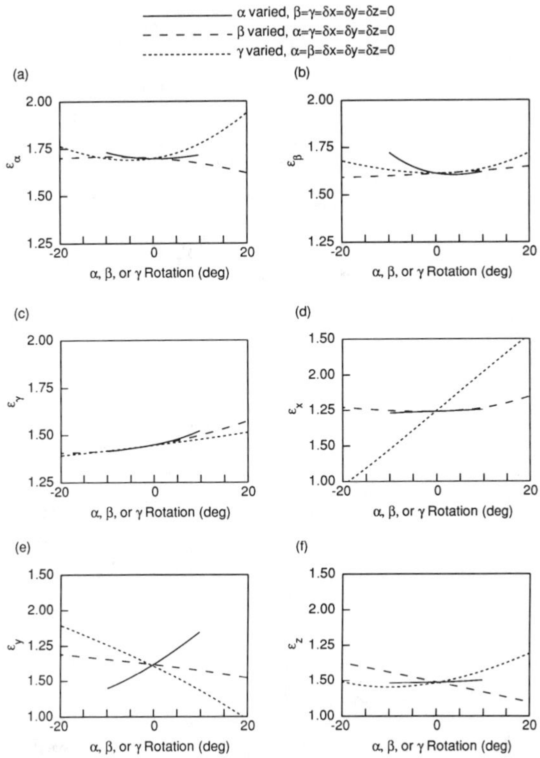

FIG. 6—*The errors in* α, β, γ, δx, δy, *and* δz *as functions of the rotations* α, β, *and* γ.

β is 1.2° at 81.5 N (for the fixtured tests β = 1.7°, sd 0.2; for the screwed tests β = 0.5°, sd 0.7). The rotation γ is less than 2.3°; the maximum difference is 2.7° at 87.5 N (for the fixtured tests γ = 0.38°, sd 0.05; for the screwed tests γ = −2.3°, sd 0.4). The maximum translation δx is 0.38 cm. There is no significant difference between the screwed and fixtured test data to about 50 N. The maximum difference of 0.12 cm occurs at 86.4 N (for the fixtured case δx = 0.37 cm, sd 0.09; for the screwed case δx = 0.25 cm, sd 0.01). The translation δy is less than 0.047 cm throughout the range of force application. The largest significant difference is 0.02 cm at 14.9 N (for the fixtured case δy = 0.03 cm, sd 0.01; for the screwed case δy = 0.01 cm, sd 0.02). The maximum translation δz is 0.52 cm for the screwed case. The difference in the screwed and fixtured measurements is insignificant to about 50 N. The largest difference is 0.16 cm at 83.1 N (for the fixtured case δz = 0.35 cm, sd 0.02; for the screwed case δz = 0.51 cm, sd 0.02).

The results from the internal-external rotation tests for the screwed case and fixtured case are shown in Fig. 9. The rotation α is less than 1.4° peak to peak. The differences in the cases are insignificant in internal rotation, and in external rotation reach 0.8° at M_z = 3.5 Nm (for the fixtured tests α = −1° sd 1; for the screwed tests α = 0.1°, sd 0.2; see Table 2). The response β is 4° peak to peak. The largest significant difference in β is 0.4° at −0.69 Nm (for the fixtured tests β = −0.7°, sd 0.3; for the screwed tests β = −0.3°, sd 0.3). The rotation γ has a peak-to-peak range of 27°. The largest difference in external rotation is 1.8° at 4.38 Nm (for the fixtured tests γ = 12.2°, sd 0.5; for the screwed tests γ = 14.0°,

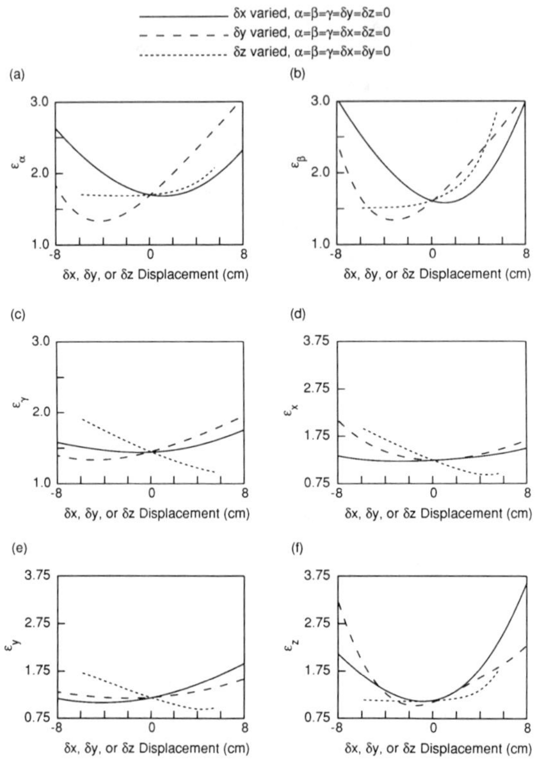

FIG. 7—*The errors in* α, β, γ, δx, δy, *and* δz *as functions of the translations* δx, δy, *and* δz.

sd 0.5). The peak-to-peak translation δx is 5 cm. There is no significant difference for internal rotation, and the maximum difference in external rotation is 0.5 cm at M_z = 3.3 Nm (for the fixtured tests δx = 2.2 cm, sd 0.5; for the screwed tests δx = 2.7 cm, sd 0.1). The peak-to-peak translation δy is 2.3 cm with no significant difference except at M_z = −0.7 Nm where it is 0.2 cm. The relative translation in the z direction has a peak-to-peak amplitude of 2.9 cm for the screwed case. The largest difference is 0.5 cm at M_z = 5.0 Nm (for the fixtured tests δz = 0.9 cm, sd 0.3; for the screwed tests δz = 1.41 cm, sd 0.07).

The differences in the screwed and fixtured test results arise from three sources: (1) a small difference in the direction of the loading exists between the cases, (2) the source platform orientation is slightly different in the two cases, and (3) tracking error occurs because of soft tissue motion. The first source was minimized by maintaining the same position of the leg for the two tests. The second source was minimized by clamping the source fixture to the chair for the screwed tests while the platform was still attached to the tracking fixtures, and then detaching the platform from the tracking fixtures. Therefore, the differences between the screwed and fixtured tests are principally attributable to tracking errors caused by soft tissue motion.

The differences in α and γ between the screwed and fixtured cases in Fig. 8 are small and sensitive to the direction of the applied load. They are not as significant in torsion in Fig. 9. The errors are larger for the anterior force tests because the anterior force applied to the calf by the experimenter deforms the calf, which then moves the tibial tracking fixture.

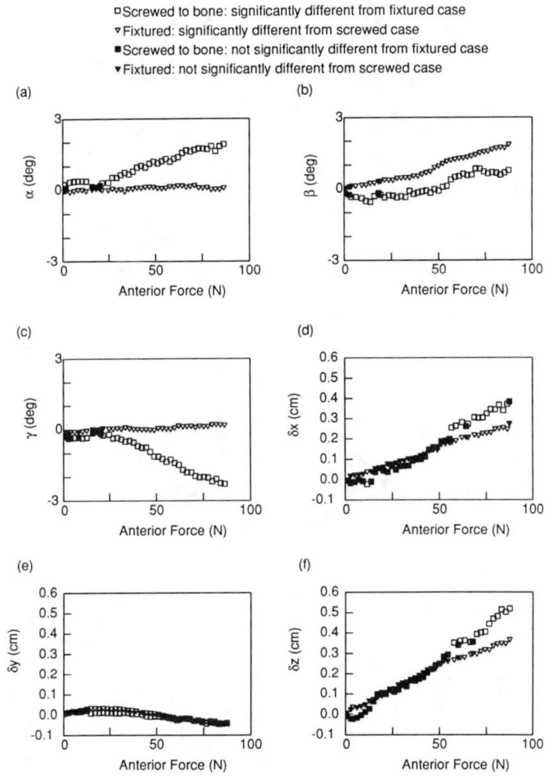

FIG. 8—*Comparison of the response to an anterior force for the screwed and fixtured cases. The two cases are significantly different if the significance level is less than 0.05. Angles α, β, and γ correspond to varus-valgus, flexion-extension, and internal-external rotations, respectively. Translations δx, δy, and δz correspond to anterior-posterior, medial-lateral, and proximal-distal translations, respectively.*

TABLE 2—*The peak-to-peak response for the applied anterior force and applied internal-external rotation and the maximum significant error caused by soft tissue motion.*

Motion	Peak-to-Peak Response	Maximum Significant Error Caused by Soft Tissue Motion
	Applied Internal-External Rotation	
α (deg)	1.4	0.8
β	4.0	0.4
γ	27.0	1.8
δ*x* (cm)	5.0	0.5
δ*y*	2.3	0.2
δ*z*	2.9	0.5
	Applied Anterior Force	
α (deg)	2.0	1.9
β	2.0	1.2
γ	2.3	2.7
δ*x* (cm)	0.38	0.12
δ*y*	0.07	0.02
δ*z*	0.5	0.16

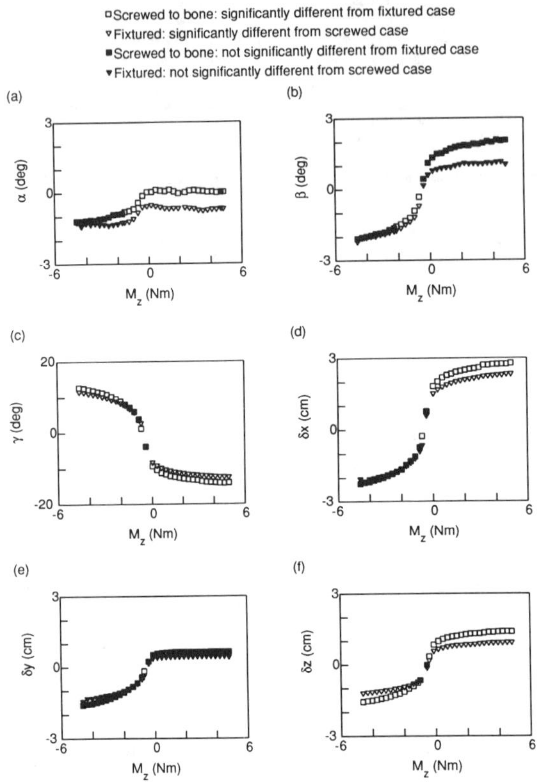

FIG. 9—*Comparison of the response to an applied internal-external rotation resulting in an applied internal-external moment,* M_z, *for the screwed and fixtured cases. The two cases are significantly different if the significance level is less than 0.05. Angles* α, β, *and* γ *correspond to varus-valgus, flexion-extension, and internal-external rotations, respectively. Translations* δx, δy, *and* δz *correspond to anterior-posterior, medial-lateral, and proximal-distal translations, respectively.*

Because the loads that cause the fixtures to move relative to the bones should be of the same magnitude in the in vivo case as they are for the cadaver specimen, the results from these tests can be used to estimate the errors caused by soft tissue motion in vivo. The soft tissue of the cadaver specimen is, however, flaccid compared to the soft tissue in the in-vivo case. Therefore, the soft tissue errors found during the cadaver experiments are likely larger than those occurring in vivo. The cadaver experiments do not account for the soft tissue motion errors as a result of muscle contraction.

Comparison to Other Techniques

This transducer has advantages when compared to linkage type measurement systems. It has better resolution than any commonly used linkage system, has no hysteresis, and has small mass. Because there is no mechanical coupling between the articulating bones and because the acoustic transducer has smaller mass than linkage systems, the transducer is better suited to dynamic measurements. (Dynamic measurements are error-prone, nonetheless.) The dynamics of the linkage system or acoustic system itself can obscure identification of the studied joint response [5]. The set-up time for a subject is substantially reduced with the acoustic transducer because there are fewer adjustments for individual subjects. The principal disadvantage of the transducer is that the data reduction process is computationally intensive, requiring a delay between the collection and viewing of the data.

The transducer directly measures the motion between the articulating bones; alternative acoustic systems discussed previously [13–22] reference the motion to a spatially fixed frame. Because of the large arrays of spatially fixed microphones used in other acoustic transducer systems, they can be difficult to use in studies where the body moves large distances (for example, snow skiing experiments). These techniques are also difficult to use outside of the laboratory environment; Engin and Peindl [18] noted the need for an anechoic environment.

Conclusions

1. A six-degree-of-freedom acoustic transducer has been developed that is lightweight and uses no mechanical linkages. Accordingly, hysteresis, backlash, and stick-slip associated with mechanical linkages are eliminated. The resolution of the transducer for translations less than 1.5 cm and rotations less than 30° around the expected operating position are 0.03 cm in translation and 0.3° in rotation. The transducer has been demonstrated in tests with a cadaver specimen for applied anterior force and applied internal-external rotation.

2. The uncertainty in the measurements, predicted by Monte Carlo simulation, depends on the measured translations and rotations. The uncertainty increases as the distance between the source and receiver platforms increases. In the worst case, the resolution of the transducer is predicted to decrease to 0.09 cm in translation and to 0.6° in rotation at an 8.0-cm translation of the platforms of the sources and receivers parallel to each other.

3. For in-vivo testing, soft tissue motion of the fixtures relative to the bone is the largest source of error. For internal-external rotation, the maximum soft tissue motion error measured in a cadaver test was 0.5 cm in translation and 1.8° in rotation. For applied anterior force, the maximum soft tissue motion error was 0.16 cm in translation and 2.7° in rotation.

References

[1] Johnson, R. J., Ettlinger, C. F., and Shealy, J. E., "Skier Injury Trends," in *Skiing Trauma and Skiing Safety: Seventh International Symposium, ASTM STP 1022*, R. J. Johnson, C. D. Mote, Jr., and M-H. Binet, Eds., American Society for Testing and Materials, Philadelphia, 1989, pp. 25–31.

[2] Quinn, T. P., Mote, C. D., Jr., and Skinner, H. B., "Three-Dimensional Loading of the Knee During Internal-External Rotation: The Effect of Ankle Constraint," in *Skiing Trauma and Skiing Safety: Seventh International Symposium, ASTM STP 1022*, R. J. Johnson, C. D. Mote, Jr., and M-H. Binet, Eds., American Society for Testing and Materials, Philadelphia, 1989, pp. 252–266.

[3] Hull, M. L. and Johnson, C., "Axial Rotation of the Lower Limb Under Torsional Loading: I. Static and Dynamic Measurements in Vivo," in *Skiing Trauma and Skiing Safety: Seventh International Symposium, ASTM STP 1022*, R. J. Johnson, C. D. Mote, Jr., and M-H. Binet, Eds., American Society for Testing and Materials, Philadelphia, 1989, pp. 277–290.

[4] Louie, J. K. and Mote, C. D., Jr., "Contribution of the Musculature to Rotatory Laxity and Torsional Stiffness at the Knee," in *Skiing Trauma and Skiing Safety: Sixth International Symposium, ASTM STP 938*, R. J. Johnson and C. D. Mote, Jr., Eds., American Society for Testing and Materials, Philadelphia, 1987, pp. 26–54.

[5] Kuo, C. Y. and Mote, C. D., Jr., "Identification of the Knee Joint in Varus-Valgus and Longitudinal Rotations in Laboratory and Snow Skiing Experiments," in *Skiing Trauma and Skiing Safety: Sixth International Symposium, ASTM STP 938*, R. J. Johnson and C. D. Mote, Jr., Eds., American Society for Testing and Materials, Philadelphia, 1987, pp. 5–25.

[6] Louie, J. K., Kuo, C. K., Gutierrez, M. D., and Mote, C. D., Jr., "Torsion of the Lower Extremity and Surface Electromyogram Measurements," in *Skiing Trauma and Safety: Fifth International Symposium, ASTM STP 860*, R. J. Johnson and C. D. Mote, Jr., Eds., American Society for Testing and Materials, Philadelphia, 1985, pp. 55–75.

[7] Ahmed, A. M., Hyder, A., Burke, D. L., and Chan, K. H., "In-Vitro Ligament Tension Pattern in the Flexed Knee in Passive Loading," *Journal of Orthopaedic Research*, Vol. 5, 1987, pp. 217–230.

[8] Isacson, J., Gransberg, L., and Knutsson, E., "Three-Dimensional Electrogoniometric Gait Recording," *Journal of Biomechanics*, Vol. 19, No. 8, 1986, pp. 627–635.

[9] Lewis, J. L., Lew, W. D., and Schmidt, J., "Description and Error Evaluation of an In Vitro Joint Testing System," *Journal of Biomechanical Engineering*, Vol. 110, 1988, pp. 238–247.

[10] Suntay, W. J., Grood, E. S., Hefzy, M. S., Butler, D. L., and Noyes, F. R., "Error Analysis of a System for Measuring Three-Dimensional Joint Motion," *Journal of Biomechanical Engineering*, Vol. 105, 1983, pp. 127–136.

[11] Blankevoort, L., Huiskes, R., and de Lange, A., "The Envelope of Passive Knee Joint Motion," *Journal of Biomechanics*, Vol. 21, No. 9, 1988, pp. 705–720.

[12] Blacharski, P. A., Somerset, J. H., and Murray, D. G., "A Three-Dimensional Study of the Kinematics of the Human Knee," *Journal of Biomechanics*, Vol. 8, 1975, pp. 375–384.

[13] Andrews, J. G. and Youm, Y., "A Biomechanical Investigation of Wrist Kinematics," *Journal of Biomechanics*, Vol. 12, 1979, pp. 83–89.

[14] Siegler, S., Chen, J., and Schneck, C. D., "The Three-Dimensional Kinematics and Flexibility Characteristics of the Human Ankle and Subtalar Joint—Part I: Kinematics," *Journal of Biomechanical Engineering*, Vol. 110, 1988, pp. 364–374.

[15] Chen, J., Siegler, S., and Schneck, C. D., "The Three-Dimensional Kinematics and Flexibility Characteristics of the Human Ankle and Subtalar Joint—Part II: Flexibility Characteristics," *Journal of Biomechanical Engineering*, Vol. 110, 1988, pp. 374–385.

[16] Engin, A. E., Peindl, R. D., Berme, N., and Kaleps, I., "Kinematic and Force Data Collection in Biomechanics by Means of Sonic Emitters—I: Kinematic Data Collection Methodology," *Journal of Biomechanical Engineering*, Vol. 106, 1984, pp. 204–211.

[17] Engin, A. E., Peindl, R. D., Berme, N., and Kaleps, I., "Kinematic and Force Data Collection in Biomechanics by Means of Sonic Emitters—II: Force Data Collection and Application to the Human Shoulder Complex," *Journal of Biomechanical Engineering*, Vol. 106, 1984, pp. 212–219.

[18] Engin, A. E. and Peindl, R. D., "On the Biomechanics of Human Shoulder Complex—I. Kinematics for Determination of the Shoulder Complex Sinus," *Journal of Biomechanics*, Vol. 20, No. 2, 1987, pp. 103–117.

[19] Peindl, R. D. and Engin, A. E., "On the Biomechanics of Human Shoulder Complex—II. Passive Resistive Properties Beyond the Shoulder Complex Sinus," *Journal of Biomechanics*, Vol. 20, No. 2, 1987, pp. 119–135.

[20] Engin, A. E. and Chen, S.-M., "Kinematic and Passive Resistive Properties of Human Elbow Complex," *Journal of Biomechanical Engineering*, Vol. 109, 1987, pp. 318–323.

[21] Engin, A. E. and Chen, S.-M., "On the Biomechanics of the Human Hip Complex In Vivo—I. Kinematics for Determination of the Maximal Voluntary Hip Complexes Sinus," *Journal of Biomechanics*, Vol. 21, No. 10, 1988, pp. 785—795.

[22] Engin, A. E. and Chen, S.-M., "On the Biomechanics of the Human Hip Complex In Vivo—II. Passive Resistive Properties Beyond the Hip Complex Sinus," *Journal of Biomechanics*, Vol. 21, No. 10, 1988, pp. 797–805.

[23] Daniel, D. M., Malcolm, L. L., Losse, G., Stone, M. L., Sachs, R., and Burks, R., "Instrumented Measurement of Anterior Laxity of the Knee," *The Journal of Bone and Joint Surgery*, Vol. 67-A, No. 5, 1985, pp. 720–726.

[24] Edixhoven, Ph., Huiskes, R., de Graaf, R., van Rens, Th. J. G., and Slooff, T. J., "Accuracy and Reproducibility of Instrumented Knee-Drawer Tests," *Journal of Orthopaedic Research*, Vol. 5, No. 3, 1987, pp. 378–387.

[25] Woltring, H. J., Huiskes, R., and de Lange, A., "Finite Centroid and Helical Axis Estimation from Noisy Landmark Measurements in the Study of Human Joint Kinematics," *Journal of Biomechanics*, Vol. 18, No. 5, 1985, pp. 379–389.

[26] Spiegelman, J. J. and Woo, S. L.-Y., "A Rigid-Body Method for Finding Centers of Rotation and Angular Displacements of Planar Joint Motion," *Journal of Biomechanics*, Vol. 20, No. 7, 1987, pp. 715–721.

[27] Panjabi, M. M., Goel, V. K., and Walter, S. D., "Errors in Kinematic Parameters of a Planar Joint: Guidelines for Optimal Experimental Design," *Journal of Biomechanics*, Vol. 15, No. 7, 1982, pp. 537–544.

[28] Panjabi, M. M., "Centers and Angles of Rotation of Body Joints: A Study of Errors and Optimization," *Journal of Biomechanics*, Vol. 12, 1979, pp. 911–920.
[29] Veldpaus, F. E., Woltring, H. J., and Dortmans, L. J. M. G., "A Least-Squares Algorithm for the Equiform Transformation from Spatial Marker Co-ordinates," *Journal of Biomechanics*, Vol. 21, No. 1, 1988, pp. 45–54.
[30] Chao, E. Y. S., "Justification of Triaxial Goniometer for the Measurement of Joint Rotation," *Journal of Biomechanics*, Vol. 13, 1980, pp. 989–1006.
[31] Grood, E. S. and Suntay, W. J., "A Joint Coordinate System for the Clinical Description of Three-Dimensional Motions: Application to the Knee," *Journal of Biomechanical Engineering*, Vol. 105, 1983, pp. 136–144.
[32] Hart, R. A., Mote, C. D., Jr., and Skinner, H. B., "The Finite Helical Axis as a Landmark for Kinematic Reference of the Knee," *Journal of Biomechanical Engineering*, 1990, in press.
[33] Suh, C. H. and Radcliffe, C. W., *Kinematics and Mechanisms Design*, Robert E. Krieger Publishing Company, Malabar, FL, 1987, pp. 378–380.
[34] Spoor, C. W. and Veldpaus, F. E., "Rigid Body Motion Calculated from Spatial Co-ordinates of Markers," *Journal of Biomechanics*, Vol. 13, No. 4, 1980, pp. 391–395.
[35] Sobol, I. M., *The Monte Carlo Method*, Popular Lectures in Mathematics, The University of Chicago Press, Chicago, 1974.

Timothy P. Quinn[1] *and C. D. Mote, Jr.*[1]

Optimal Design of an Uncoupled Six-Degree-of-Freedom Dynamometer

REFERENCE: Quinn, T. P. and Mote, C. D., Jr., "**Optimal Design of an Uncoupled Six-Degree-of-Freedom Dynamometer,**" *Skiing Trauma and Safety: Eighth International Symposium, ASTM STP 1104*, C. D. Mote, Jr. and Robert J. Johnson, Eds., American Society for Testing and Materials, Philadelphia, 1991, pp. 94–111.

ABSTRACT: A design analysis of a class of six-degree-of-freedom strain-gage dynamometers that are virtually uncoupled in each force and moment component is presented. The method of design is detailed, and an optimal design algorithm is implemented. The dynamometer is made of six or more T-sections with thin webs and flanges called shear panel elements (SPE). Complete stress and buckling analyses are carried out for the SPE, and experiments confirm the predictions of the analyses. The optimal design method is illustrated with several case studies. A dynamometer has been built and used in laboratory and field experiments.

KEY WORDS: dynamometer, six degree of freedom, uncoupled, shear panel element, optimal design, cantilever plate, skiing injury

Nomenclature

b, c	Dimensions of the cantilever plate in the ξ and ζ directions
d, f_w, f_f, t_w, t_f	Geometry of the SPE, see Fig. 1
D	Flexural rigidity
E, ν	Young's modulus and Poisson's ratio
$\bar{e}$	Shear strain in (ξ, ζ) coordinates at the center of the cantilever plate ($b/2$, $c/2$)
$\bar{e}_w$	Shear strain at the center of the web; $\bar{e}_w = \bar{e}$ with $L = P$, $b = f_w$, $c = d$, and $t = t_w$
f_{ij}, g_{ij}	Coefficients in the approximation of u and v
F_X, F_Y, F_Z	External force components applied to the cage
$F_{Y'}$	External force applied to the cage of the Y' direction (for example, $F_{Y'} = F_X$ if Y' is aligned with X)
$K_{X'}$, $K_{Y'}$, $K_{Z'}$	Stiffnesses of a SPE for forces applied to the ends of the flange in the X', Y', Z' directions, respectively
K_1	Torsional stiffness of the web
K_2	Bending stiffness of one arm of the flange
K_{min}	Minimum allowable design stiffness of the SPE in the Y' direction
K_t	Torsional stiffness of the SPE about the X' axis

[1]Graduate student and professor and chairman, respectively, Department of Mechanical Engineering, University of California, Berkeley, CA 94720.

l Distance from the moment axis of the reference coordinates to the flange of the SPE, see Fig. 1
L Force applied at the end of the cantilever plate; see Fig. 5
$\overline{L}$ The force L at the onset of buckling
$\overline{L}_f$ The buckling force in the flange; $\overline{L}_f = \overline{L}$ with $b = f_f/2$, $c = d$, and $t = t_f$
$\overline{L}_w$ The buckling force in the web; $\overline{L}_w = \overline{L}$ with $b = f_w$, $c = d$, and $t = t_w$
M_X, M_Y, M_Z External moment components applied to the cage
$M_{Z'}$ External moment applied to cage in the Z' direction (for example, $M_{Z'} = M_Y$ if Z' is aligned with Y)
p_{ij}, q_{ij} Coefficients in the approximation of w
P Total external force applied to the SPE
$r_1 - r_3$ Minimum allowable stiffness ratios
S The set of all possible $\mathbf{X}$
S1–S7 SPEs of the dynamometer in Fig. 3
S_y Yield strength
$\sigma_\zeta, \sigma_\xi, \sigma_{\xi\zeta}$ Stresses in the cantilever plate
$\sigma'_\zeta, \sigma'_\xi, \sigma'_{\xi\zeta}$ Nondimensional stresses in the cantilever plate
$\overline{\sigma}$ Maximum von Mises stress in the cantilever plate;

$$\overline{\sigma} = \max_{\substack{0 \le \xi \le b \\ 0 \le \zeta \le c}} (\sigma_\xi^2 + \sigma_\zeta^2 - \sigma_\xi \sigma_\zeta + 3\,\sigma_{\xi\zeta}^2)^{1/2}$$

$\overline{\sigma}_f$ Maximum von Mises stress in the flange; $\overline{\sigma}_f = \overline{\sigma}$ with $L = P/2$, $b = f_f/2$, $c = d$, and $t = t_f$
$\overline{\sigma}_w$ Maximum von Mises stress in the web $\overline{\sigma}_w = \overline{\sigma}$ with $L = P$, $b = f_w$, $c = d$, and $t = t_w$
t Thickness of the cantilever plate
T Shear traction applied at the end of the cantilever plate, see Fig. 5
T1–T6 SPEs in a six-degree-of-freedom dynamometer
u, v Displacements of the cantilever plate along ξ and ζ
$\overline{v}$ $= v(c, b/2)$
$\overline{v}_f$ $= \overline{v}$ with $L = 1/2$, $b = f_f/2$, $c = d$, and $t = t_f$
$\overline{v}_w$ $= \overline{v}$ with $L = 1$, $b = f_w$, $c = d$, and $t = t_w$
w Transverse displacement of the cantilever plate
X–Y–Z Coordinates at the center of the dynamometer
X'–Y'–Z' Coordinates at the base of the SPE
$\mathbf{X}$ $= [l, d, f_w, f_f, t_w, t_f]$
Π Potential energy functional for the cantilever plate
ξ, ζ Local coordinate system for the cantilever plate

Introduction

Multicomponent dynamometers have been used to measure the force and moment components applied to a skier's foot [*1–3*] and have been incorporated into designs of the ski binding [*4–6*]. Many designs of multicomponent strain-gage dynamometers have been reported [*7–15*], but few authors discuss the design process. Reuber et al. [*16*] illustrated the usefulness of symbolic processing techniques in selection and design of single-degree-of-freedom dynamometers. Hou and Twu [*17*] presented an automated, optimal design scheme for strain-gage balances for wind tunnel testing using repeated evaluations with finite elements. Lin and Beadle [*18*] studied optimum placement of strain gages when a structure is used as its own force transducer. Sinden and Boie [*19*] described a design method for capacitive force sensors.

The purpose of this paper is to present a complete design method for a class of virtually uncoupled, linear, six-degree-of-freedom, strain-gage dynamometers. Within limits, the designer can control the sensitivities of the loading component measurements. The dynamometer is analyzed, and design data and methods of optimal design are presented. Verification tests are performed on a prototype dynamometer. The optimal design procedure maximizing the sensitivity of the dynamometer is implemented in several case studies.

The class of dynamometers studied offers several advantages. Because the dynamometer is uncoupled and linear in all components, the output signals can be directly used for feedback control or analog recording; calibration is simple. Compact and relatively lightweight designs are possible.

Shear Panel Element Dynamometer

A shear panel element (SPE) has a T-shaped cross section with a thin web and flange built in at the base of the "T" (Fig. 1). The geometry of an SPE is specified by six design variables, l, d, f_w, f_f, t_w, t_f, as seen in Fig. 1. Four strain gages are mounted at $\pm 45°$ to the X' axis at the center of the web, two gages, one on top of the other, on each side (Fig. 2). The output of the bridge is a measurement of the shear strain in the $X'-Y'$ plane.

The dynamometer design is a combination of six or more SPEs each built into a common base. An example of a seven-SPE dynamometer is shown in Fig. 3. The measured force and moment are applied to the cage, which is pinned to the base frame through the ends of the flanges of each SPE. Figure 4 shows a generic six SPE dynamometer design.

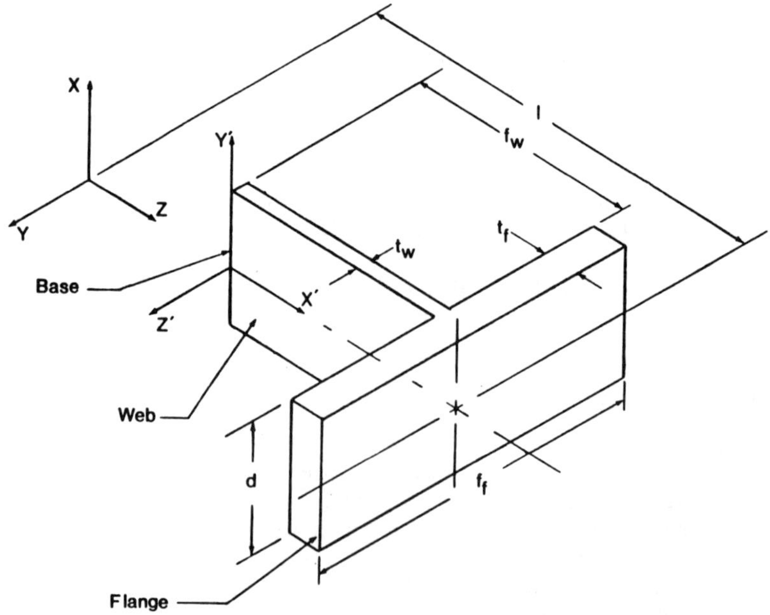

FIG. 1—*A shear panel element: it is built in at the base, and load is applied through pins on the ends of the flange.*

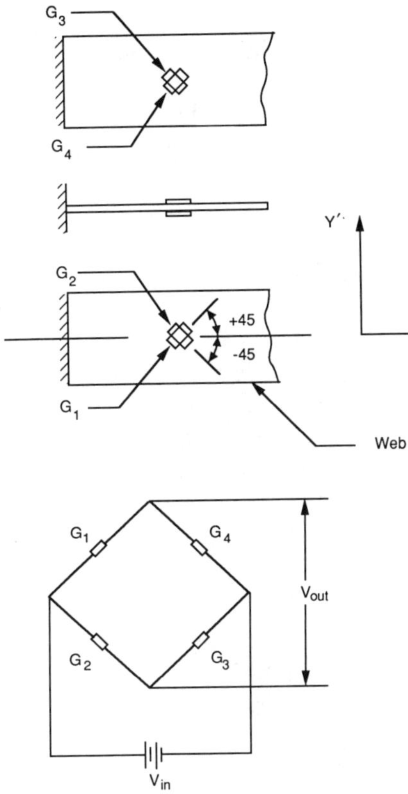

FIG. 2—*Placement of the strain gages,* $G_1 - G_4$, *on the web of the shear panel element and in the Wheatstone bridge.* G_1 *and* G_3 *are at* $+45°$ *to the* X′ *axis, and* G_2 *and* G_4 *are at* $-45°$. V_{in} *is the excitation voltage, and* V_{out} *is the output voltage. Arrows indicate the directions of the* X′–Y′ *axes.*

The ratios of the stiffnesses, $(K_{Y'}/K_{Z'})$, $(K_{Y'}/K_{X'})$, $(K_{Y'}l/K_t)$, for a SPE in Fig. 1 are all normally designed to be at least 500. Accordingly, a force F_Z and a moment M_y in Fig. 4 are effectively supported by elements T1 and T2 only. Because each pair of SPEs in Fig. 4 essentially supports single components of the force and moment, the SPE pairs T1 and T2, T3 and T4, and T5 and T6 may be designed independently. The six-SPE dynamometer is statically determinant and is virtually mechanically uncoupled. The strain-gage positions on the web and in the bridge circuit ensure that only shear in the plane of the web is measured.

The shear in the web is proportional to the force applied in the Y' direction at the end of the SPE in Fig. 1. In Fig. 4 the force in the X or Y or Z direction is proportional to the sum of the signals from the appropriate SPE pair, and the moment in the Z or X or Y directions is proportional to the difference of those signals. The external forces in T1 and T2 are f'' and f', respectively:

$$\left.\begin{matrix} f' \\ f'' \end{matrix}\right\} = \frac{1}{2}\left(F_Z \pm \frac{M_Y}{l}\right) \tag{1}$$

The external force applied to each SPE is denoted P in the subsequent discussion.

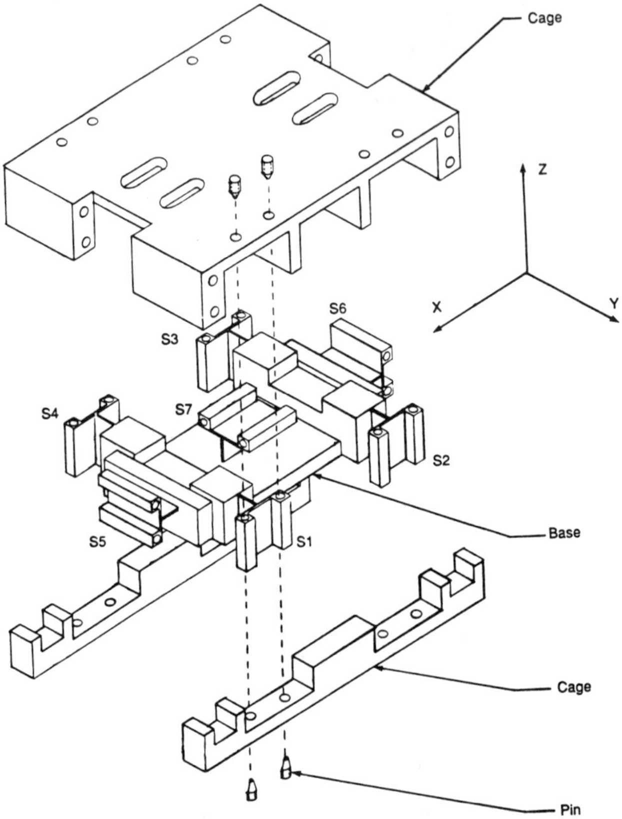

FIG. 3—*A six-degree-of-freedom shear-panel dynamometer. The load is applied to the cage, which is supported by several shear panel elements through pins at the ends of the flanges. The base is connected to ground. Arrows indicate the directions of the* X–Y–Z *axes.*

Using elementary design analysis, Levin and Mote [*20*] designed and built the SPE dynamometer shown in Fig. 3. Four SPE (S1–S4) support F_Z (4000 N max) and M_X and M_Y (100 Nm max). Elements S5 and S6 support F_Y (1000 N max) and M_Z (60 Nm max). Element S7 supports F_X (1300 N max). The overall dimensions of the dynamometer are $14 \times 9.5 \times 3.2$ cm.

The load is applied to the SPE through pins at the ends of the flanges (Fig. 3). The pins are Allen head screws whose ends are tapered to a point. The SPE flanges are terminated in square ends with detents for the pins. The pins are threaded through the cage, and a small compressive preload is applied to the flange. The pins must ensure each SPE supports load in its "stiff" direction to prevent yielding other SPE in their "soft" directions. To maintain the configuration under load, the base and the cage are very stiff, virtually rigid. To minimize hysteresis, sliding surfaces and bolted joints are avoided to the extent possible (for example, SPE pairs S2, S3, and S1, S4 are machined from a single block).

Levin and Mote found the dynamometer to have coupling between the six loading components of less than 1% of full scale and to be linear in all components with correlation coefficients greater than 0.999. Hysteresis was less than 2% of full scale for the moment

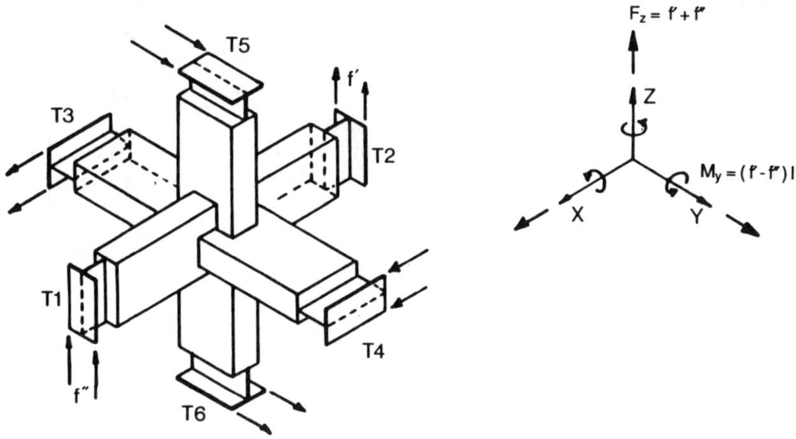

FIG. 4—*Ideal shear panel element six-degree-of-freedom dynamometer configuration. Element pairs (for example, T1 and T2) support single force and moment components.* f′ *and* f″ *are external forces applied to elements T2 and T1. Arrows indicate the directions of the* X–Y–Z *axes.*

components with typical values substantially less than 2%. The dynamometer has root mean square accuracies of 1, 1, and 4 N for F_X, F_Y, and F_Z and 0.2, 0.5 and 0.2 Nm for M_X, M_Y, and M_Z, respectively. The dynamometer is the principal, multicomponent dynamometer used in all laboratory and snow skiing experiments [*21*].

Modeling

For design, it is necessary to calculate the strength and stiffness of the SPE to loads in the Y' (stiff) direction and the stiffnesses of the SPE to loads in the X' and Z' directions. For loading in the Y' direction, the web and each arm of the flange are modeled as cantilever plates in plane stress (Fig. 5). The boundary conditions require the displacements $u(\xi,\zeta)$ and $v(\xi,\zeta)$ vanish at $\xi = 0$ and the shear traction, T, at $\xi = b$ is uniform. Edges $\zeta = 0$ and $\zeta = c$ are traction free. The boundary traction is $T = L/tc$ where L is the applied force. For the web, $L = P$, and for each arm of the flange, $L = P/2$.

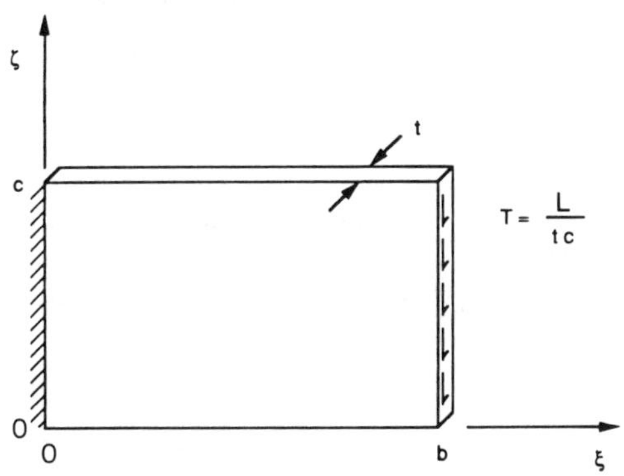

FIG. 5—*The cantilever plate model for the web and each arm of the flange of the SPE.*

The plate can fail in two ways: the yield strength of the material can be exceeded at some point or the plate can buckle laterally. To analyze buckling, the boundary conditions are modeled as simple supports on edges $\xi = 0, b$ and free on edges $\zeta = 0, c$.

The material is homogeneous and linearly elastic, and infinitesimal strain theory is appropriate. Because the plate has a small span-to-depth ratio, end effects can be important and Euler–Bernoulli (E–B) beam formulas are not necessarily reliable. The solution to the plane stress problem is approximated by minimizing the discretized potential energy functional, Π:

$$\Pi = \frac{E}{4(1 - \nu^2)} \int_0^c \int_0^b [2(u,_\xi^2 + v,_\zeta^2) + 4\,\nu\, u,_\xi\, v,_\zeta + (1 - \nu)(u,_\zeta^2 + v,_\xi^2) + 2(1 - \nu)u,_\zeta v,_\xi]d\xi\, d\zeta + \int_0^c T\, v|_{\xi = b} d\zeta \tag{2}$$

The components of the displacement field are each represented by

$$\left.\begin{matrix} u \\ v \end{matrix}\right\} = \sum_{i=1}^{N1} \sum_{j=1}^{M1} f_{ij} \sin\left(\frac{i\pi\xi}{2b}\right) \sin\left(\frac{j\pi\zeta}{2c}\right) + \sum_{i=1}^{N2} \sum_{j=0}^{M2} g_{ij} \sin\left(\frac{i\pi\xi}{2b}\right) \cos\left(\frac{j\pi\zeta}{2c}\right) \tag{3}$$

The coefficients f_{ij} and g_{ij}, minimizing the discretized Π, are determined following the Ritz method [*22*], giving an approximation to u and v. The stresses are then

$$\begin{aligned} \sigma_\xi &= \frac{E}{1 - \nu^2} (u,_\xi + \nu\, v,_\zeta) \\ \sigma_\zeta &= \frac{E}{1 - \nu^2} (v,_\zeta + \nu\, u,_\xi) \\ \sigma_{\xi\zeta} &= \frac{E}{2\,(1 + \nu)} (u,_\zeta + v,_\xi) \end{aligned} \tag{4}$$

The stiffness of the SPE in Fig. 1 in the Y' direction is the reciprocal of the displacement of the center line of the flanged at its ends when a unit load is applied to the SPE; each arm of the flange is assumed to support half this unit load. This gives

$$K_{Y'} = \frac{1}{\bar{v}_f + \bar{v}_w} \tag{5}$$

where $\bar{v}_w$ is the deflection of the web under a unit load and $\bar{v}_f$ is the deflection of the flange (alone) under a half unit load.

In the Z' direction, the stiffness of the web, modeled as the bending of a cantilever E–B beam with large width-to-span ratio [*23*], is

$$K_{Z'} = \frac{d\, t_w^3}{4\, f_w^3} \frac{E}{(1 - \nu^2)} \tag{6}$$

Deformation of the flange is neglected in the Z' stiffness prediction. The stiffness of the flange in the X' direction is

$$K_{X'} = \frac{4\,d\,t_f^3}{f_f^3} \frac{E}{(1 - \nu^2)} \tag{7}$$

Here, deflection is predicted from bending of a cantilever beam of large width-to-span ratio having half of the total load applied at each of the flange. The deformation of the web is neglected in the X' stiffness prediction.

For torsion about the X' axis, the web is modeled as a beam in torsion and the flange is modeled as two plates in plane stress as described above. Let the torsional stiffness of the web be K_1 and the bending stiffness of one arm of the flange be K_2. The torsional stiffness of the web is calculated using the formula for a beam of narrow rectangular cross section given in Timoshenko and Goodier [*24*]:

$$K_1 = \frac{E\,t_w^3}{6(1 + \nu)} \frac{d}{f_w} \left(1 - 0.630 \frac{t_w}{d}\right) \tag{8}$$

K_2 is given by $K_2 = 1/\bar{v}$ where $\bar{v}$ is calculated for a plate with $t = t_f$, $b = f_f/2$, $c = d$, and $L = 1$. The torsional stiffness of the SPE is then

$$K_t = \frac{f_f^2\,K_1\,K_2}{K_1 + f_f^2\,K_2} \tag{9}$$

The force at the onset of buckling of a Kirchhoff plate is determined from stationarity of

$$\Lambda[w] \triangleq \frac{D \int_0^c \int_0^b \left\{ \left(\frac{\partial^2 w}{\partial \xi^2} + \frac{\partial^2 w}{\partial \zeta^2} \right)^2 - 2(1 - \nu) \left[\frac{\partial^2 w}{\partial \xi^2} \frac{\partial^2 w}{\partial \zeta^2} - \left(\frac{\partial^2 w}{\partial \xi\, \partial \zeta} \right)^2 \right] \right\} d\xi\, d\zeta}{- \int_0^c \int_0^b \left[\sigma'_\xi \left(\frac{\partial w}{\partial \xi} \right)^2 + \sigma'_\zeta \left(\frac{\partial w}{\partial \zeta} \right)^2 + 2\sigma'_{\xi\zeta} \frac{\partial w}{\partial \zeta} \frac{\partial w}{\partial \xi} \right] d\xi\, d\zeta} \tag{10}$$

where

$$D = \frac{E\,t^3}{12(1 - \nu^2)},$$

$$\begin{aligned} \sigma_\xi &= \sigma'_\xi \left(\frac{L}{tc}\right), \\ \sigma_\zeta &= \sigma'_\zeta \left(\frac{L}{tc}\right), \\ \sigma_{\xi\zeta} &= \sigma'_{\xi\zeta} \left(\frac{L}{tc}\right), \end{aligned} \tag{11}$$

and w is the transverse displacement of the plate [25]. The stresses are determined in Eq 4, and the approximate expansion for w is

$$w = \sum_{i=1}^{R1} \sum_{j=1}^{Q1} p_{ij} \sin\left(\frac{i\pi\xi}{b}\right) \sin\left(\frac{j\pi\zeta}{2c}\right) + \sum_{i=1}^{R2} \sum_{j=0}^{Q2} q_{ij} \sin\left(\frac{i\pi\xi}{2b}\right) \cos\left(\frac{j\pi\zeta}{2c}\right) \tag{12}$$

The coefficients p_{ij} and q_{ij} are chosen to render $\Lambda[w]$ in Eq 10 stationary. The approximate eigenvalue $\overline{L}/c = \Lambda[w]$ is evaluated at the extremal of Eq 10.

The optimal design maximizes the shear strain at the center of the web of an SPE pair (for example, T1 and T2 in Fig. 4) for a unit applied force. This design maximizes the sensitivity of the dynamometer subject to constraints on the SPE design for strength and stiffness and for constraints on the admissible ranges of the design variables. The design problem is to find $\mathbf{X} = [l, d, f_w, f_f, t_w, t_f]$, $\mathbf{X} \in S$ such that

$$\overline{e}_w(\mathbf{X}) \text{ is a maximum} \tag{13}$$

subject to

$$\begin{gathered}
\frac{K_{Y'}}{K_{Z'}} > r_1 \\
\frac{K_{Y'}}{K_{X'}} > r_2 \\
\frac{K_{Y'}l}{K_t} > r_3 \\
K_{Y'} > K_{\min} \\
\overline{\sigma}_w < S_y \\
\overline{\sigma}_f < S_y \\
P < \overline{L}_w \\
\frac{P}{2} < \overline{L}_f
\end{gathered} \tag{14}$$

The shear strain for a given load is maximized using an augmented Lagrangian method with all derivatives computed numerically [26]. The displacements u and v, giving the stresses in Eq 4, are parameterized by Poisson's ratio ν and the aspect ratio, b/c. They are linear in L/Et. The buckling solutions of the discrete eigenvalue problem are also parameterized by ν and b/c. The buckling and stress analyses are carried out for candidate aspect ratios in advance of the optimization. The results needed in the optimization, $\overline{\sigma}$, $\overline{\nu}$, and $\overline{e}$, are tabulated for $L/Et = 1$, $\nu = 0.3$, and $b/c < 1.5$ (Table 1). Piece-wise cubic splines with continuous first derivatives are then fit to the tabulated values, and the splines are used in the optimization procedure to reduce greatly the number of computations.

TABLE 1—*Design table for a cantilever, rectangular plate with constant in-plane shear traction, L/tc, applied to the free end.*

$\frac{b}{c}$	$\bar{\sigma}$ $\left(\frac{L}{tc} = 1\right)$	$\bar{e}$ $\left(\frac{L}{Etc} = 1\right)$	$\bar{v}$ $\left(\frac{L}{tE} = 1\right)$	$\frac{\overline{Lc}}{D}$
0.05	3.35	1.30	0.13	6219.97
0.10	4.11	1.32	0.26	1174.31
0.15	4.37	1.35	0.40	510.52
0.20	4.58	1.39	0.55	292.73
0.25	4.77	1.47	0.71	189.43
0.30	4.95	1.56	0.89	131.84
0.35	5.13	1.65	1.09	96.43
0.40	5.33	1.73	1.32	73.05
0.45	5.54	1.80	1.57	56.81
0.50	5.76	1.86	1.85	45.13
0.55	5.99	1.90	2.16	36.52
0.60	6.23	1.93	2.51	30.05
0.65	6.47	1.96	2.89	25.09
0.70	6.71	1.97	3.31	21.24
0.75	6.96	1.99	3.77	18.19
0.80	7.20	2.00	4.28	15.74
0.85	7.45	2.00	4.84	13.75
0.90	7.70	2.01	5.44	12.12
0.95	7.95	2.01	6.10	10.76
1.00	8.19	2.01	6.82	9.62
1.05	8.44	2.01	7.59	8.66
1.10	8.69	2.01	8.43	7.83
1.15	8.93	2.01	9.33	7.12
1.20	9.18	2.01	10.30	6.50
1.25	9.43	2.01	11.34	5.97
1.30	9.67	2.01	12.46	5.49
1.35	9.92	2.01	13.65	5.08
1.40	10.17	2.01	14.92	4.71
1.45	10.41	2.01	16.28	4.38
1.50	10.66	2.01	17.72	4.08

Verification and Experiments

The shear strains $\bar{e}_w$ in elements S5 and S6 in the dynamometer in Fig. 3 were measured and compared to predictions. The nominal dimensions of the web in both elements are $f_f = 0.914$ cm, $d = 2.54$ cm, $f_w = 0.914$ cm, $l = 5.64$ cm, and $t_w, t_f = 0.041 \begin{Bmatrix} +0.003 \\ -0.000 \end{Bmatrix}$ cm. The base of the dynamometer was fixed with the Y axis directed vertically. The Wheatstone bridges for elements S5 and S6 were balanced. A shunt resistor was used to calibrate both bridges [*27*]. A cable was then pinned to the cage at the S6 element, and known weights were suspended from it. The suspended weights were 222.4, 266.9, 311.4, and 355.9 N.

Results

The predicted $\bar{v}$ is seen in Fig. 6(*a*) for $\nu = 0.3$ and $L/Et = 1$. The $\bar{v}$ for 20 to 80 terms in Eq 3 differ by less than 4% over the b/c range evaluated. The 80-term solution for $\bar{v}$ is

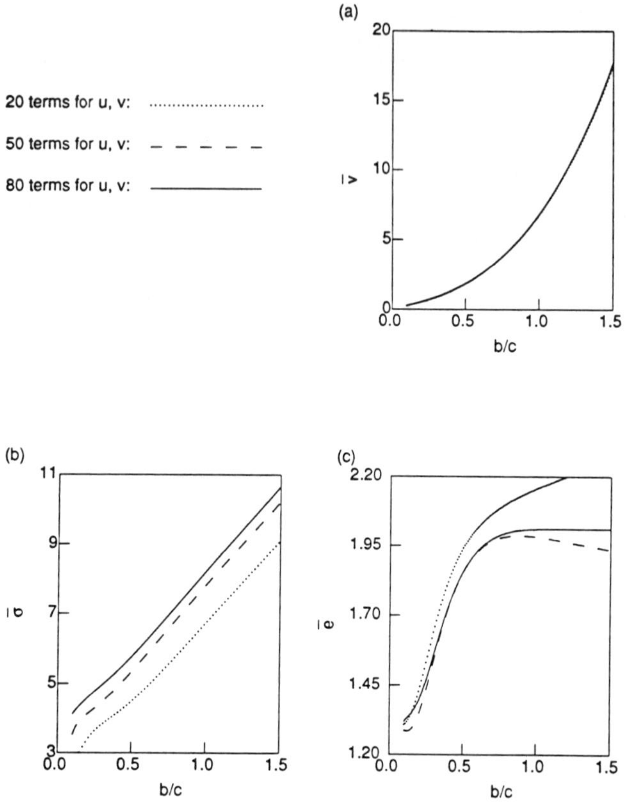

FIG. 6—*Ritz analysis for* (a) *the displacement* $\overline{v}$, (b) *the maximum von Mises stress* $\overline{\sigma}$, *and* (c) *the shear strain* $\overline{e}$ *of a cantilever, rectangular plate subject to a constant in-plane shear traction at its free end.*

within 3% of that obtained by E–B theory for $4 < b/c < 5$. For $b/c > 5$, the difference between the 80-term solution and E–B theory is negligible.

The stress field in the plate depends on the aspect ratio b/c and Poisson's ratio; it is linear in L/tc. The maximum von Mises stress $\overline{\sigma}$ is located at $(\xi,\zeta) = (0,0)$ and $(0,c)$. The plot of $\overline{\sigma}$ in Fig. 6(*b*) is for $\nu = 0.3$ and $L/tc = 1$. For the 80-term expansions

$$\overline{\sigma} = (4.95 \frac{b}{c} + 3.31) \frac{L}{tc}, \tag{15}$$

a more conservative estimate than that given by E–B beam theory ($\overline{\sigma} = 6\ b/c\ L/tc$) for $b/c < 3$.

The shear strain at the center of the plate $\overline{e}$ depends on b/c, ν and is linear in L/Etc. A plot of $\overline{e}$ for $\nu = 0.3$ and $L/Etc = 1$ is shown in Fig. 6(*c*). The solution converges for $b/c < 1$, and the error is estimated to be less than $\pm 3\%$ for $b/c > 1$. The 80-term expansions give $\overline{e} \cong 2.01$ for $b/c > 1$; for $L/Etc = 1$ and $\nu = 0.3$, E–B beam theory predicts $\overline{e} = 1.95$, independent of aspect ratio. This result shows that any web with $b/c \geq 1$, for the intents and purposes here, is an optimal one.

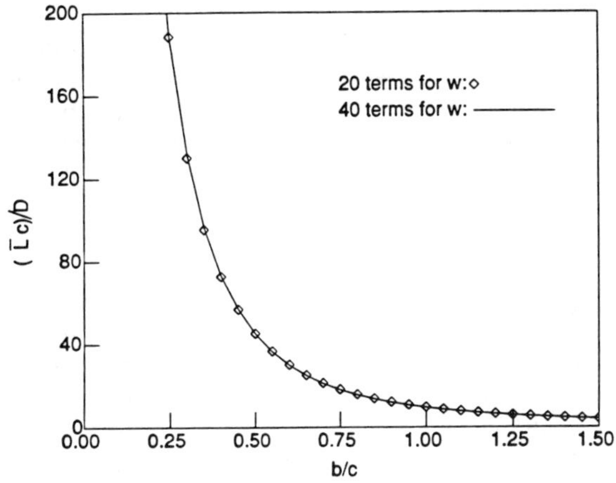

FIG. 7—*Ritz analysis for lateral buckling of a cantilever, rectangular plate in Fig. 5. The plate is pinned at* $\xi = 0$ *and* $\xi = b$ *and free at* $\zeta = 0$ *and* $\zeta = c$.

To understand the effect of choosing the distribution of the traction as uniform on the boundary at $\zeta = b$, the solutions for $\overline{v}$, $\overline{\sigma}$, and $\overline{e}$ for a parabolic distribution were also computed with the 80-term expansions in u and v. The results were within 3% of those shown in Fig. 6 for a uniform traction.

When tested against the exact buckling solution in Ref *28* for $\sigma'_{\xi\zeta} = \sigma'_{\xi} = 0$ and $\sigma'_{\zeta} = -1$, the buckling algorithm reproduced the exact buckling load with less than 0.5% error for a 40-term expansion in Eq 12. The nondimensional buckling load for the cantilever plate is given in Fig. 7 for 20- and 40-term expansions in w.

Table 1 summarizes the 80-term solutions for $\overline{\sigma}$, $\overline{e}$, and $\overline{v}$ and the 40-term solution of $\overline{L}c/D$ for aspect ratios less than 1.5 that are useful for design purposes.

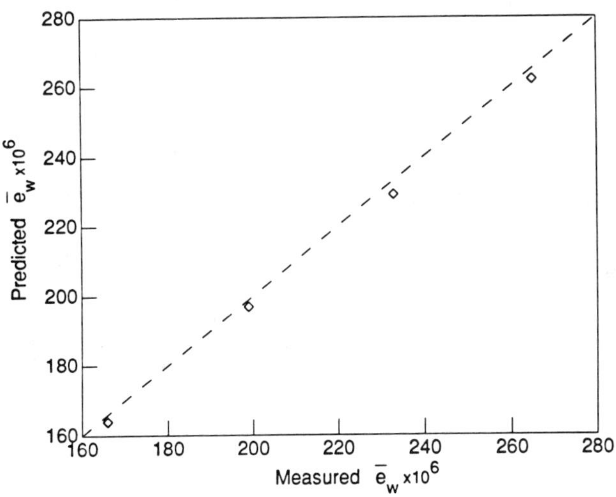

FIG. 8—*Comparison of the measured shear strain* $\overline{e}$ *in an SPE to the theoretically predicted value.*

The shear strain $\bar{e}_w$ measured in element S6 of Fig. 3 was measured to be a constant 16.9 ± 0.6 times greater than the shear strain measured in element S5 for all suspended weights. Element S6 carried 96.4% of the load. The theoretically predicted and measured shear strains $\bar{e}_w$ in S6 are shown in Fig. 8. The maximum difference between predicted and measured values is 2%; note that the tolerance in the thickness of the web leads to a ±4% uncertainty on the predicted value of $\bar{e}_w$.

Optimization

The SPE S5 and S6 in the dynamometer in Fig. 3 are analyzed, and the results are shown in Table 2. Elements S5 and S6 have relatively thick flanges and webs (t_w,t_f = 0.041 cm) and are therefore stiff in the Y' direction ($K_{Y'}$ = 64.1 kN/mm). The short span of the flange (f_f = 0.914 cm) leads to a small $K_{Y'}/K_{X'}$ = 31.7. In this dynamometer, element S7 has the same dimensions as S5 and S6. Therefore, a force applied in the X direction in Fig. 3 is supported by elements S5 and S6 at about 3% each. The dynamometer, however, is uncoupled and linear as long as deflections of S5 and S6 remain small. The factor of safety for elements S5 and S6 is 1.35 for yield in the web under $F_{Y'}$ = 1.0 kN and $M_{Z'}$ = 60.0 Nm.

An optimal design for the elements S5 and S6 (Case Study 1) in Fig. 3 is given in Table 3. The allowable ranges of the design variables, **X**, are chosen so that the dynamometer can be manufactured. The optimal web thickness is unchanged from the Table 2 value, but the aspect ratio f_w/d is larger for the optimal design (0.43 instead of 0.36), and the flange is thinner and longer increasing $K_{Y'}/K_{X'}$. The element stiffness in the Y' direction is $K_{Y'}$ = 35.2 kN/mm. The active constraints are the yield strength of the web, the stiffness ratio $K_{Y'}/K_{X'}$ = 750, and the buckling loads of the web and flange. The minimum values of l and t_f are optimal. The sensitivity of the optimally designed SPE is 2.0 times the sensitivity in the existing elements S5 and S6. However, the optimally designed SPE has a decreased factor of safety (1.0) and is more difficult to manufacture because of the decreased thickness of the flange and the increased yield strength.

TABLE 2—*Analysis of elements S5 and S6 of the dynamometer in Fig. 3.*

<table>
<tr><td colspan="4">Load Applied to Dynamometer</td><td colspan="4">F_Y = 1.0 (kN)</td><td colspan="4">M_Z = 60 (Nm)</td></tr>
<tr><td colspan="4">Load Applied to S5 and S6</td><td colspan="4">P = 1.03 (kN)</td><td colspan="4">$\frac{P}{2}$ = 0.516 (kN)</td></tr>
<tr><td colspan="3">Material Properties</td><td colspan="3">E = 207 (GPa)</td><td colspan="3">ν = 0.3</td><td colspan="3">S_y = 0.6895 (GPa)</td></tr>
<tr><td rowspan="5">Analysis</td><td>l (cm)</td><td>d (cm)</td><td>f_w (cm)</td><td>f_f (cm)</td><td>t_w (cm)</td><td>t_f (cm)</td><td>l - w (cm)</td><td>$K_{Y'}$ (kN/mm)</td><td>$\frac{K_{Y'}}{K_{Z'}}$</td><td>$\frac{K_{Y'}}{K_{X'}}$</td><td>$\frac{K_{Y'}\,l}{K_t}$</td></tr>
<tr><td>5.639</td><td>2.54</td><td>0.914</td><td>0.914</td><td>0.041</td><td>0.041</td><td>4.72</td><td>64.1</td><td>442</td><td>31.7</td><td>4.46×10^6</td></tr>
<tr><td colspan="6">$\bar{L}_w$ = 4.99 (kN)</td><td colspan="5">$\bar{L}_f$ = 19.455 (kN)</td></tr>
<tr><td colspan="6">$\bar{\sigma}_w$ = 0.511 (GPa)</td><td colspan="5">$\bar{\sigma}_f$ = 0.225 (GPa)</td></tr>
<tr><td colspan="11">$\bar{e}_w$ = 792 μ</td></tr>
</table>

TABLE 3—*Case Study 1. Optimal design of elements S5 and S6 of the dynamometer in Fig. 3.*

Load Applied to Dynamometer				$F_{Y'} = 1.0$ (kN)					$M_{Z'} = 60$ (Nm)		
Material Properties			E = 207 (GPa)				$\nu = 0.3$			$S_y = 1.034$ (GPa)	
Design Limits	l (cm)	d (cm)	f_w (cm)	f_f (cm)	t_w (cm)	t_f (cm)	$l - w$ (cm)	$K_{Y'}$ (kN/mm)	$\frac{K_{Y'}}{K_{Z'}}$	$\frac{K_{Y'}}{K_{X'}}$	$\frac{K_{Y'}\,l}{K_t}$
Maximum	6.00	4.00	4.50	3.50	0.635	0.635	-	-	-	-	-
Minimum	1.5	1.27	0.635	0.635	0.033	0.033	0.00	0.175	750	750	750
Optimal Design	1.5	3.22	1.38	2.82	0.041	0.033	0.120	35.2	756	750	1956
	Load Applied to Each SPE					$P = 2.49$ (kN)				$\frac{P}{2} = 1.25$ (kN)	
			$\bar{L}_w = 2.50$ (kN)					$\bar{L}_f = 1.28$ (kN)			
			$\bar{\sigma}_w = 1.034$ (GPa)					$\bar{\sigma}_f = 0.642$ (GPa)			
						$\bar{e}_w = 1627\ \mu$					

Tables 4 through 7 show the results for different case studies. In Case Study 2, the load is $F_{Y'} = 2.0$ kN and $M_{Z'} = 120$ Nm, two times the Table 3 values. A minimum $l - w = 0.67$ cm is specified, but otherwise the design limits and material are those in Case Study 1. The same constraints are encountered with the addition that the $l - w$ equals its assigned minimum 0.67 cm. None of the other design variables reached its limit. The optimal aspect ratio in the web is again 0.43, which leads to the same shear strain under maximum load.

The load in Case Study 3 shown in Table 5 is four times that in Case Study 1, 4.0 kN and 240 Nm. The maximum values of the design parameters were increased, and the same material was used. The same constraints as in Case Study 3 are active. The optimal aspect ratio for the web is again 0.43.

Case Study 4 in Table 6 has the same loading and design limits as in Case 1, but the yield strength of the material is decreased. The active constraints are yield of the web, buckling of the web and flange, and $K_{Y'}/K_{X'} = 750$. The design variable t_f is at its limit. The optimal aspect ratio for the web is again 0.43. The yielding constraint of the web drives the optimal aspect ratio of the web to 0.43.

Case Study 5 in Table 7 has one tenth the load of Case Study 1. The lower limits on **X** have been relaxed because of the small load. The active constraints are $K_{Y'}/K_{Z'} = 750$ and $K_{Y'}/K_{X'} = 750$. The minimum limits of t_w and t_f have been reached as well as the maximum value of f_f. The yielding constraint of the web is not active, giving an optimal aspect ratio of 0.71.

Discussion

All information needed to design an SPE pair that meets constraints of Eq 14 is contained in Eqs 1 and 5 through 9, and Table 1. If this calculation is not implemented through an

TABLE 4—*Case Study 2. Optimal design with the design limits, constraints, and material properties of Case Study 1 with two times the applied load.*

Load Applied to Dynamometer				$F_{Y'}$ = 2.0 (kN)					$M_{Z'}$ = 120 (Nm)		
Material Properties			E = 207 (GPa)			ν = 0.3			S_y = 1.034 (GPa)		
Design Limits	l (cm)	d (cm)	f_w (cm)	f_f (cm)	t_w (cm)	t_f (cm)	l - w (cm)	$K_{Y'}$ (kN/mm)	$\frac{K_{Y'}}{K_{Z'}}$	$\frac{K_{Y'}}{K_{X'}}$	$\frac{K_{Y'}\,l}{K_t}$
Maximum	6.00	4.00	4.50	3.50	0.635	0.635	-	-	-	-	-
Minimum	1.5	1.27	0.635	0.635	0.033	0.033	0.670	0.175	750	750	750
Optimal Design	2.33	3.86	1.660	3.261	0.049	0.038	0.670	42.5	761	750	3326
	Load Applied to Each SPE				P = 3.57 (kN)				$\frac{P}{2}$ = 1.79 (kN)		
	$\overline{L}_w$ = 3.57 (kN)						$\overline{L}_f$ = 1.79 (kN)				
	$\overline{\sigma}_w$ = 1.034 (GPa)						$\overline{\sigma}_f$ = 0.656 (GPa)				
	$\overline{e}_w$ = 1627 μ										

TABLE 5—*Case Study 3. Optimal design with the constraints and material properties of Case Study 1 with four times the applied load. The maximum design limits have been increased.*

Load Applied to Dynamometer				$F_{Y'}$ = 4.0 (kN)					$M_{Z'}$ = 240 (Nm)		
Material Properties			E = 207 (GPa)			ν = 0.3			S_y = 1.034 (GPa)		
Design Limits	l (cm)	d (cm)	f_w (cm)	f_f (cm)	t_w (cm)	t_f (cm)	l - w (cm)	$K_{Y'}$ (kN/mm)	$\frac{K_{Y'}}{K_{Z'}}$	$\frac{K_{Y'}}{K_{X'}}$	$\frac{K_{Y'}\,l}{K_t}$
Maximum	6.00	4.45	5.08	3.81	0.635	0.635	-	-	-	-	-
Minimum	1.5	1.27	0.635	0.635	0.033	0.033	0.670	0.175	750	750	750
Optimal Design	4.57	4.39	1.889	3.713	0.056	0.044	2.681	48.3	761	750	9853
	Load Applied to Each SPE				P = 4.63 (kN)				$\frac{P}{2}$ = 2.31 (kN)		
	$\overline{L}_w$ = 4.63 (kN)						$\overline{L}_f$ = 2.31 (kN)				
	$\overline{\sigma}_w$ = 1.034 (GPa)						$\overline{\sigma}_f$ = 0.655 (GPa)				
	$\overline{e}_w$ = 1627 μ										

TABLE 6—*Case Study 4. Optimal design with the design limits, constraints, and applied load of Case Study 1 with decreased yield strength.*

Load Applied to Dynamometer				$F_{Y'} = 1.0$ (kN)				$M_{Z'} = 60$ (Nm)			
Material Properties			$E = 207$ (GPa)				$\nu = 0.3$		$S_y = 0.861$ (GPa)		
Design Limits	l (cm)	d (cm)	f_w (cm)	f_f (cm)	t_w (cm)	t_f (cm)	$l - w$ (cm)	$K_{Y'}$ (kN/mm)	$\frac{K_{Y'}}{K_{Z'}}$	$\frac{K_{Y'}}{K_{X'}}$	$\frac{K_{Y'} l}{K_t}$
Maximum	6.00	4.00	4.50	3.50	0.635	0.635	-	-	-	-	-
Minimum	1.5	1.27	0.635	0.635	0.033	0.033	0.00	0.175	750	750	750
Optimal Design	1.76	3.48	1.50	2.91	0.040	0.033	0.264	35.9	940	750	7865
	Load Applied to Each SPE				$P = 2.21$ (kN)				$\frac{P}{2} = 1.10$ (kN)		
			$\overline{L}_w = 2.21$ (kN)					$\overline{L}_f = 1.35$ (kN)			
			$\overline{\sigma}_w = 0.861$ (GPa)					$\overline{\sigma}_f = 0.512$ (GPa)			
					$\overline{e}_w = 1356\ \mu$						

TABLE 7—*Case Study 5. Optimal design with the constraints and material properties of Case Study 1 with one tenth the applied load. The minimum design limits have been decreased.*

Load Applied to Dynamometer				$F_{Y'} = 0.1$ (kN)				$M_{Z'} = 6.0$ (Nm)			
Material Properties			$E = 207$ (GPa)				$\nu = 0.3$		$S_y = 1.034$ (GPa)		
Design Limits	l (cm)	d (cm)	f_w (cm)	f_f (cm)	t_w (cm)	t_f (cm)	$l - w$ (cm)	$K_{Y'}$ (kN/mm)	$\frac{K_{Y'}}{K_{Z'}}$	$\frac{K_{Y'}}{K_{X'}}$	$\frac{K_{Y'} l}{K_t}$
Maximum	6.00	4.00	4.50	3.50	0.635	0.635	-	-	-	-	-
Minimum	0.635	0.635	0.635	0.635	0.033	0.033	0.635	0.175	750	750	750
Optimal Design	2.03	1.95	1.39	3.50	0.033	0.033	0.635	11.14	750	750	3530
	Load Applied to Each SPE				$P = 0.198$ (kN)				$\frac{P}{2} = 0.099$ (kN)		
			$\overline{L}_w = 0.713$ (kN)					$\overline{L}_f = 0.426$ (kN)			
			$\overline{\sigma}_w = 0.208$ (GPa)					$\overline{\sigma}_f = 0.118$ (GPa)			
					$\overline{e}_w = 294\ \mu$						

optimal design algorithm, several iterations will probably be necessary to achieve an optimal design. The Case Studies in Tables 2 through 7 may be useful for initiating the search. For example, if an SPE pair is to support a 5-kN force and 300-Nm moment, the optimal l, d, f_w, f_f, t_w, and t_f of Case Study 3 (Table 5) could be used to start the iteration process.

SPE configurations other than the pairs shown in Fig. 4 can also be designed by modifying the process. Elements that support only a force component and no moment component, such as S7 in Fig. 3, are designed by replacing Eq 1 with $P = F_{Y'}$. To design a four-element set, such as S1–S4 in Fig. 3, the design scheme is modified to include the loading from the second moment component (S1–S4 support F_Z, M_Y, and M_X).

Conclusions

1. The design and design analysis of a class of six-degree-of-freedom strain-gage dynamometers are described. These dynamometers have the advantage that they are linear and virtually uncoupled in all components. The size and configuration of the dynamometer are widely variable and often depend on the application. The sensitivities of the dynamometer in different loading directions are tunable within limits through design of the SPE.
2. An optimal design procedure is presented and illustrated in several case studies. The optimal design maximizes the shear strain at the strain gages in the center of the web subject to constraints imposed on the geometry, stiffnesses, yielding, and buckling of the SPE.

Acknowledgment

The authors thank the National Institutes of Health for the partial sponsorship of this research program and Salomon SA and Tyrolia for their continued support and interest.

References

[*1*] Asang, E., Grimm, C., Krexa, H., and Wittmann, G., "Ski-Telemetrie," IAS Scientific Report, 1974.

[*2*] Mote, C. D., Jr. and Hull, M. L., "Laboratory and Field Research on Ski Bindings," in *Skiing Safety II*, J. M. Figueras, Ed., International Series in Sports Sciences, Vol. 5, University Park Press, Baltimore, 1978, pp. 244–270.

[*3*] Kuo, C. Y., Louie, J. K., and Mote, C. D., Jr., "Control of Torsion and Bending of the Lower Extremity During Skiing," in *Skiing Trauma and Safety: Fifth International Symposium, ASTM STP 860*, R. J. Johnson and C. D. Mote, Jr., Eds., American Society for Testing and Materials, Philadelphia, 1985, pp. 91–110.

[*4*] Lieu, D. K. and Mote, C. D., Jr., "An Electronic Ski Binding Design with Biofeedback," *Journal of Mechanical Design*, Vol. 102, 1980, pp. 677–682.

[*5*] Wunderly, G. and Hull, M. L., "A New Electromechanical Binding/Dynamometer for Actively Controlled Snow Ski Binding Systems," in *Skiing Trauma and Safety: Sixth International Symposium, ASTM STP 938*, C. D. Mote, Jr. and R. J. Johnson, Eds., American Society for Testing and Materials, Philadelphia, 1987, pp. 249–259.

[*6*] Wunderly, G. S., Hull, M. L., and Maxwell, S., "A Second Generation Microcomputer Controlled Binding System for Alpine Skiing Research," *Journal of Biomechanics*, Vol. 21, No. 4, 1988, pp. 299–318.

[*7*] Beckwith, T. G., Buck, N. L., and Maragoni, R. D., *Mechanical Measurements*, Addison Wesley, Reading, 1982, pp. 427–428.

[*8*] Ono, K. and Hatamura, Y., "A New Design for 6-Component Force/Torque Sensors," in *Mechanical Problems in Measuring Force and Mass*, H. Wieringa, Ed., Martinus Nijhoff, Dordrecht, 1986, pp. 39–48.

[*9*] Chaplin, ..., Lueders, M., and Zhao, Y., "Three-Point Hitch Dynamometer Design and Calibration," *Applied Engineering in Agriculture*, Vol. 3, No. 1, 1987, pp. 10–13.

[*10*] Watson, P. C. and Drake, S. H., "Method and Apparatus for Six Degree of Freedom Force Sensing," U. S. Patent No. 4 094 192, 13 June 1978.
[*11*] Molland, A. F., "A Five-Component Strain Gauge Wind Tunnel Dynamometer," *Strain*, Vol. 14, No. 1, 1978, pp. 7–13.
[*12*] Goodwin, R. J., "An Extended Octagonal Ring Transducer for Use in Tillage Studies," *Journal of Agricultural Engineering Research*, Vol. 20, 1975, pp. 347–352.
[*13*] Millward, A. and Rossiter, J., "The Design of a Multi-Purpose Multi-Component Strain Gauge Dynamometer," *Strain*, Vol. 19, 1983, pp. 27–30.
[*14*] Regan, K. and Reuber, M., "3-D Force-Sensing Robot Hand," in *Proceedings of the 1985 ASME International Computers in Engineering Conference and Exhibition*, R. Raghavan and S. M. Rohde, Eds., Vol. 1, ASME, New York, 1985, pp. 165–167.
[*15*] Girard, D., "Development of Multicomponent Force Transfer Standards by ONERA for French BNM," in *Mechanical Problems in Measuring Force and Mass*, H. Wieringa, Ed., Martinus Nijhoff, Dordrecht, 1986, pp. 1–12.
[*16*] Reuber, M., Kornegay, J., Melehy, W., and Panjabi, C., "Symbolic Processing as an Aid to the Solution of Inverse Design Problems: Applications," in *Proceedings of Second International Conference on Inverse Design Concepts and Optimization in Engineering Science*, G. S. Dulikravich, Ed., 1987.
[*17*] Hou, J. W. and Twu, S. L., "Optimum Design of Internal Strain Gage Balances: An Example of Three-Dimensional Shape Optimization," *Journal of Mechanisms, Transmissions, and Automation in Design*, Vol. 109, June, 1987, pp. 257–262.
[*18*] Lin, C.-T. and Beadle, C. W., "The Optimal Design of Force Transducers Which Are Cross-Axis Sensitive," in *Sensors and Controls for Automated Manufacturing and Robotics*, K. A. Stelson and L. M. Sweet, Eds., ASME, New York, 1984, pp. 179–191.
[*19*] Sinden, F. W. and Boie, R. A., "A Planar Capacitive Force Sensor with Six Degrees of Freedom," in *Proceedings of 1986 IEEE International Conference on Robotics and Automation*, Vol. 3, IEEE Computer Society Press, Washington, DC 1986, pp. 1806–1814.
[*20*] Levin, A. and Mote, C. D., Jr., "An Uncoupled Six Degree of Freedom Dynamometer," University of California, Department of Mechanical Engineering Report, 1983.
[*21*] Kuo, C. Y., Louie, J. K., and Mote, C. D., Jr., "Field Measurements in Snow Skiing Injury Research," *Journal of Biomechanics*, Vol. 16, No. 8, 1983, pp. 609–624.
[*22*] Reddy, J. N., *Applied Functional Analysis and Variational Methods in Engineering*, McGraw-Hill, New York, 1986, pp. 258–285.
[*23*] Timoshenko, S., "Mathematical Determination of the Modulus of Elasticity," *Mechanical Engineering*, Vol. 45, No. 4, April 1923, pp. 259–260.
[*24*] Timoshenko, S. P. and Goodier, J. N., *Theory of Elasticity*, McGraw-Hill, New York, 1970, pp. 309–313.
[*25*] Timoshenko, S. P. and Gere, J. M., *Theory of Elastic Stability*, McGraw-Hill, New York, 1961, pp. 348–351.
[*26*] Gill, P. E., Murray, W., and Wright, M. H., *Practical Optimization*, Academic Press, London, 1981, pp. 225–233.
[*27*] Dally, J. W. and Riley, W. F., *Experimental Stress Analysis*, McGraw-Hill, New York, 1978, pp. 251–253.
[*28*] Woinowsky-Krieger, S., "Uber die Beulsicherheit von Reckteckplatten mnit querverschieblichen Rändern," *Ingenieur-Archiv*, Vol. 19, 1951, pp. 200–207.

Markku Järvinen[1] *and Pekka Kannus*[2]

Conservative Treatment of Acute Knee Ligament Injuries—Long-Term Results

REFERENCE: Järvinen, M. and Kannus, P., "**Conservative Treatment of Acute Knee Ligament Injuries—Long-Term Results,**" *Skiing Trauma and Safety: Eighth International Symposium, ASTM STP 1104*, C. D. Mote, Jr. and Robert J. Johnson, Eds., American Society for Testing and Materials, Philadelphia, 1991, pp. 112–121.

ABSTRACT: A total of 221 patients were treated conservatively for acute knee ligament injuries at the Tampere University Central Hospital in Finland between 1975 and 1981. Ninety-eight patients had an acute tear of the anterior cruciate ligament (ACL), alone (37) or in combination with the medial collateral ligament (MCL) (61). Ninety-six had an isolated MCL injury, and 27 had an isolated injury of the lateral ligament compartment (LAT) of the knee.

The patients were immobilized in plaster cast, posterior splint, or knee bandage, and no attempts were made to correct ligamentous instability. The patients started isometric exercises of the quadriceps and hamstrings during the first one to two weeks of the immobilization period. Straight leg raises were usually instituted within the first two to four weeks. Walking with crutches with partial weight-bearing was allowed approximately one to two weeks after injury, and full weight-bearing was allowed after two to five weeks. Increasing mobilization and rehabilitation of the injured knee was usually begun immediately after the immobilization period, and the rehabilitation continued under supervision of the attending surgeon for at least six months.

The follow-up study of the patients (average, eight years after the injury; range four to twelve years) included a questionnaire; clinical examination; functional tests; radiological examination; knee strength measurements by a isokinetic testing device; the Lysholm and Marshall scales for subjective, clinical, and functional evaluations; and the authors' scales for radiological and muscle strength evaluations.

The multidimensional follow-up analysis revealed that the long-term outcome after a Grade II sprain (partial tear) of the ACL, MCL, or LAT was good and acceptable even if residual mild or moderate laxity was often demonstrable. In Grade III sprains (complete tears), the long-term results were poor, involving an unstable knee with thigh muscle weakness, post-traumatic osteoarthritis, and severe subjective symptoms.

KEY WORDS: skiing injuries, knee ligament injuries, anterior cruciate ligament, medial collateral ligament, lateral ligament compartment, surveys

Knee injuries are relatively frequent in skiing. Although the incidence of skiing injuries in general has decreased during the last two decades, the corresponding decrease has not been found in knee ligament injuries sustained in skiing [*1*]. Knee ligament injuries in skiing are most often associated with downhill skiing; cross-country skiing is regarded to be a relatively safe sport [*2–5*].

Analysis of knee ligament injuries treated operatively at Tampere University Central Hospital in Finland between 1975 and 1981 showed that half of the injuries occurred in sports activities and half of these were sustained in cross-country skiing (Fig. 1 and Table

[1]Chief Surgeon, Division of Orthopaedics, Department of Surgery, University Central Hospital of Tampere, 33520 Tampere, Finland.

[2]Resident physician, Tampere Research Station of Sports Medicine, Kaupinpuistonkatu 1, SF-33500 Tampere, Finland.

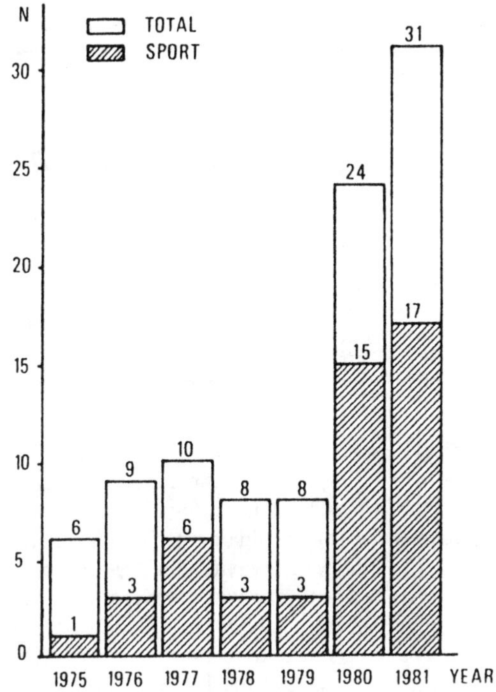

FIG. 1—*Distribution of the patients operated on because of acute knee ligament injury according to year of operation and the role of sports as a cause of the injury (reprinted with permission from Ref* 6).

1) [*6,7*]. Because of a relatively small number of patients treated operatively in the first few years of the observation period, we decided to analyze all the patients treated nonsurgically during the years 1975 to 1981 [*8–11*].

Patients and Methods

Patients

A total of 221 patients, who were treated conservatively for acute knee ligament injuries at Tampere University Central Hospital during the years 1975 to 1981 and who met all the inclusion criteria of the study, were accepted to the follow-up investigation. The initial entrance criteria of the study were that the injured structure was the anterior cruciate ligament (ACL) (alone or in combination with the medial collateral ligament [MCL]), MCL (alone), or lateral ligament compartment (LAT) (alone); no previous knee injuries, knee operations, or general illnesses; and no simultaneous fractures of the injured knee (simultaneous meniscus tears were accepted).

In addition, all patients had to have a positive clinical diagnosis at the initial clinical examination after the injury, that is, all the examining physicians confirmed the same positive diagnosis, and further examinations (ordinary or stress radiographs, arthrography, examination under anesthesia, arthroscopy, arthrotomy) had no discrepancy with, but possibly confirmed the initial clinical diagnosis. In the great majority of the included patients, the clinical diagnosis was confirmed (and other injuries were excluded) by examination under anesthesia, arthrotomy, arthroscopy, or a combination of these modalities.

TABLE 1—*Distribution of patients treated operatively according to cause of sports injury. Competitive athletes are indicated in parentheses.*

Cross-country skiing	23 (2)
Soccer	8 (6)
Volleyball	4
Ice hockey	3 (2)
Track and field sports	2 (2)
Motor sport	2 (2)
Boxing	1 (1)
Cycling	1
Gymnastics	1
Slalom skiing	1
Weight lifting	1 (1)
Wrestling	1 (1)
TOTAL	48 (17)

The American Medical Association classification system of injuries to the knee ligaments was used. Only Grade II or III injuries were included in this study. A Grade II injury was a moderate acute knee distortion leading to local tenderness and swelling and moderate disability caused by partial tear of the ligament. In clinical stress tests, the knee showed mild (1+) to moderate (2+) abnormal laxity, but a hard end point when compared with the uninjured knee. A Grade III injury was a severe knee distortion leading to marked tenderness and swelling and severe disability as a result of a complete tear of the ligament in question. In clinical stress tests, the knee showed severe (3+) abnormal laxity with soft end point when compared with the uninjured knee.

According to these criteria, 98 patients had an acute tear of the ACL, alone (37) or in combination with the MCL (61). Ninety-six had an isolated MCL injury, and 27 had an isolated injury of the LAT of the knee. The Grade II and III ratios were in ACL injuries 44/54 (in isolated ACL injuries 14/23 and in combined ACL and MCL injuries 30/31, respectively), in isolated MCL injuries 65/31, and in isolated LAT injuries 13/14.

Table 2 lists the general initial characteristics of the patients. Ninety-nine patients (45%), sustained their injury in sport, and 20 (21%) of these were skiing injuries.

Treatment

In the primary treatment, no attempts were made to correct ligament instability. The great majority of the arthrotomies performed were undertaken on suspicion of accompanying meniscus rupture or intra-articular loose body. Only in some cases were procedures other than arthrotomy actually performed because the menisci were intact or no loose bodies were found. Of the ACL injuries, there were eleven medial, two lateral, and one bilateral primary meniscectomies. Of the MCL injuries, there were twelve medial and three lateral meniscectomies, and three removals of loose bodies. Among the LAT injuries, there were two lateral meniscectomies.

All patients were immobilized in plaster cast, posterior splint, or knee bandage. The median time of immobilization was in the ACL and MCL groups in Grade II sprains four weeks (range one to seven weeks) and in Grade III sprains five weeks (two to eight weeks) and in the LAT injuries three weeks (two to five weeks) and four weeks (two to seven weeks), respectively.

The patients started isometric exercises of the quadriceps and hamstrings during the first one to two weeks of the immobilization period. Straight leg raises were usually instituted within the first two to four weeks. Walking with crutches with partial weight-bearing was

TABLE 2—*Initial characteristics of the basic populations of the long-term follow-up after conservative treatment of acute knee ligament injuries.*

	ACL (N = 98)	MCL (N = 96)	LAT (N = 27)
Age[a] years	32 ± 13	36 ± 15	34 ± 17
Sex			
Men	71	46	12
Women	27	50	15
Injured knee			
Right	44	57	5
Left	54	39	22
Accident			
Sports	47	38	14
Work	22	22	4
Traffic	16	12	4
Home, leisure, etc.	13	24	5

[a]Mean ± standard deviation.

ACL = anterior cruciate ligament; MCL = medial collateral ligament; LAT = lateral compartment of the knee.

allowed approximately one to two weeks after injury, and full weight-bearing was allowed after two to five weeks. Increasing mobilization and rehabilitation of the injured knee was usually begun immediately after the immobilization period, and the rehabilitation continued under supervision of the attending surgeon for at least six months.

Follow-up

The patients were reviewed at an average of 8 years (range four to twelve years) after their injury. The follow-up examination consisted of a questionnaire, a clinical examination with functional tests, a radiological evaluation, and muscle strength measurements. In all measurements, the opposite knee served as a control.

The results were evaluated using four different scales: Lysholm and Marshall scales for subjective, functional, and clinical evaluation and the authors' scales for radiological [*12*] and isokinetic and isometric strength evaluation [*13*].

Results

Grade II Sprains

The follow-up scores of patients with Grade II sprains were excellent or good (Table 3). None of these patients required an operation because of chronic ligament insufficiency during the follow-up period. Three medial and one lateral meniscectomies were the only operative procedures undertaken during the follow-up.

At the time of review, all 54 patients with Grade II MCL injury, 82% of patients with LAT injury, and 66% of patients with ACL injury reported that their physical activity was still at least at the preinjury level. Three patients in the ACL group had to change occupation because of the knee, but in the other groups no changes were observed.

At the clinical follow-up examination, the most usual pathological finding was persistent mild to moderate laxity of the injured knee (Tables 4 and 5). However, gross one-plane

TABLE 3—*Follow-up scores of patients having Grade II sprain of the anterior cruciate ligament, medial collateral ligament, or lateral compartment. E = excellent, G = good, F = fair, P = poor.*

Scale		ACL (N = 41)	MCL (N = 54)	LAT (N = 11)
Lysholm	median (range)	90 (17–100) (G)	94 (62–100) (E)	88 (62–100) (G)
Marshall	median (range)	42 (20–49) (G)	45 (35–50) (G)	41 (32–46) (G)
Radiological	median (range)	98 (73–100) (G)	99 (92–100) (G)	98 (94–100) (G)
Strength	median (range)	90 (22–100) (E)	94 (68–100) (E)	94 (68–100) (E)

(≥16-mm separation of joint surfaces in clinical stress tests with soft end point) or rotatory (severe tibial subluxation in relation to femur without spontaneous reduction) laxities occurred in only three cases.

The median (range) relative extension and flexion deficits of strength in the injured thigh were in the ACL group 3 (0 to 46%) and 1% (0 to 44%); in the MCL group 2 (0 to 28%) and 0% (0 to 20%); and in the LAT group 1 (0 to 21%) and 0% (0 to 4%), respectively. The median quadriceps muscle atrophy in the same groups, measured as a difference in the circumferences of the thighs 15 cm proximal of the medial joint line, was minimal: in the ACL group 0.5 cm (0 to 2.0 cm), MCL group 0 cm (0 to 1.5 cm), and LAT group 0 cm (0 to 1.5 cm).

Grade III Sprains

The follow-up scores of patients with Grade III sprains were in sharp contrast to those of patients with Grade II sprains, and the final results were mostly poor (71%) or fair (15%) (Table 6). During the follow-up, 9 of the 49 patients in the ACL group had undergone ACL reconstruction because of persisting instability and giving-way symptoms. For the same reasons, at follow-up, 8 additional patients in this ACL group had decided to have a reconstruction operation of the ACL. These 8 operations were performed within 6 months after the follow-up examinations. No patient in the MCL or LAT groups required a reconstruction of knee ligaments.

The second most common operation during the follow-up was meniscectomy (in the ACL group eight medial and one lateral, MCL group three medial, and LAT group two lateral).

The physical activity of the patients was clearly reduced due to the injured knee (in the ACL group in 80%, in the MCL group in 63%, and in the LAT group in 75% of the patients). The numbers of occupational changes for the same reason were 25, 22, and 17% of the patients, respectively. Partial or total pensions were eventually granted to 18 and 10% of patients in the ACL group, 22 and 4% in the MCL group, and 17 and 0% in the LAT group, respectively.

Injuries to the opposite knee occurred in only three patients during the follow-up, but later injuries to the index knee were frequent. During the follow-up, 38% of the patients in the ACL group, 22% in the MCL group, and 25% in the LAT group suffered several (at least three) distortions of the injured knee. The majority of subsequent injuries were mild or moderate and were treated conservatively.

At the clinical follow-up examination, the most frequent pathological finding was persistent abnormal laxity of the injured knee. The amounts and directions of the follow-up laxities are summarized in Tables 7 and 8.

TABLE 4—*Distribution of patients having Grade II sprain of the anterior cruciate ligament, medial collateral ligament, or lateral compartment according to the gradation of one-plane follow-up laxities of the injured knee.*

	ACL (N = 41)					MCL (N = 54)					LAT (N = 11)				
Laxity	0	1+	2+	3+	4+	0	1+	2+	3+	4+	0	1+	2+	3+	4+
Anterior	2	7	12	18	2	29	12	9	4	0	4	2	2	3	0
Medial	9	7	12	13	0	5	13	25	11	0	8	1	1	1	0
Lateral	37	1	1	2	0	54	0	0	0	0	0	2	5	4	0
Posterior	39	1	0	1	0	53	1	0	0	0	10	1	0	0	0

Laxity gradation:
0 = No laxity
1+ = Mild laxity (1–5 mm)
2+ = Moderate laxity (6–10 mm)
3+ = Severe laxity with hard end point (11–15 mm)
4+ = Gross laxity with soft end point (≥16 mm)

TABLE 5—*Distribution of patients having Grade II sprain of the anterior cruciate ligament, medial collateral ligament, or lateral compartment according to the gradation of rotatory follow-up laxities of the injured knee.*

	ACL (N = 41)				MCL (N = 54)				LAT (N = 11)			
Laxity	0	1+	2+	3+	0	1+	2+	3+	0	1+	2+	3+
Anteromedial	4	19	16	2	14	24	16	0	6	3	1	1
Anterolateral	13	21	5	2	42	10	2	0	4	5	2	0
Posterolateral	40	1	0	0	54	0	0	0	5	6	0	0

Laxity gradation:
0 = No rotatory laxity
1+ = Mild rotatory laxity
2+ = Moderate rotatory laxity
3+ = Severe or gross rotatory laxity

According to the strength analysis, the median (range) relative extension and flexion deficits of strength in the injured knee were 17% (0 to 80%) and 14 (0 to 60%) in the ACL group; 21 (0 to 82%) and 16% (0 to 67%) in the MCL group; and 22 (0 to 70%) and 12% (0 to 52%) in the LAT group, respectively. The median quadriceps muscle atrophy in the same groups was 1.5 (0 to 4.0 cm), 1.5 (0 to 3.0 cm), and 1.0 cm (0 to 3.0 cm), respectively.

Discussion

Multidimensional analysis with the aid of the standardized knee scoring scales showed great similarity in all our present studies involving the long-term results of conservatively treated Grade II and III sprains of the knee ligaments. In Grade II sprains, the follow-up scores were mainly good and acceptable in every type of injury studied. Conversely, the conservative treatment in Grade III sprains was in every aspect clearly poorer, leading in a great number of cases not only to chronic, symptomatic instability, but also to post-traumatic osteoarthritis. In addition, many of these patients suffered from moderate or severe strength deficit and a significant number of reinjuries to the index knee.

One of the most common follow-up findings was the persistent laxity of the injured knee when compared to the opposite knee. We should, however, keep in mind that because diagnostic problems always exist in acute-phase examination, the weight of these retrospective findings as evidence for definitive conclusions is limited.

However, conservative therapy in Grade II sprains seems acceptable and seems to be the method of choice if it is accepted that residual 1+ to 3+ abnormal laxity is often demon-

TABLE 6—*Follow-up scores of patients having Grade III sprain of anterior cruciate ligament, medial collateral ligament, or lateral compartment. E = excellent, G = good, F = fair, P = poor.*

Scale		ACL (N = 40)	MCL (N = 27)	LAT (N = 12)
Lysholm	median (range)	60 (7–95) (F)	66 (25–100) (F)	64 (32–100) (F)
Marshall	median (range)	26 (14–39) (P)	26 (16–44) (P)	28 (19–42) (P)
Radiological	median (range)	85 (48–99) (P)	86 (57–100) (P)	90 (59–100) (F)
Strength	median (range)	64 (9–100) (F)	56 (20–98) (F)	58 (10–100) (F)

TABLE 7—*Distribution of patients having Grade III sprain of the anterior cruciate ligament, medial collateral ligament, or lateral compartment according to the gradation of one-plane follow-up laxities of the injured knee.*

	ACL (N = 40)					MCL (N = 27)					LAT (N = 12)				
Laxity	0	1+	2+	3+	4+	0	1+	2+	3+	4+	0	1+	2+	3+	4+
Anterior	0	0	3	11	26	0	3	8	8	8	0	1	2	5	4
Medial	2	3	3	24	8	0	0	2	12	13	6	1	5	0	0
Lateral	24	3	5	6	2	21	4	2	0	0	0	0	1	8	3
Posterior	35	2	1	2	0	25	1	1	0	0	11	1	0	0	0

Laxity gradation:
0 = No laxity
1+ = Mild laxity (1–5 mm)
2+ = Moderate laxity (6–10 mm)
3+ = Severe laxity with hard end point (11–15 mm)
4+ = Gross laxity with soft end point (≥16 mm)

TABLE 8—*Distribution of patients having Grade III sprain of the anterior cruciate ligament, medial collateral ligament, or lateral compartment according to the gradation of rotatory follow-up laxities of the injured knee.*

	ACL (N = 40)				MCL (N = 27)				LAT (N = 12)			
Laxity	0	1+	2+	3+	0	1+	2+	3+	0	1+	2+	3+
Anteromedial	1	6	9	24	0	1	13	13	6	2	2	2
Anterolateral	4	8	13	15	10	7	4	6	1	3	3	5
Posterolateral	37	3	0	0	26	1	1	0	4	5	3	0

Laxity gradation:
0 = No rotatory laxity
1+ = Mild rotatory laxity
2+ = Moderate rotatory laxity
3+ = Severe or gross rotatory laxity

strable years after the injury. The critical point may be between 3+ and 4+ laxity. Only the latter laxity is gross enough to cause symptomatic rotatory subluxations of the tibia in relation to femur during activity. With sufficient muscular performance, knees with Grade II sprain of the ACL, MCL, or LAT seem to remain functionally stable and almost asymptomatic.

It has been suggested that mild medial abnormal laxity is more important than mild or moderate sagittal abnormal laxity as regards to symptoms. In contrast with this conception, the subjective and functional outcome of patients with Grade II MCL injury as slightly better than cases with Grade II ACL injury. The apparent reason for this discrepancy was that in this study the knees with Grade II MCL injury had much fewer 3+ or 4+ abnormal laxities than the knees with Grade II ACL injury (Tables 4 and 5).

In Grade III sprains, the muscle function is not normally sufficient to compensate the complete loss of integrity of a particular knee ligament. Only in top level athletes with extremely high muscular performance has an ACL insufficiency been reported to be amenable to masking by muscles, and also in our material there was one Olympic gold medal winner in cross country skiing with total loss of ACL but good function in the involved knee.

Thigh muscle atrophy after knee ligament injury may indirectly increase the dynamic knee instability and patellofemoral malalignment, which, in turn, may not only accelerate the osteoarthritic process but also cause ligamentous and meniscal lesions, and may—by discomfort and disuse of the knee—increase atrophy of the thigh musculature itself.

Thus, atrophy of the thigh muscles is not entirely an independent reason for prolonged dysfunction of the injured knee; in failures, it is always a question of a sum effect of the whole vicious circle. However, muscle atrophy is almost the only possible factor to be influenced nonoperatively.

In conclusion, in Grade II sprains of knee ligaments, early, intensive, and supervised rehabilitation of the injured knee seems to be an adequate primary method; Grade III sprains obviously call for an operative approach.

References

[*1*] Howe, J. and Johnson, R. J., "Knee Injuries in Skiing," *Clinics in Sports Medicine*, Vol. 1, 1982, pp. 277–288.

[*2*] Boyle, J. J., Johnson, R. J., Pope, M. H., Pierce, J. C., and Brady, M. M., "Cross-Country Skiing Injuries," in *Skiing Trauma and Safety: Fifth International Symposium, ASTM STP 860*, R. J.

Johnson and C. D. Mote, Jr., Eds., American Society for Testing and Materials, Philadelphia, 1985, pp. 411–422.

[3] Kannus, P., Niittymaki, S., and Jarvinen, M., "Cross-Country Skiing Injuries: Has the Change of Skiing Style Affected the Frequency and Types of Skiing Injuries Treated at an Outpatient Sports Clinic?" *Scandinavian Journal of Sports Science*, Vol. 10, 1988, pp. 17–21.

[4] Sandelin, J., Kiviluoto, O., and Santavirta, S., "Injuries of Competitive Skiers in Finland: A Three Year Survey," *Annales Chirurgiae et Gynaecologiae*, Vol. 69, 1980, pp. 97–101.

[5] Westlin, N. E., "Injuries in Long Distance, Cross Country and Downhill Skiing," *Orthopedic Clinics of North America*, Vol. 7, 1976, pp. 55–58.

[6] Jarvinen, M. and Kannus, P., "Clinical and Radiological Long-Term Results After Primary Knee Ligament Surgery," *Archives of Orthopaedic and Traumatic Surgery*, Vol. 104, 1985, pp. 1–6.

[7] Kannus, P. and Jarvinen, M., "Role of Sports in Etiology and Prognosis of Surgically Treated Acute Knee Ligament Injuries," *International Journal of Sports Medicine*, Vol. 7, 1986, pp. 39–43.

[8] Kannus, P., "Long-Term Results of Conservatively Treated Medial Collateral Ligament Injuries of the Knee Joint," *Clinical Orthopaedics and Related Research*, Vol. 226, 1988, pp. 103–112.

[9] Kannus, P., "Nonoperative Treatment of Grade II and III Sprains of the Lateral Ligament Compartment of the Knee," *American Journal of Sports Medicine*, Vol. 17, 1989, pp. 83–88.

[10] Kannus, P., "Conservative Treatment of Acute Knee Distortions—Long-Term Results and Their Evaluation Methods," *Acta Universitatis Tamperensis*, Ser. A, Vol. 250, 1988, pp. 1–110.

[11] Kannus, P. and Jarvinen, M., "Conservatively Treated Tears of the Anterior Cruciate Ligament. Long-Term Results," *Journal of Bone Joint Surgery. American Volume*. Vol. 69-A, 1987, pp. 1007–1012.

[12] Kannus, P., Jarvinen, M., and Paakkala, T., "A Radiological Knee Scoring Scale for Evaluation of Post-traumatic Osteoarthritis After Knee Ligament Injuries," *International Orthopaedics*, Vol. 12, 1988, pp. 291–297.

[13] Kannus, P., Jarvinen, M., and Latvala, K., "Knee Strength Evaluation. A Standardized Test Protocol and Scoring Scale for Isokinetic and Isometric Strength Measurement of the Knee Joint for Evaluation of Long-Term Healing Results of Various Knee Problems and Their Treatment Procedures," *Scandinavian Journal of Sports Science*, Vol. 9, 1987, pp. 9–13.

Skiing Injury Statistics

Laurence R. Young[1] *and Shirley M. Lee*[1]

Alpine Injury Pattern at Waterville Valley—1989 Update

REFERENCE: Young, L. R. and Lee, S. M., "**Alpine Injury Pattern at Waterville Valley—1989 Update,**" *Skiing Trauma and Safety: Eighth International Symposium, ASTM STP 1104*, C. D. Mote, Jr. and Robert J. Johnson, Eds., American Society for Testing and Materials, Philadelphia, 1991, pp. 125–132.

ABSTRACT: The 1988/1989 Waterville Valley, NH, injury patterns show a further decline in lower leg injuries and a trend toward a reduction in knee and thumb injuries. Advanced skiers are now far more likely to injure the upper body, especially shoulder, thumb, or head, than the lower body. The introduction of a high-speed quadruple lift at Waterville Valley in 1988/1989 was associated with only a modest increase in injury rate.

KEY WORDS: skiing, injuries, statistics, epidemiology, injury patterns

Ski patrol records of reported injuries at Waterville Valley (WV), New Hampshire, have been maintained and analyzed over the 25 years of full operation [*1–3*]. Uncontrolled factors such as reportability and diagnosis make it difficult to attach significance to the absolute level of injuries or the relative frequency [*4,5*]. However, the relatively constant reporting conditions and population at risk (monitored by periodic control studies) makes long-term longitudinal studies of this type valuable for detection of trends in injury patterns and influences of changes in equipment or operations. For example, we were able to verify the predicted reduction of lacerations of the face and head when ski brakes began to replace restraining leashes.

The 1988/1989 winter season saw the introduction of the first high-speed, base-to-summit four-person (quad) chairlift at WV. The increased time spent skiing after introduction of the quad lift was expected to contribute to a higher injury rate per skier day and to more skier fatigue, which could manifest itself in either a change in the type of injuries or a tendency for injuries to occur earlier in the day.

Methods

The injury data were gathered from reports on standard National Ski Areas Association accident forms, completed by a ski patroller or nurse shortly after the accident. Skiing-related accidents were included separately in this study. Skier days were reported by the Ticket Department, based on daily sales and estimates of number of season pass holders present. The personnel involved in reporting both accidents and attendance was the same from 1987 to 1989. Computer analyses of the data were conducted using MacIntosh Excel at the Massachusetts Institute of Technology (MIT) Man-Vehicle Laboratory. For the 1987/1988 season, before the quad lift, there were 838 injuries for 808 skiing cases based on

[1]Professor and student assistant, respectively, Man-Vehicle Laboratory, Massachusetts Institute of Technology, Room 37-219, Cambridge, MA 02139.

264 210 skier days. For the 1988/1989 season, there were 1047 injuries for 954 skiing cases based on 288 396 skier days. For both seasons, there was heavy reliance on artificial snow to supplement minimal natural snowfall.

Results

Overall Injury Rate

Despite the introduction of the high-speed quad chairlift and the observed but not quantified large increase in total number of descents, the injury rate increased only about 10 to 15%, depending on the metric used. All cases were up from 3.16 (per thousand skier days) in 1987/1988 to 3.37 in 1988/1989. Skiing cases were up from 3.06 to 3.31. Skiing injuries (including multiple injuries per case) were up from 3.17 to 3.63. The "all cases" injury rate was higher than for any year since 1981/1982 (Fig. 1). However, given the fluctuations in this rate over the last 25 years, it is premature to identify a definite effect of the increased exposure.

Time of Injuries

The distribution of time of day of injuries remained virtually unchanged, despite the introduction of the quad chairlift. The injuries were distributed almost uniformly between 1100 and 1600 h, with a mean time of 1236 (Fig. 2). (As previously reported, this distribution lags the skiing exposure by 1 to 2 h and supports the contribution of fatigue to injuries.) The distribution of arrival and departure times was not measured. However, the impression of ski area management was that many of the season pass holders left earlier in the day after introduction of the quad chairlift, or took a long break in the middle of the day. Sales of afternoon lift tickets were only 4% of the total ticket sales; this percentage barely increased in 1989 relative to the past season.

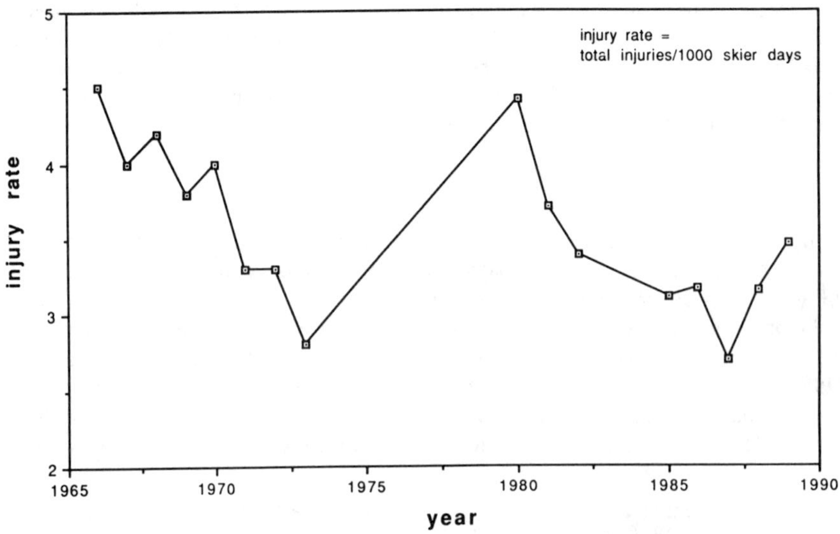

FIG. 1—*Ski injury rate.*

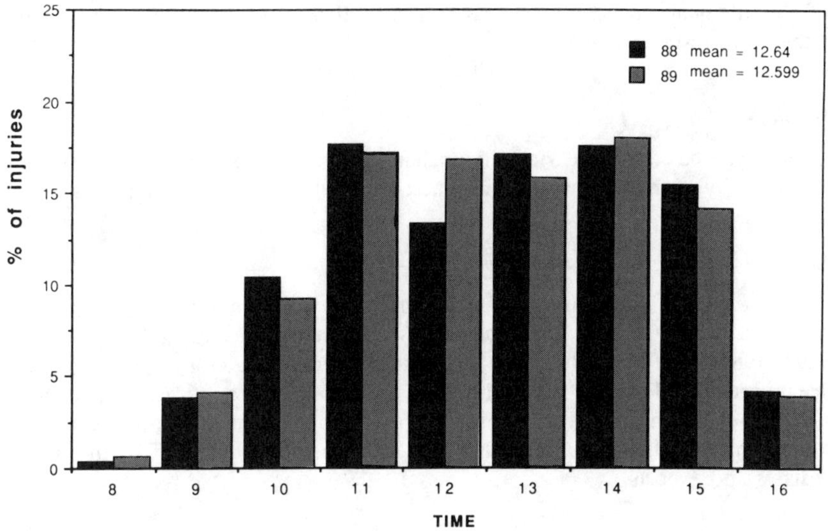

FIG. 2—*Comparison of ski injury rates in the 1987/1988 and 1988/1989 seasons.*

Relative Incidence of Injuries to Different Parts of the Body

The continued prominence of knee injuries is still noted and accounted for 25% of all injuries in the latest year, but there is a hint of slight decline in this rate since its high of 30% in 1985/1986. Thumb injuries have also declined somewhat over the past five years, from their high point of 17% in 1981/1982 to the current level of 10% (Fig. 3). Lower leg injuries continue the decline of the past fifteen years from 13%, and are now only 5% of

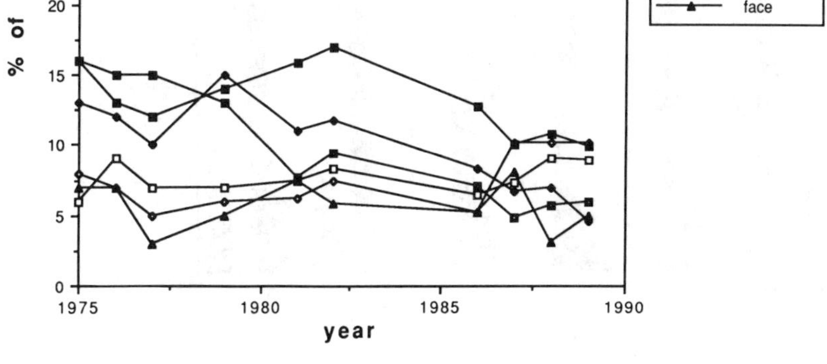

FIG. 3—*Comparison of injuries to different parts of the body.*

the total. Shoulder and head injuries have risen to 10% (up from 7%) and 9% (up from 6%) of the total, respectively.

Type of Injury

The injury type has remained virtually unchanged over the past eight years. Sprains and strains, principally of the knee and thumb, account for more than half the total (Fig. 4).

Distribution of Injured Body Part According to Ability

A consistent variation in injury pattern is seen with reported ability, as illustrated by the comparisons in Figs. 5, 6, and 7 (for beginners, intermediates, and experts, respectively) for the 1987/1988 and 1988/1989 seasons, and summarized in Fig. 8 for the 1988/1989 season. The knee injuries that dominate the beginner pool (38 to 42%) drop successively with ability, to only 22% of expert injuries. The difference is made up in upper body injuries, particularly shoulder, thumb, and head injuries, which account for roughly 60% of all the injuries to intermediates and experts.

Binding Release

One or both ski bindings released in the fall associated with the accident in 54% of the cases. (Records did not indicate whether the binding that released was on the same side of the body as the injury, nor whether the binding released before or after the injury occurred.) The binding released in 56% of the intermediate and expert group injuries but only in 47% of the beginner injuries. For lower extremity injuries (ankle, lower leg, knee), the binding released in 49% of the cases; whereas for upper body and thigh injuries, the binding released 62% of the time.

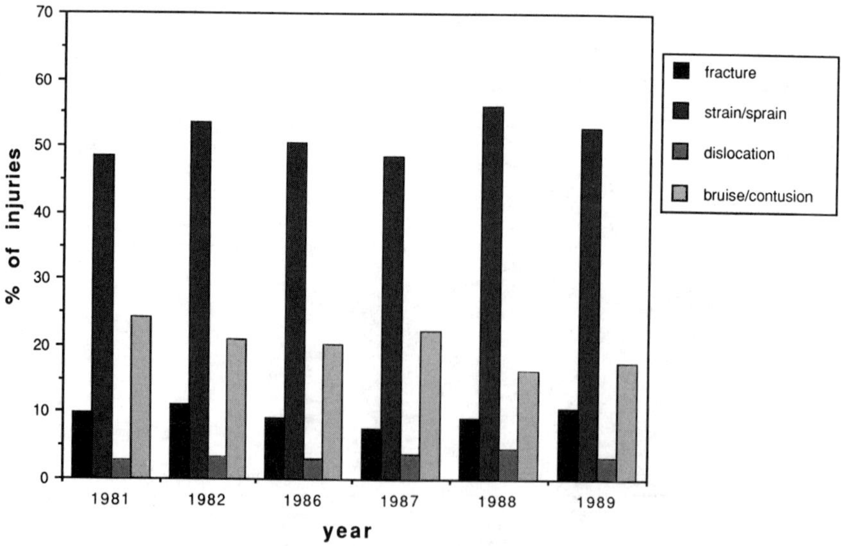

FIG. 4—*Distribution of kinds of injuries.*

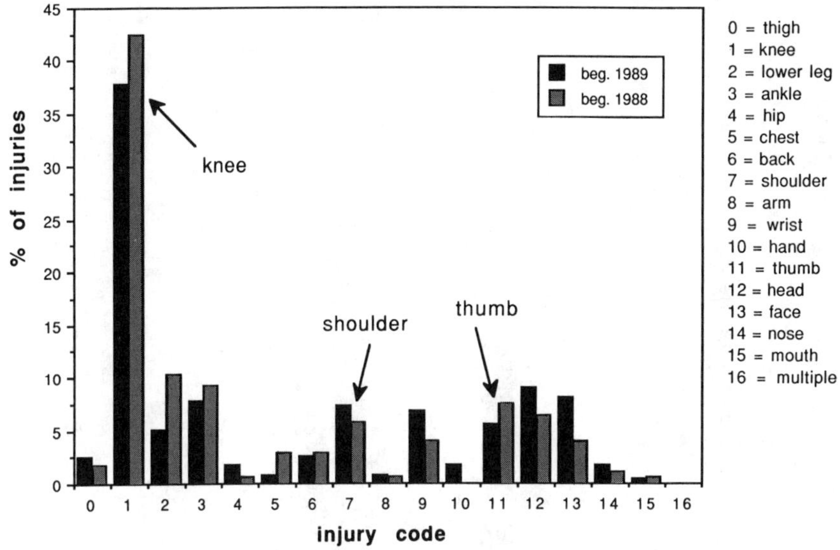

FIG. 5—*Comparison of beginner skiers' injuries.*

Discussion

The shift in relative injury to different parts of the body, along with the influence of ability on this distribution, suggests several explanations. The continuing decline in lower leg injuries is probably attributable to both the continuing improvements in ski bindings and the increasing attention to proper adjustment and testing of the bindings [*6*]. The possible trend

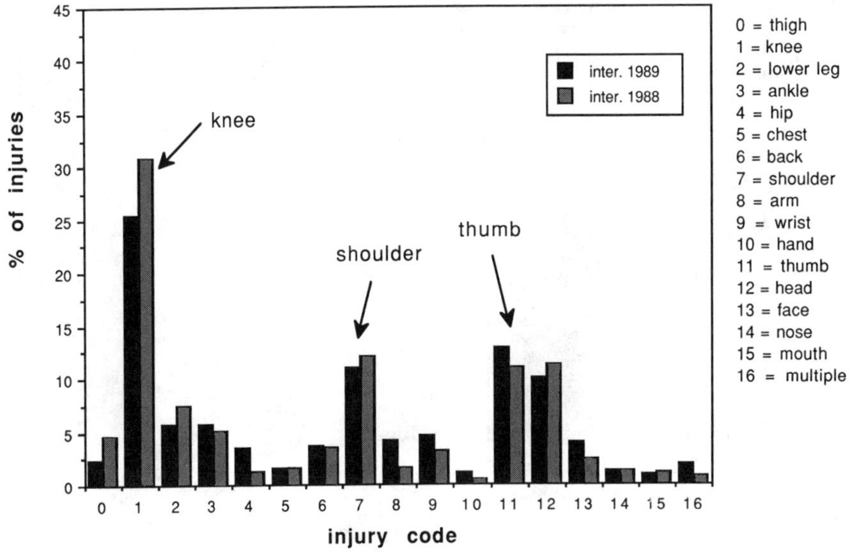

FIG. 6—*Comparison of intermediate skiers' injuries.*

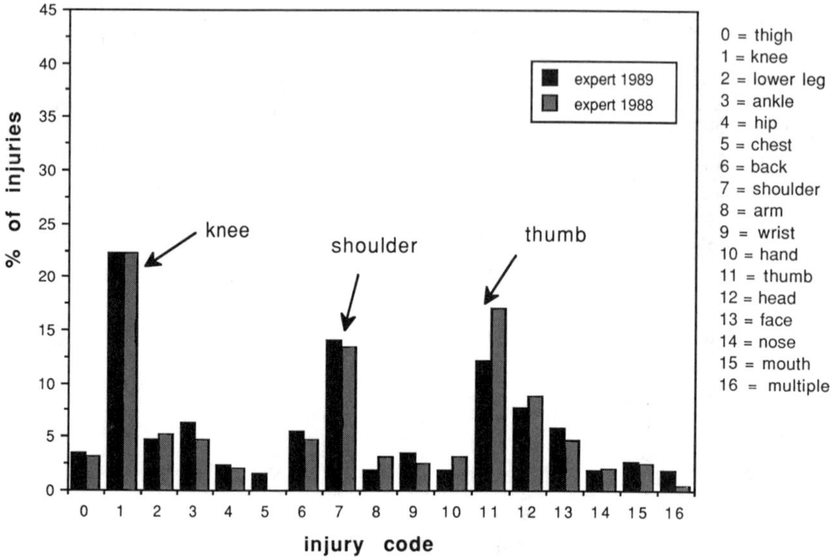

FIG. 7—*Comparison of expert skiers' injuries.*

toward decreasing knee injuries might have the same explanation, but is not evident in any radical changes in boot design.

In an independent study of the efficacy of bindings that release upward at the toe, we found an insufficient usage to draw any conclusions regarding this factor. The change in pattern of injuries with ability clearly suggests the relationship between skiing style and injury. The current study did not concentrate on binding releases, but it did indicate the

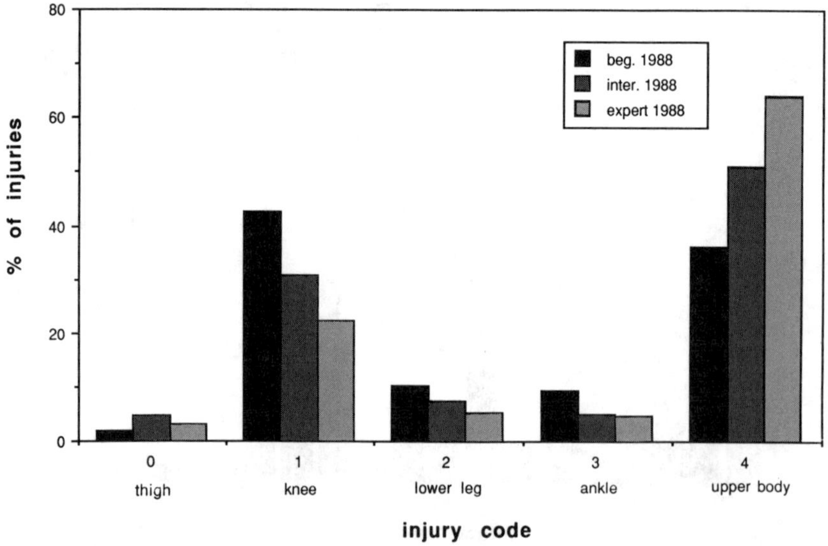

FIG. 8—*Comparison of injuries to different areas of the body among skiers of various abilities.*

high frequency with which an injury occurs despite release of one or both bindings. The beginning skier is still the victim of the slow forward twisting fall, in which the binding may or may not release, and the knee is injured because of the torque exerted by the ski as a lever or perhaps by the boot itself [*7,8*]. The advanced skier is more likely to be skiing faster, release from his or her bindings, and fly forward with arms extended to impact the snow, a tree, or another skier, injuring the thumb, shoulder, or head.

The quad chairlift began operation shortly after the season opened and was in use almost daily. The combination of a longer run, shorter uphill ride time, and reduced waiting time meant a vast increase in the percentage of time a typical skier actually spent skiing, as opposed to waiting for or riding the lift. The absence of a more substantial increase in the injury rate with the increased exposure to risk each hour is surprising. With the absence of data concerning the actual vertical distance traveled, one can only speculate as to the explanation. Certainly one possibility, which is borne out by discussion with numerous uninjured skiers, is that the total number of runs is only slightly increased, and that the skiers are skiing for only part of the day. Many more skiers appear to leave early or arrive late, so that the total exposure to risk per day may not be elevated even if the risk per hour is higher. The absence of any shift in the temporal distribution of injuries argues against any change in fatigue as a factor and furthermore suggests that any tendency to ski a shorter day is balanced among early and late skiers. Both of these speculations require verification by a specific control population study.

Skier injury rates have traditionally been expressed by the metric "injuries per thousand skier days" or equivalently its inverse, "mean days between injuries." This estimate of exposure to risk is based largely on the convenience of counting daily lift tickets and estimating crowd size by other confirming methods (including number of cars in the parking lot and amount of food sold in the restaurants). It has been recognized that the skier who takes only one run and then retires to the bar is at less risk of incurring a skiing injury than the one who skis all day. Furthermore, although rare collisions injure a skier waiting on line, almost all of the injuries occur to a skier who is moving on the snow or standing on the slopes. Consequently, it has often been suggested that a more appropriate measure of exposure would be present if injuries were calculated as incidence per 1000 vertical meters skied. At least one extensive study from Switzerland has been reported using the number of accidents per 10 000 vertical meters skied as the metric [*9*]. This involves additional work for lift attendants, however, and has rarely been accomplished. (The 1988/1989 WV study also did not count total vertical descent but relied on the observation that the total skiing time and distance appeared to increase dramatically.) Probably the most meaningful measure of exposure is the number of hours spent on skis or on the slopes (as opposed to on the lifts or waiting for them).

Acknowledgments

This research was supported by Waterville Valley, M.I.T., and by Look ski bindings. We are particularly grateful to the Waterville Valley Professional Ski Patrol, especially Robert Eames, Director, and Ellen Ederscheim, William Cushing, Director of Safety, and to William Rathman, Waterville Corporation.

References

[*1*] Young, L. R., Oman, C. M., and Crane, H., *Orthopedic Clinics of North America*, Vol. 7, No. 1, Jan. 1976.

[*2*] Crane, H. D., Young, L. R., and Cushing, W., "The Influence of Equipment and Ski Factors on Ski Injuries with an Update—13-Year Study," in *Ski Trauma and Skiing Safety III*, Publications Series of TÜV-Edition, Munich, 1981.

[3] Young, L. R., "Skier Fall Modes and Injury Patterns," in *Ski Trauma and Skiing Safety IV*, Publications Series of TÜV-Edition, Munich, 1982.

[4] Knipschild, P. G. and Bouter, L. M., "Risk Factors for Ski Injuries: A Crash Course of Epidemiologic Methods and Emphasis on Comparability in Experiments and Case-Control Studies," in *Skiing Trauma and Safety: Seventh International Symposium, ASTM STP 1022*, R. J. Johnson, C. D. Mote, Jr., and M.-H. Binet, Eds., American Society for Testing and Materials, Philadelphia, 1989.

[5] Shealy, J. E., "Two-Year Statistical Analysis of Skiing Injuries at 13 Selected Areas in the U.S.A.," in *Ski Trauma and Skiing Safety IV*, Publication Series of TÜV-Edition, Munich, 1982.

[6] Johnson, R. J., Ettlinger, C. F., and Shealy, J. E., "Skier Injury Trends," in *Skiing Trauma and Safety: Seventh International Symposium, ASTM STP 1022*, R. J. Johnson, C. D. Mote, Jr., and M.-H. Binet, Eds., American Society for Testing and Materials, Philadelphia, 1989.

[7] Lystad, H., "A Five-Year Survey of Skiing Injuries in Hemsedal, Norway," in *Skiing Trauma and Safety: Seventh International Symposium, ASTM STP 1022*, R. J. Johnson, C. D. Mote, Jr., and M.-H. Binet, Eds., American Society for Testing and Materials, Philadelphia, 1989.

[8] Ekeland, A., Holtmoen, Å., and Lystad, H., "Skiing Injuries in Alpine Recreational Skiers," in *Skiing Trauma and Safety: Seventh International Symposium, ASTM STP 1002*, R. J. Johnson, C. D. Mote, Jr., and M.-H. Binet, Eds., American Society for Testing and Materials, Philadelphia, 1989.

[9] Bally, A. and Bonjour, F., "An Investigation into Ski Injuries and Equipment in Switzerland: Objectives, Means, and Observations," in *Skiing Trauma and Safety: Seventh International Symposium, ASTM STP 1002*, R. J. Johnson, C. D. Mote, Jr., and M.-H. Binet, Eds., American Society for Testing and Materials, Philadelphia, 1989.

Jasper E. Shealy[1] *and David A. Miller*[1]

A Relative Analysis of Downhill and Cross-Country Ski Injuries

REFERENCE: Shealy, J. E. and Miller, D. A., "**A Relative Analysis of Downhill and Cross-Country Ski Injuries,**" *Skiing Trauma and Safety: Eighth International Symposium, ASTM STP 1104*, C. D. Mote, Jr. and Robert J. Johnson, Eds., American Society for Testing and Materials, Philadelphia, 1991, pp. 133–143.

ABSTRACT: This retrospective analysis of cross-country (XC) and downhill (DH) injuries is based on the Consumer Product Safety Commission (CPSC) National Electronic Injury Surveillance System (NEISS) data files and a survey of XC and DH skiing population demographics conducted by the National Ski Retailers Association (NSRA). The study finds that within each sport, the injury population and population at risk demographics are quite similar, but there are significant differences between the two sports in terms of the injury patterns and between the two populations at risk. There are significant interactions between the two sports with respect to gender. The mean levels of severity of injury are not significantly different. There are implications with regard to injury mechanisms as well as hardware factors.

KEY WORDS: ski injuries, downhill injuries, cross-country injuries, severity, knee injuries, gender differences

Cross-country (XC) skiing injuries have not been subjected to the same degree of analysis as have downhill (DH) skiing injuries. Relatively few researchers [*1–9*] have reviewed XC injuries. Only two studies [*3,8*] have compared XC and DH injuries. From a research viewpoint, it is much more difficult to gather data on XC injuries than DH injuries. DH skiing is generally more organized than XC; it typically takes place at an area designated for DH skiing, where there is usually a ski patrol that operates a first aid facility. XC skiing, on the other hand, is commonly done in a less organized manner. Only recently have XC skiing centers become popular in the United States. The low daily utilization rate of the XC skiing centers and the relative rarity of a ski patrol facility make the use of ski patrol data for analytical purposes impractical.

The injury data for this paper are based on the analysis of skiing injury reports gathered by the Consumer Product Safety Commission (CPSC) through the National Electronic Injury Surveillance System (NEISS). Before September 1979, all injury reports in which the product used at the time of injury was listed as ski equipment were coded 1216. From October 1979 through December 1982 (three ski seasons), ski injuries were broken into several categories, among these were 3232 (informal downhill) and 3281 (informal cross-country). Since January 1983, all skiing-related injuries have been merged back into one category.

The NEISS intake system consists of approximately 100 hospital emergency rooms and departments (ER/ED) across the United States. Any time an injured person comes to that facility for treatment from a product-related (meaning that a product, or equipment, was

[1]Professor and research assistant, respectively, Rochester Institute of Technology, 425 French Road, Rochester, NY 14618.

in use at the time of the injury) incident, information on the victim, the product, and the injury is submitted by ER/ED personnel to the CPSC headquarters for statistical treatment. Based on the sample construction, CPSC can use the NEISS numbers to project what the national numbers would be for any given product. An earlier paper [*8*] was based on preliminary projected figures from 1979 through 1981. This paper is based on the actual reported cases rather than projected numbers for the entire period when the coding allowed for clear discrimination between DH and XC injuries. During the span of time in question, the CPSC NEISS system gathered over 9000 actual injuries. Of these, 1018 were specifically noted as recreational DH and 119 as recreational XC injuries. The remaining reports were not recreational or were not clearly classified as to a specific sport or activity. According to the CPSC weighting procedures, this is equivalent to over 50 000 DH injuries and about 7000 XC injuries. This gives a ratio of about 7 DH injuries for every XC injury reported. A 1984 NSRA study of the skiing population found 12.9 million skiers, 8.4 million DH skiers, 4.5 million XC skiers, or a ratio of about 2 DH skiers for every XC skier. The injury analysis that follows is based on the sample of 1137 actual reported injuries.

The NEISS database has been criticized for a variety of reasons, but, the fact remains, this is the only national database for product-related injuries. It has been in place since 1970. CPSC epidemiologists have gone to great lengths to determine the proper weighting factors to compensate for over- and underrepresentation on a variety of factors, including socioeconomic stratification, urban/suburban/rural population distribution, and so forth. It has many strengths. There is a consistency over the years with terms and definitions, the medical diagnoses are made by medical personnel, and the data auditing is done by professional statisticians and epidemiologists.

For the purpose of this study, the greatest strength of the database is that it treats DH and XC injuries in the same way (that is, the same method of diagnosis, with the same terminology, same definitions, and so forth). There are two weaknesses: first, the number of XC injuries is small, only 119. But so far, all XC studies in the literature are small, they have sample sizes that range from 11 to 283. Second, many of the approximately 100 hospitals that serve as intake sources for the data are not necessarily ideally located for skiing injuries. This is a necessary fact of life if one wishes to have a nationwide sampling process. Because of this potential problem, comparisons have been made wherever possible with other studies to see if there are any inconsistencies in the findings.

The NEISS database does not contain measures of exposure to risk or control groups and, thus, cannot make estimates of the actual rate of injuries in terms of injuries per exposure to risk based on these data. Speculation as to the actual rates has been done previously [*2–4,8*]. Those estimates of the XC rate (not actual calculations) range from 0.1 to 0.5 injuries per 1000 skier visits (SV) [*4*] to an estimate that the XC rate might be as high as one half that of DH [*8*]. The only prospective study to date [*2*] that has been done with XC injuries found a rate of 1.5 injuries per 1000 SV for the first season and 0.48 the second, for a two-season average of 0.72 injuries per 1000 SV.

All the analyses in this report are done on a relative or percentage basis and not on a rate per thousand skier visits or mean days between injuries as done in other reports. This study does not make any estimate as to what the rate of injuries might be in terms of injuries per 1000 SV.

One of the major problems facing all XC injury studies has been the lack of a large injury database and information about the population at risk. This study is no exception, and, thus, it is not an ideal situation for an epidemiological study. On the other hand, it is the only database known to the authors in which the intake mechanism is such that direct comparability between DH and XC injuries can be reasonably assumed. In this instance, the evaluation of the injuries was the same regardless of the source of the injured person (that is, by emergency medical personnel). Because of the smallness of the numbers, one must be very careful in drawing conclusions from the results. It is suggested that the results of this analysis be seen more as a basis for formulating hypotheses for future work than as representing the final word on the issue.

The use of this database is particularly advantageous because the diagnoses are done by medically qualified personnel as opposed to ski patrol or first aid trained personnel making diagnoses of the injury. This gives confidence in the accuracy of the medical aspects of the data. Another advantage is that the same personnel, reporting terminology, and definitions have been used for both sports, so the results for the two sports are comparable.

The population-at-risk data were obtained from the National Ski Retailers Association. While the injury data are from 1979 through 1983, the control or population-at-risk data are from January to December of 1986. There is no reason to believe that the demographics of the sport underwent significant changes during the 1980s.

Results

Age

The median ages for males and females and for DH and XC skiing are given in Table 1. There is no significant difference between the male and female ages within each sport, nor is there a significant difference between the injured and control groups within each sport, but there is a significant difference (t-test, $p < 0.05$) between the DH and XC populations (injured as well as control). The median age of 27 for XC skiers compares well with an average age of 27 in the study by Hodgdon [*6*] but is somewhat lower than in other studies, such as 33 in Boyle et al. [*2*] and 36 in Paus et al. [*10*].

Gender

Table 2 shows that the relative percentages of male to female skiers differs significantly (Chi-square test, $p < 0.05$) between the DH and the XC injured population as well as in the control population. But the relative frequency of males to females (M:F ratio) within each sport is approximately the same in the injured as in the control group. Considering the differences between the two data sources, the similarity of the age distributions and the relative distributions of males and females are quite remarkable. This agrees with findings of Boyle [2] in that the M:F ratio is the same for the injured group as for the control group.

Diagnosis

The diagnoses of injuries (Table 3 and Fig. 1) for the two types of skiing (DH and XC) are not significantly different (Chi-square tests). The main apparent differences seem to be that DH injuries include more abrasions and bruises and fewer fractures than XC, but, as previously noted, this is not a significant difference. Other studies [*2,6,9,10,12*] have found the percentage of injuries that are fractures range from 14.1 to 54%.

TABLE 1—*Median age (years) at time of injury.*

	DH		XC	
Group	Male	Female	Male	Female
Control (NSGA)	20	20	26	27.5
Injured (NEISS)	20	19	27	28

TABLE 2—*Percentage of male and female skiers.*

Group	DH		XC	
	Male	Female	Male	Female
Control (NSGA)	60.9	39.1	45.4	54.6
Injured (NEISS)	61.5	38.5	43.7	56.3

TABLE 3—*Distribution of injuries.*

Diagnosis	DH, %	XC, %
Strain/sprain	42.7	42.9
Abrasion/bruise	23.4	17.7
Fracture	21.7	25.2
Laceration	5.0	7.6
Dislocation	2.6	5.0
Concussion/head injury	2.6	1.7
All others	2.1	0.0

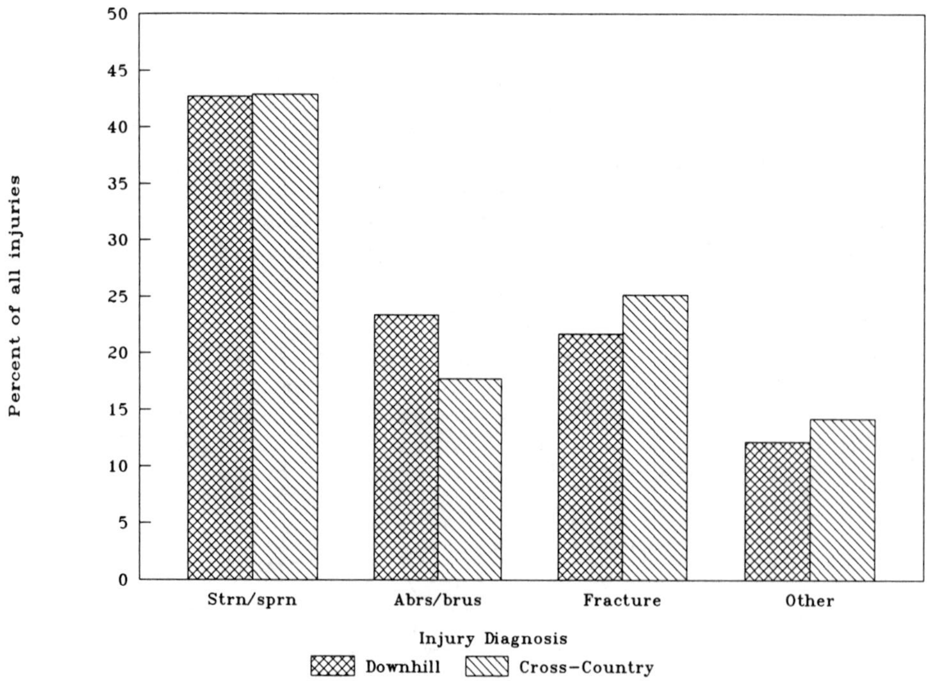

FIG. 1—*Injury diagnosis by sport.*

TABLE 4—*Body part injured.*

Body Part	DH	XC	Ratio (DH:XC)
Head/face/neck	9.5	5.9	1.6
Shoulder	7.7	10.1	0.8
Hand/wrist/arm/elbow	7.5	13.4	0.6
Finger/thumb	17.0	10.9	1.6
Torso	7.8	10.1	0.8
Upper leg	1.7	0.8	2.1
Knee	26.5	26.1	1.0
Lower leg	11.2	4.2	2.7
Ankle	9.0	11.8	0.8
Foot/toe	2.1	6.7	0.3

Part of Body Injured

The analysis of the part of the body injured as a function of the sport (Table 4 and Fig. 2) reveals some significant differences. Injuries to the knee are the most common in both sports. Face and head injuries are 1.6 times more common in DH than XC. The same is true for finger and thumb injuries. Lower leg (tibia) injuries are 2.7 times higher in DH than XC. XC has a higher percentage of shoulder, hand, wrist, arm, elbow, ankle, foot, and toe injuries. The percentage of all XC injuries that were knee injuries was 26%; Boyle [2] found knees constituted 24.5% of all XC injuries.

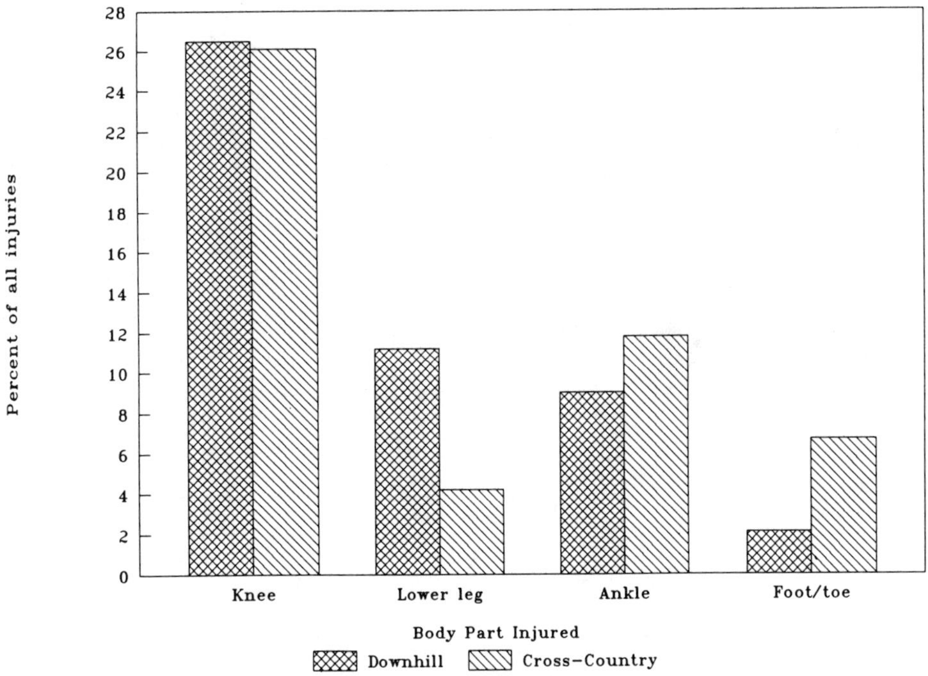

FIG. 2—*Body part injured by sport.*

TABLE 5—*Severity of injury using CP & C Severity Rating Scale.*

Severity	DH %	DH Cum%	XC %	XC Cum%
1	23.5	23.5	30.2	30.2
2	35.1	58.6	27.7	57.9
3	27.5	86.1	23.5	81.4
4	9.9	96.0	15.1	96.5
5	3.2	99.2	1.7	98.2
6	0.8	100.0	1.7	99.9

Severity

The severity as rated by the CPSC (Table 5 and Fig. 3) on a scale from 1 to 8 (1 = negligible, 8 = death) reveals no significant difference (Kolmogorov-Smirnov test) between the two sports. Both have a median value of 2 (minor).

Diagnosis by Gender by Type of Skiing

When the diagnosis is considered as a function of gender, between the two sports (Table 6), interesting interactions are found. The primary ones are for strain/sprain and fracture diagnoses. Males have a higher strain/sprain percentage for XC than DH (48.1 versus 39.6); for females, it is just the opposite (38.8 versus 47.7). For fracture diagnoses, the same type of interaction exists. Males have a higher fracture percentage in DH than XC (24.1 versus 19.2), while females have a lower percentage (17.9 versus 29.9).

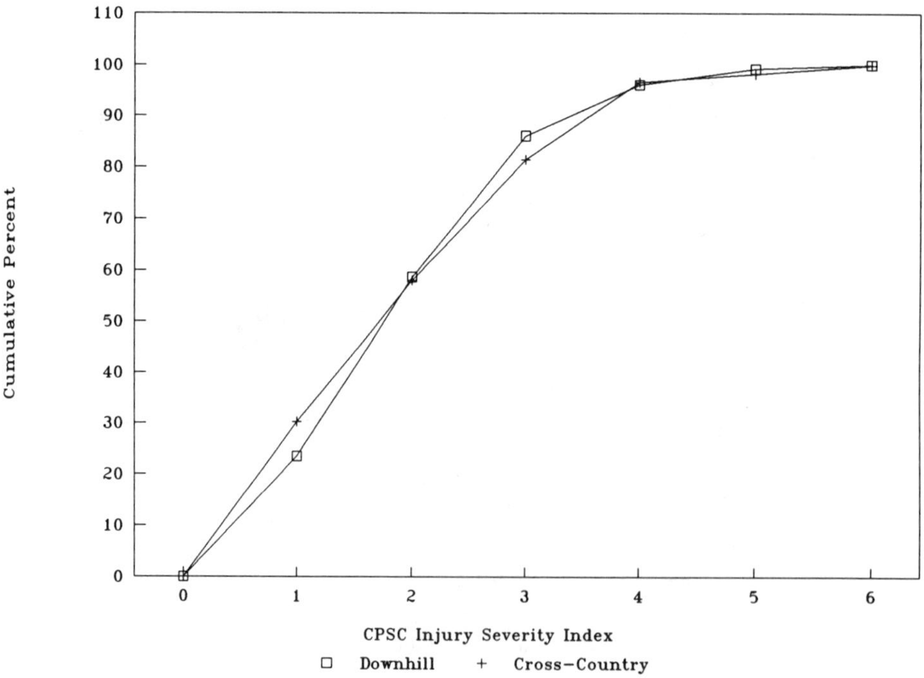

FIG. 3—*Severity of injury by sport.*

TABLE 6—*Nature of injury by gender by sport.*

Diagnosis	Male		Female	
	DH, %	XC, %	DH, %	XC, %
Strain/sprain	39.6	48.1	47.7	38.8
Abrasion/bruise	23.2	19.2	23.7	16.4
Fracture	24.1	19.2	17.9	29.9
Laceration	5.8	3.9	3.8	10.5
Dislocation	3.0	7.7	1.8	3.0
Head injury	2.2	1.9	3.1	1.5
All others	2.3	0.0	2.1	0.0

Body Part Injured by Gender by Type of Skiing

When the part of the body that was injured is controlled for gender for the two types of skiing (Table 7), a significant (Chi-square test, $p < 0.05$) interaction (Fig. 4) appears. The male knee injury percentage is higher for XC than DH (30.8 versus 21.6); for females, the percentage is higher for DH than XC (34.3 versus 22.4). In no other case does the gender difference exhibit any significant interaction with type of skiing.

Discussion

Based on the analysis of these data, there are interesting similarities and differences between the injuries sustained in DH and XC skiing. There are differences in body part injured and diagnosis between the two genders as a function of skiing and as a function of the interaction between the genders and the type of skiing. The interactions of gender with sport and nature of injury and body part are in most cases the same as noted by Paus [*10*].

Age and Gender

In each sport, the age and gender distribution of the injured population is very similar to the respective population at risk. In other words, the fact that the XC injured skier tends to be older and more likely female than male merely reflects the fact that the population at risk is older and has a higher proportion of females than males. The typical age of the injured skier is not different for males and females within the two sports. There is a difference

TABLE 7—*Body part injured by gender by sport.*

Body Part	Male		Female	
	DH, %	XC, %	DH, %	XC, %
Knee	21.6	30.8	34.4	22.4
Finger/thumb	18.5	11.5	14.5	10.5
Head/neck/face	7.5	1.9	12.2	9.0
Ankle	9.7	13.5	7.9	10.5
Shoulder	9.3	15.4	5.1	6.0
Arm	7.3	7.7	7.7	17.9
Torso	9.3	11.5	5.6	9.0
Lower leg	13.3	5.8	7.9	3.0
Femur	1.1	1.9	2.6	0.0
Miscellaneous	2.1	0.0	2.0	11.9

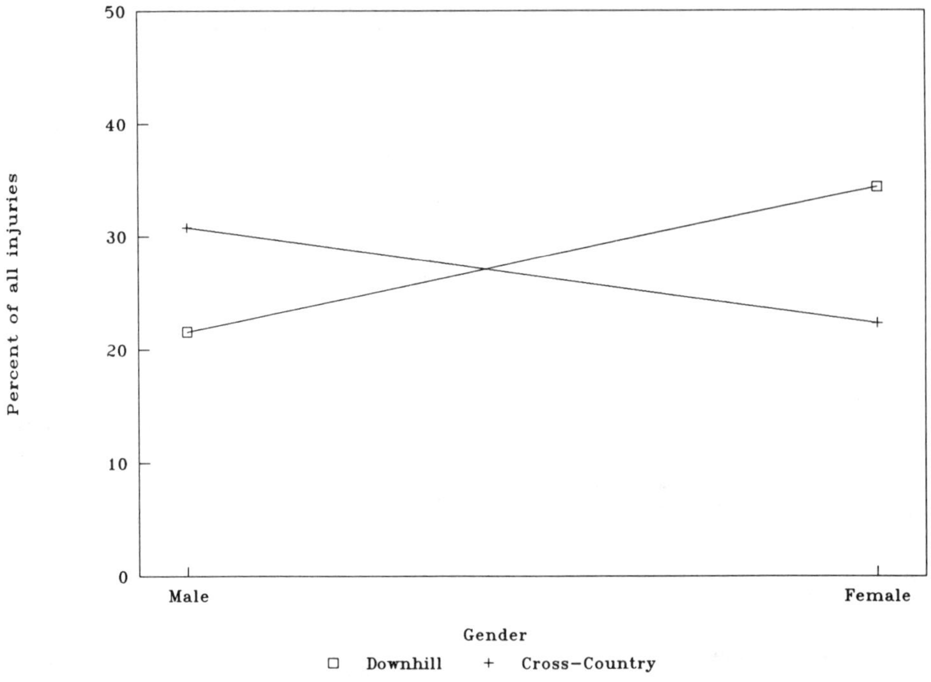

FIG. 4—*Knee injuries by gender by sport.*

between the ratio of male to female within the injured population for the two sports. Males are the dominant fraction in DH, females are dominant in XC. This is due to differences in the populations at risk.

Diagnosis

The diagnosis cannot be considered without taking gender into account because there are significant interactions. Specifically, we note that the diagnoses for strain/sprain and fracture for the two sports are affected by the gender of the victim.

Strain/sprain injuries are the most common diagnosis in both sports. Males have a higher incidence in XC than DH; the opposite is true for females.

Within the two sports, fractures are the third most common injury in DH and second most common injury in XC (21.7 versus 25.2%). A relatively high fracture rate in XC skiing has been noted by many researchers [*2,3,6,7,9*], with values ranging from 14 to 27% of all injuries. The abrasion, bruise, contusion injury is the second most common in DH and third most common in XC (23.4 versus 17.7%). This is somewhat surprising because DH skiing is generally perceived to be a higher velocity sport than XC, which means there would be more kinetic energy to be disposed of in a fall and, hence, presumably a greater propensity toward fractures. Also, there is a more rigid fixation (the boot-binding system) in DH than XC, which would seem to make for a less yielding system. Renstrom and Johnson [*11*] indicate that with the advent of synthetic materials such as fiber glass for the skis, more rigid coupling systems, and deep hardpacked tracks, the speeds and the potential for serious injuries have increased. The high percentage of fractures and other serious injuries noted in many of the studies would seem to support that conclusion.

The diagnosis of the injury also exhibits an interaction with gender and type of skiing. The female fracture percentage is higher for XC than DH; for males it is just the opposite. The strain/sprain injury has the opposite trend: a higher percentage of males injured in XC and a higher percentage of females injured in DH. In magnitude, these trends are offsetting (that is, if the two diagnoses were combined, there would not be any significant differences between the two sports or the two genders). The abrasion/bruise injury does not exhibit any interaction with gender.

This suggests that there may be a trade-off between the two sports and the genders for strain/sprain and for fracture injuries. For some reason, females appear to be at greater risk than males for fractures in XC and strain/sprains in DH. Alternatively, one could view the results as saying males are at greater risk for strain/sprains in XC and fractures in DH than are females.

Body Part

The knee is the most commonly reported injured body part in both sports: 26.5% in DH, 26.1% in XC. The finger/thumb is the second most common body part to be injured in DH (17.0%), but the fourth most common body part injured in XC (10.9%). Arms are the second most common body part injured in XC (13.4%); they are fourth most common body part injured in DH (7.5%). Lower leg (or tibia) is the third most common body part injured in DH (11.2%), but lower leg is ninth (out of nine categories) in XC (4.2%).

Only knee injuries demonstrate a significant gender-driven interaction. Males experience a higher percentage of knee injuries in XC than do females (30.8 versus 22.4%), females have a higher percentage in DH than do males (34.4% versus 21.6%). None of the other major categories exhibit any tendency to interact with gender.

These findings are of particular interest. To find that the knee is the most commonly reported part of the body to be injured in XC suggests that the rigid boot-ski coupling in DH skiing is not a necessary requirement for a knee injury, because the boot-coupling in XC is far less rigid. In fact, XC binding systems typically have a free heel and a torsionally flexible boot, while DH boots are just the opposite. The DH boot essentially locks the ankle in a fixed or narrow range of flexion, whereas the XC boot does not. Unfortunately, the data in this study are not sufficiently detailed to reveal a specific diagnosis in terms of severity (Grade I, II, or III) or specific ligament(s). As has been noted elsewhere [*2,3,9,12*], however, Grade III knee sprains account from 24 to 50% of all knee sprains in some studies. Studies that have identified specific ligaments [*2,7,12*] show that medial collateral ligaments (MCL) and anterior cruciate ligaments (ACL) are commonly involved. Renstrom and Johnson [*11*] and Boyle et al. [*2*] indicate that the injury mechanisms are often the same, that is, external rotation and adduction of the lower extremity.

The percentage of tibial injuries is higher in DH than XC (11.2 versus 4.2%). This is most likely due to the differences in equipment; the DH equipment provides for a rigid coupling that would allow bending and twisting loads to be applied to the tibial shaft. It would seem that there would be a trade-off of ankle injuries for tibial injuries. To a minor degree, this seems to be true; the XC ankle injury rate is 11.8 versus 9.0% for DH. Clearly this is in the expected direction but does not completely offset the noted difference in tibial shaft injuries.

Injuries to the arm, shoulder, and torso are common in XC skiing. These three categories together account for 33.6% of XC injuries but only 23.1% of DH injuries. Finger and thumb injuries account for 17.0% of reported DH injuries, but only 10.9% of XC injuries. Face, head, and neck injuries comprise 9.5% of the reported DH injuries; the comparable figure for XC was only 5.9%.

Severity

Severity ratings of injuries are controversial. The authors do not endorse or condemn the severity rating method used by CPSC analysts using the hospital emergency room data. In this matter, there is no reason to believe that there would be any bias in its application. For the sake of comparison between the two sports, this severity rating should be as good as any other.

The analysis found no significant severity differences between the two sports or the genders. In each case, the median severity was 2 (minor). This may be surprising to some because the general perception is that XC skiing is less dangerous than DH skiing.

When the findings of this study and the others referred to in this paper are carefully examined, it is clear that XC skiing is characterized by a fracture rate that rivals that of DH skiing in relative percentages. XC skiing has many severe knee injuries, as well. Spiral fractures of the femur have been recorded [*7*]. Numerous deaths have also been noted [*1,6*].

The analysis of Boyle [*2*] shows that over 88% of the injuries take place during the downhill portion of XC skiing, where the velocities are greatest and control is least. All the above lead the authors to conclude that the similar severity index ratings of the two activities are neither coincidental nor due to a statistical reporting artifact, but rather they are most likely a reflection of the reality of the situation. While the rate of injuries may be less on the basis of number of injuries per 1000 SV, there is no reason to believe that the severity is any less.

Conclusions

1. This paper points out several significant differences between the two types of skiing (DH versus XC). The injury patterns are similar in that they both are dominated by the strain/sprain injury, with the knee being the most commonly reported part of the body to be injured. The intriguing aspect of this is that the knee injury dominates both sports, even though the equipment is so different between the two sports. This shows that the current DH release systems should not be viewed as the major cause (or means of prevention) of the knee injury, to the extent that a rigid coupling with a fixed ankle joint or a failure to release causes the injury, because in XC skiing, one does not have a rigid coupling and the ankle is relatively free to flex and yet XC has a knee injury potential that rivals DH in relative frequency as well as severity. Clearly, more in-depth study and analysis are needed here, and especially more specific diagnoses as to which ligaments and what injury mechanisms are at work. This study also points out that there are some interesting differences between male and female skiers in terms of injury modes.

2. The reported median level of severity of injury between the two sports is identical, suggesting (as did Lyons [*7*]) that XC injuries may not be as benign as many people seem to believe.

3. The typical XC injured skier is older than the typical DH skier. This reflects an older population at risk. Males dominate the DH injured group, females dominate the XC group; both findings are reflections of the population at risk gender distribution.

References

[*1*] Berghold, F., "Fatal Skiing Accidents in Austria—Epidemiology and Analysis," in *Skiing Trauma and Safety: Seventh International Symposium, ASTM STP 1022*, R. J. Johnson, C. D. Mote, Jr., and M.-H. Binet, Eds., American Society for Testing and Materials, Philadelphia, 1989, pp. 63–68.

[2] Boyle, J. J., Johnson, R. J., Pope, M. H., Pierce, J. C., and Brady, M. M., "Cross-Country Skiing Injuries," in *Skiing Trauma and Safety: Fifth International Symposium, ASTM STP 860*, R. J. Johnson and C. D. Mote, Jr., Eds., American Society for Testing and Materials, Philadelphia, 1985, pp. 411–422.

[3] Eriksson, E., *Orthopedics Clinics of North America*, Vol. 7, 1976, pp. 3–6.

[4] Gamble, W. E., "Cross-Country Skiing Injuries," American Academy of Orthopaedic Surgeons Course on Winter Sports Injuries, Arthroscopy, and Arthrography of the Knee, Aspen, CO, 30 March 1978.

[5] Gillette, N., *Nordic 1981—2nd Annual Trade Publication*, Nordic Skiing Inc., West Brattleboro, VT, Vol. 2, 1980, pp. 8–11.

[6] Hodgdon, D. P., *Nordic Ski Accident Data, 1973–1978*, National Ski Patrol System, Denver, CO, 1978.

[7] Lyons, J. W. and Porter, R. E., "Cross-Country Skiing: A Benign Sport?" *JAMA*, Vol. 239, No. 4, Jan. 1978, pp. 334–335.

[8] Shealy, J. E., "A Comparison of Downhill and Cross-Country Skiing Injuries," in *Skiing Trauma and Safety: Fifth International Symposium, ASTM STP 860*, R. J. Johnson and C. D. Mote, Jr., Eds., American Society for Testing and Materials, Philadelphia, 1985, pp. 423–432.

[9] Westlin, N. E., "Injuries in Long-Distance, Cross-Country, and Downhill Skiing," *Orthopedic Clinics of North America*, Vol. 7, 1976, pp. 55–58.

[10] Paus, A., Tuveng, J. M., Nilssen, A., and Halter, I., "Skiing Injuries, Alpine Sports," in *Ski Trauma and Skiing Safety: Fourth International Symposium*, TUV Publication Series, TÜV, Munich, 1982, pp. 194–201.

[11] Renstrom, P. and Johnson, R. J., "Cross-Country Skiing," Draft copy of chapter, c. 1980.

[12] Johnson, R. J., Ettlinger, C. F., and Shealy, J. E., "Skier Injury Trends," in *Skiing Trauma and Safety: Seventh International Symposium, ASTM STP 1022*, R. J. Johnson, C. D. Mote, Jr., and M.-H. Binet, Eds., American Society for Testing and Materials, Philadelphia, 1989, pp. 25–31.

Arne Ekeland,[1] Åge Holtmoen,[2] and Harald Lystad[3]

Alpine Skiing Injuries in Scandinavian Skiers

REFERENCE: Ekeland, A., Holtmoen, Å., and Lystad, H., "**Alpine Skiing Injuries in Scandinavian Skiers,**" *Skiing Trauma and Safety: Eighth International Symposium, ASTM STP 1104*, C. D. Mote, Jr. and Robert J. Johnson, Eds., American Society for Testing and Materials, Philadelphia, 1991, pp. 144–151.

ABSTRACT: The skiing injuries and skiing behavior of skiers from Norway, Sweden, and Denmark were studied in 4 Norwegian ski resorts during the winter of 1985/1986. A total of 328 injured skiers were recorded and compared with a randomly selected control population of 316 uninjured skiers.

The skiing injury ratio—injured skiers (%)/uninjured skiers (%)—was significantly higher for Danes (2.0) than for Norwegians (0.9) and Swedes (1.0) ($P < 0.01$). This national difference was also observed after correction for skiing ability and skiing experience, which are the main determinants of injury risk in alpine skiing. In accordance with this, Danish beginners had an injury ratio about four times those for Norwegian and Swedish beginners. Present or previous skiing instruction reduced the injury ratio significantly only for the Norwegians; no significant differences were observed between the skiers from the three countries regarding binding testing.

The previously reported higher injury risk for Norwegian compared to Swedish alpine skiers no longer exists. This may be due to more information about skiing safety in Norway in the 1980s. The relatively higher injury ratio for the Danes may be due to shorter skiing seasons, but less public information about skiing safety may also have contributed.

KEY WORDS: age factors, athletic injuries, binding tests, head injuries, knee injuries, nationalities, release bindings, skiing, skiing instruction, skiing safety, skiing trauma, sports

Public information on alpine skiing safety has been organized differently in the Scandinavian countries. The Swedish National Board for Consumer Policies became engaged in skiing safety during the 1970s. The Board provided information about skiing safety to the public, initiated binding testing campaigns, and made the sports shops stop marketing skiing equipment not approved according to the German standards, Deutsches Institut für Normung (DIN) [*1–3*]. The information on skiing safety given to Norwegian skiers was more casual at that time, and a study of skiing injuries in comparable populations of Norwegian and Swedish skiers in the period 1976 to 1978 disclosed a much higher injury rate among Norwegians than among Swedes [*4*]. The study also revealed that many more Swedes than Norwegians had tested their bindings for release. A later study showed that twice as many Swedes (30%) as Norwegians (15%) on the slopes had bindings that released at recommended setting, and the Norwegians were overrepresented among skiers with too tight bindings [*5*]. The results of these and other studies initiated the formation of an Alpine Skiing Safety Council in Norway [*6*]. Thus, the Norwegians have been increasingly informed about skiing safety in the 1980s.

[1]Senior orthopedic surgeon, Orthopedic Service, Surgical Department, Ullevaal Hospital, University of Oslo, N-0407 Oslo 4, Norway.

[2]Master in sport science, The Norwegian College of Physical Education and Sport, N-0807 Oslo 8, Norway.

[3]Medical officer of health, Hemsedal Health Center, N-3560 Hemsedal, Norway.

This study compares the injury risk for Norwegian and Swedish skiers in the mid-1980s by which time skiers from both countries should have received considerable public information about skiing safety. In addition, the injury risk in a small population of Danish skiers was studied. Denmark has mild winters with poor snow, and no organized public information about skiing safety.

Material and Methods

The skiing injuries in four popular Norwegian ski resorts (Hemsedal, Hovden, Oppdal, and Trysil) were recorded during the winter season 1985/1986. The registration was carried out by local physicians at each resort's single medical center. A skiing injury was defined as any injury occurring in a skiing accident that resulted in the skier being brought to the medical center or voluntarily seeking medical assistance. A control population of 316 uninjured skiers was selected randomly from lift lines in the same skiing areas throughout the season. These skiers were asked a series of questions about sociological and skiing data, and were thereafter allowed to bypass the lift line. Thus, the response to the study among the randomly selected control population of skiers was very hearty. Data were collected on forms designed to assist in computer processing.

The skiing injury ratio for each group was calculated as the percentage of injured skiers in that group divided by the percentage of uninjured skiers in the group. The injury ratio was related to the skier's nationality, to type of injury, to age and sex, to skiing ability and skiing experience, to skiing instruction, and to binding adjustment and testing. Regarding skiing ability, the skiers were classified by their performance of turns [*4,7*].

The results are presented as median and range, as percentage of the population of skiers, and as injury ratios. Differences were evaluated statistically by the two-sided Wilcoxon [*8*] or Fisher-Irwin [*9*] tests and were considered significant when $P < 0.05$.

Results

The skiing population (control population) consisted of 59% Norwegians, 33% Swedes, 6% Danes and 3% of other nationalities. The latter 3% of skiers are not considered further in this study.

Injury-Related Factors

Risks for Different Injuries—The skiing injury ratio was significantly higher for Danes than for Norwegians and Swedes (Fig. 1). The difference was even higher when lower extremity equipment-related (LEER) injuries were considered (Fig. 2).

The type and location of the injuries have been published previously [*10*]. The injured Norwegians suffered more head injuries (21%) than Swedes (7%) and Danes (5%) ($P <$ 0.002). Corresponding observations were made regarding the head injury ratios for the three nationalities (Fig. 3). In contrast, only 17% of the injured Norwegians suffered knee injuries, compared to 30% of the Swedes and 40% of the Danes ($P < 0.02$). The relative difference among the three countries was even higher when injury ratios were considered (Fig. 4).

Causes of Injury—Collisions accounted for 19% of the injuries, but no significant differences were observed in the frequency of collision-induced injuries for the Scandinavian skiers. Other injury causes were also similar for skiers from the three countries.

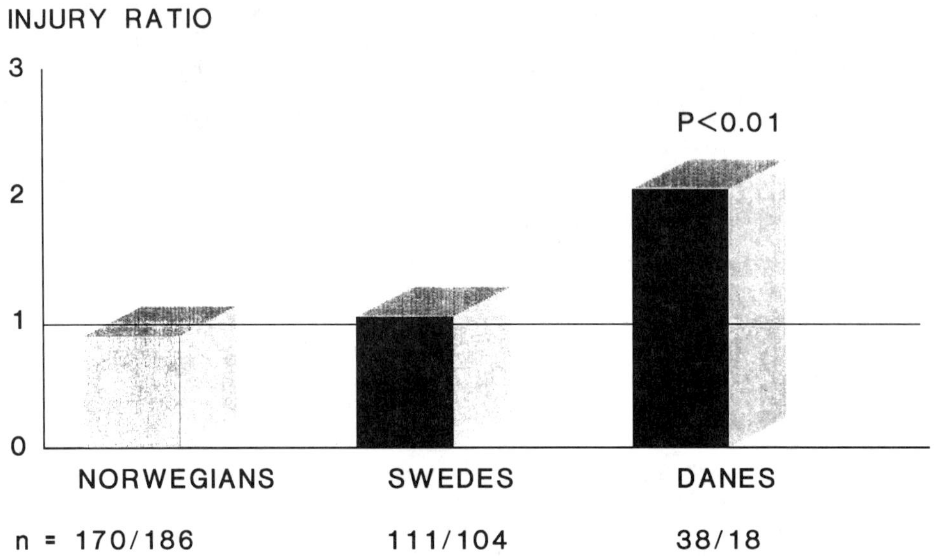

FIG. 1—*Injury ratios—injured skiers (%)/uninjured skiers (%)—for Scandinavian recreational skiers. A significant difference between Danish and Norwegian and Swedish skiers is indicated* (n = *number of injured/uninjured skiers).*

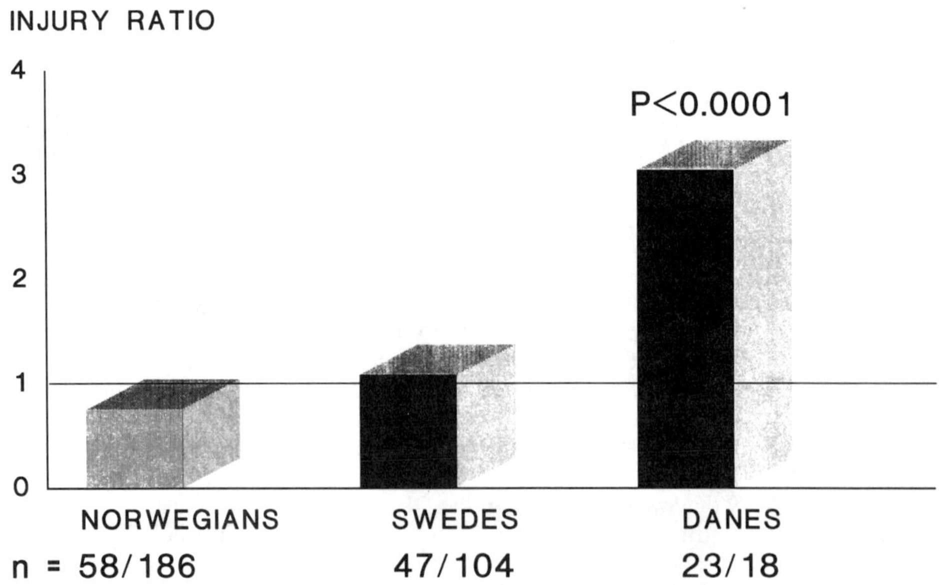

FIG. 2—*Lower extremity equipment-related skiing injury ratios—injured skiers (%)/uninjured skiers (%)—for Scandinavian recreational skiers. A significant difference between Danish and Norwegian and Swedish skiers is indicated* (n = *number of injured/uninjured skiers).*

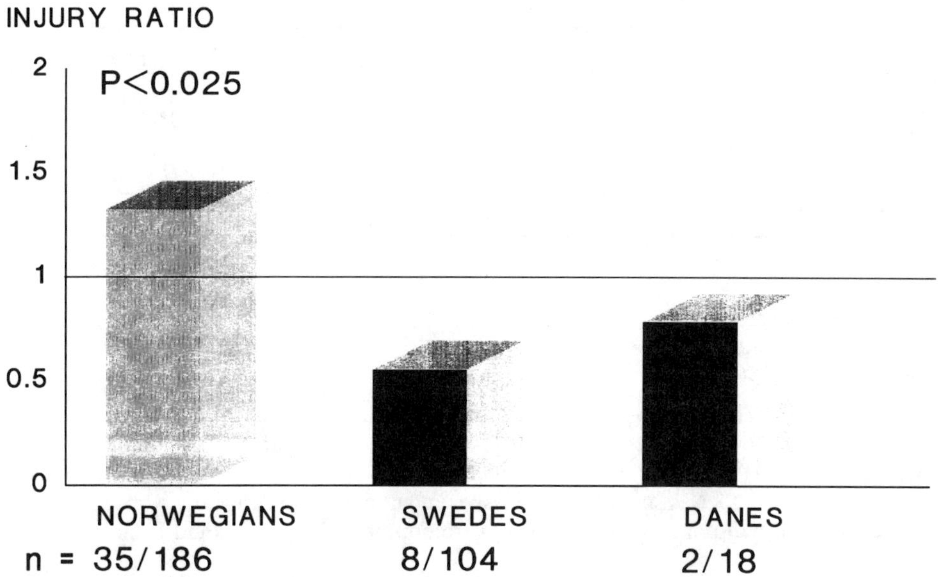

FIG. 3—*Head injury ratios—injured skiers (%)/uninjured skiers (%)—for Scandinavian recreational skiers. A significant difference between Norwegian and Swedish and Danish skiers is indicated* (n = *number of injured/uninjured skiers).*

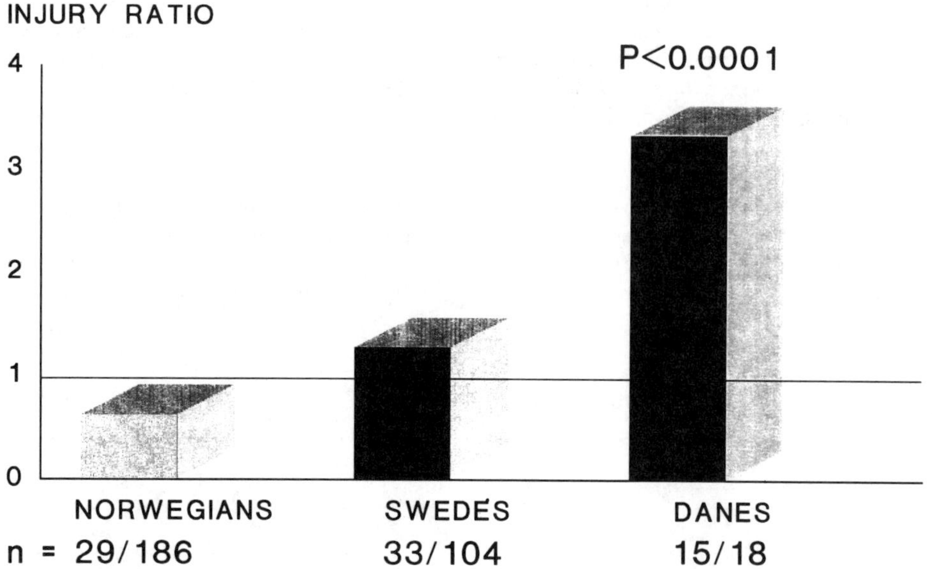

FIG. 4—*Knee injury ratios—injured skiers (%)/uninjured skiers (%)—for Scandinavian skiers. A significant difference between Danish and Norwegian and Swedish skiers is indicated* (n = *number of injured/uninjured skiers).*

TABLE 1—*Age of recreational Scandinavian skiers. Significant differences between injured and uninjured skiers are indicated (median with range;* n = *number of skiers).*

Skiers	*n*	Injured		Uninjured
Norwegians	356	20 (2–57)	$P < 0.05$	24 (6–53)
Swedes	215	24 (6–70)		24 (5–61)
Danes	56	29 (5–46)		20 (8–57)

Skier-Related Factors

Age and Sex—The age and sex distributions were similar for skiers from the three countries, but injured skiers were significantly younger than uninjured skiers among the Norwegians (Table 1). This was mainly a result of the age group 15 to 19 years old, which with an injury ratio of 2.3 was significantly at risk compared to the average for Norwegian skiers ($P < 0.005$). Corresponding observations were not made for Swedes and Danes.

Skiing Ability and Experience—The skiing ability for Norwegians and Swedes was similar; Danes had a lower ability. Corresponding observations were made for skiing experience, with a median number of six skiing seasons for Norwegians and Swedes, and two for the Danes. These figures were equal for the populations of injured and uninjured skiers.

The skiing injury risk is related to skiing ability and skiing experience [*10,11*]. When corrected for ability and experience by standardization, the injury ratios for the Danes was reduced by about 25%, whereas the corresponding ratios for Norwegian and Swedes only disclosed minor changes. In accordance with this, injured Danish beginners were significantly overrepresented among the injured beginners ($P < 0.02$) with an injury ratio (13.2) about four times higher than those for Norwegian (3.0) and Swedish (3.3) beginners. Corresponding observations ($P < 0.05$) were made for skiers with zero to two skiing seasons in which the injury ratio for the Danes was 1.9 compared to 1.4 for Norwegians and Swedes.

Skiing Instruction—Significantly more uninjured than injured Norwegians had attended ski school classes, giving them a lower injury ratio than uninstructed skiers (Table 2). This difference was not significant for skiers from the two other countries, where the percentage skiers who had received instruction was higher both for injured and uninjured skiers.

TABLE 2—*Skiing instruction for Norwegians. Significant differences between injured and uninjured skiers are indicated (*n = *number of skiers).*

Skiers	*n*	Present or Previous Skiing Instruction, %		No Skiing Instruction, %
Injured	143	29	$P < 0.005$	71
Uninjured	181	45		55
Injury ratio[a]		0.64		1.29

[a]Injury ratio = injured skiers (%)/uninjured skiers (%).

Equipment-Related Factors

Bindings—Most of the bindings of uninjured skiers were adjusted in a ski shop, but more Norwegians adjusted the bindings themselves (30%) compared to Swedes (16%) and Danes (11%) ($P < 0.02$).

No significant differences were observed among skiers from the three countries regarding binding testing. About 40% of the skiers had never tested their bindings, and few had used a binding test instrument (Table 3). Less than 25% had self-release tested their bindings during the week preceding their involvement in the study.

Discussion

This study reveals that the relatively increased risk for alpine skiing injuries for Norwegians compared to Swedes reported in studies from the period 1976 to 1980 [*4,5,12*] no longer exists. This may be related to the increased public information about skiing safety disseminated in Norway during the 1980s. The Norwegian Alpine Skiing Safety Council was formally established in 1984. The main skiing-related organizations and the Norwegian Product Control Authority are members of the council. Besides providing information on skiing safety directly to the public, the council has also launched binding testing campaigns, arranged skiing safety conferences, inhibited trade of poor skiing equipment, and acted to promote the work for skiing safety in each of the participating organizations [*6*].

The data in this case control study are presented as injury ratios. Many epidemiologists prefer to calculate odd ratios with 95% confidence intervals, and this mode of calculation confirmed the significant findings in the study (data not shown).

The study disclosed higher injury ratios for Danes than for Norwegians and Swedes even after correcting for skiing ability and skiing experience. The Danish skiing population was small in this study, and the figures should, therefore, be interpreted with care. A high injury risk for Danish skiers has, however, also been reported in other studies [*13,14*]. The injury ratio for the Danes was especially high for LEER injuries and knee injuries (see Figs. 2 and 4). This is probably related to the lower skiing ability of the Danes, because beginners are more prone to these types of injuries [*15–17*]. Also, Danish studies have reported a high percentage of knee injuries in alpine skiers [*18,19*].

The relatively increased risk for head injuries among Norwegian skiers (see Fig. 3) was primarily due to increased exposure to head injuries in the age group 15 to 19 years old [*10*]. Many of these injuries may be prevented by the use of protective helmets. Helmets are seldom used by recreational skiers over 10 to 12 years of age. The Norwegian Alpine Skiing Safety Council has, therefore, launched a campaign to increase the use of skiing helmets also among adolescents.

Beginners are most at risk on the slopes [*10,15,16*]. Skiing instruction may reduce the time spent on the slope as a beginner, and current or previous instruction reduced the injury

TABLE 3—*Binding testing for uninjured Scandinavian skiers* (n = *number of skiers*).

Testing Behavior	Norwegians, % (n = 180)	Swedes, % (n = 104)	Danes, % (n = 18)
Test instrument/ self-release test	5	12	6
Self-release test alone	54	50	50
Not tested	41	39	44

risk for Norwegian skiers (see Table 2). This was, however, not observed significantly for skiers from Sweden and Denmark. This may be due to the fact that the majority of the skiers from the latter countries had attended ski school classes some time in their skiing career. Any effect of instruction on the skiing injury risk for these skiers may, therefore, be difficult to detect without further information about the instruction given.

More Norwegians had adjusted their bindings themselves than Swedes and Danes. It is important that skiers who adjust the setting of their bindings themselves are conscious of what they are doing. It is, therefore, reassuring that this group of skiers performed frequent binding tests [*7*].

About 40% of the skiers had not tested their bindings. Thus, the mode and frequency of binding testing have remained unchanged for the Norwegians but have deteriorated for the Swedes compared to previous studies [*4,5*]. Even though the figures for binding testing were about 10 percentage points higher when skiers from several other areas in Norway were included [*7*], the public information about binding testing ought to be repeated steadily to keep a high frequency of testing.

In conclusion, the risk for a skiing injury was similar for Norwegian and Swedish alpine recreational skiers. The relatively higher skiing injury ratios for Danes compared to Norwegians and Swedes even after correcting for skiing ability and experience may be related to shorter skiing seasons for the Danes [*18*], to less information about skiing safety, to poor skiing equipment, or other factors. The mode and frequency of binding testing should be improved for all Scandinavian skiers, because skiers with tested bindings are less prone to LEER injuries [*10,20*].

Acknowledgments

The authors wish to thank Sivert R. Asphaug, M.D. (Oppdal), Dag S. Skagestad, M.D. (Bykle), and Jon A. Sparby, M.D. (Trysil), who treated many of the injured skiers and kindly collected some of the data for this study. District leader Hjalmar Hansen and other members of the Red Cross Rescue Service provided part of the data for the control population of uninjured skiers. Marit Eriksen, graduate student, the Norwegian College of Physical Education and Sport, and Per Ludvigsen, engineer, Sophies Minde Orthopaedic Hospital, provided technical help.

The study has been financially supported by grants from the Norwegian Confederation of Sport and the Norwegian Research Council for Science and the Humanities.

References

[*1*] Danielsson, K., "Swedish Measures for Reduction of Skiing Accidents with Special Reference to Children," *Orthopedic Clinics of North America*, Vol. 7, No. 1, 1976, pp. 59–61.

[*2*] Danielsson, K., "Prevention of Skiing Accidents by Action of the National Swedish Board for Consumers Policies," in *Skiing Safety II*, J. M. Figueras, Ed., *International Series on Sport Sciences*, Vol. 5, University Park Press, Baltimore, 1978, pp. 156–169.

[*3*] Eriksson, E. and Danielsson, K., "A National Ski Injury Survey," in *Skiing Safety II*, J. M. Figueras, Ed., *International Series on Sport Sciences*, Vol. 5, University Park Press, Baltimore, 1978, pp. 47–55.

[*4*] Ekeland, A., "Injuries to Advanced and Expert Skiers During Summer Skiing," in *Ski Trauma and Skiing Safety III*, R. J. Johnson, W. Hauser, J. Karlsson, and M. K. Lamont, Eds., Publication Series of TÜV-Edition, Munich, 1982, pp. 119–125.

[*5*] Ekeland, A. and Lund, Ø., "Functional Control of Release Bindings in Uninjured Scandinavian Skiers," in *Ski Trauma and Skiing Safety IV*, W. Hauser, J. Karlsson, and M. Magi, Eds., Publication Series of TÜV-Edition, Munich, 1982, pp. 59–68.

[*6*] Ekeland, A., Larsen, S. R., Tuxen, A. G., and Nygaard, P., "Organization of Skiing Safety in Norway," in *Skiing Trauma and Safety: Seventh International Symposium, ASTM STP 1022*,

R. J. Johnson, C. D. Mote, Jr., and M.-H. Binet, Eds., American Society for Testing and Materials, Philadelphia, 1989, pp. 342–353.

[7] Ekeland, A., Holtmoen, Å., and Lystad, H., "Skiing Behavior of Alpine Recreational Skiers," in *Skiing Trauma and Safety: Seventh International Symposium, ASTM STP 1022*, R. J. Johnson, C. D. Mote, Jr., and M.-H. Binet, Eds., American Society for Testing and Materials, Philadelphia, 1989, pp. 85–93.

[8] Diem, K. and Lentner, C., Eds., Documenta Geigy. *Scientific Tables*, 7th ed., Ciba-Geigy Ltd., Basel, 1975, p. 172.

[9] Bhattacharyya, G. K. and Johnson, R. A., *Statistical Concepts and Methods*, Wiley, New York, 1977, pp. 441–444.

[10] Ekeland, A., Holtmoen, Å., and Lystad, H., "Skiing Injuries in Alpine Recreational Skiers," in *Skiing Trauma and Safety: Seventh International Symposium, ASTM STP 1022*, R. J. Johnson, C. D. Mote, Jr., and M.-H. Binet, Eds., American Society for Testing and Materials, Philadelphia, 1989, pp. 41–50.

[11] Shealy, J. E., "Overall Analysis of NSAA/ASTM Data on Skiing Injuries for 1978 Through 1981," in *Skiing Trauma and Safety: Fifth International Symposium, ASTM STP 860*, R. J. Johnson and C. D. Mote, Jr., Eds., American Society for Testing and Materials, Philadelphia, 1985, pp. 302–313.

[12] Nilssen, A., Tuveng, J. M., Paus, A., and Holter, I., "Skiing Injuries, Alpine Sports," in *Skiing Trauma and Skiing Safety IV*, W. Hauser, J. Karlsson, and M. Magi, Eds., Publication Series of TÜV-Edition, Munich, 1982, pp. 187–194.

[13] Nielsen, K., "Vintersportsskader" (Wintersport Injuries), *Ugeskrift for Læger*, Vol. 148, 1986, pp. 480–481.

[14] Krogsgaard, M. R., "Danske skiskader" (Danish Skiing Injuries), *Ugeskrift for Læger*, Vol. 149, 1987, pp. 185–187.

[15] Johnson, R. J. and Ettlinger, C. F., "Alpine Ski Injuries: Changes Through the Years," *Clinics in Sports Medicine*, Vol. 1, No. 2, 1982, pp. 181–197.

[16] Hauser, W., Asang, E., and Müller, B., "Injury Risk in Alpine Skiing," in *Skiing Trauma and Safety: Fifth International Symposium, ASTM STP 860*, R. J. Johnson and C. D. Mote, Jr., Eds., American Society for Testing and Materials, Philadelphia, 1985, pp. 338–348.

[17] Ekeland, A., Holtmoen, Å., and Lystad, H., "Lower Extremity Equipment Related Injuries in Alpine Recreational Skiers," *American Journal of Sports Medicine* (submitted for publication).

[18] Ravn, H., Langkilde, N. C., Ovesen, P. G., Busch, F., Christensen, K., et al., "Skiskademønsteret i Vejle Amt (Ski Injury Pattern in Vejle Province), *Ugeskrift for Læger*, Vol. 150, 1988, pp. 1148–1151.

[19] Lauridsen, K., Boel, J., and Jørgensen, U., "Ætiologi og profylakse ved skiskader—en dansk skadestueopgørelse" (Etiology and Prophylaxis for Skiing Injuries—A Danish Emergency Room Registration), *Nordisk Medicin*, Vol. 103, 1988, pp. 19–20.

[20] Ascherl, R., Schlemmer, H., Lechner, F., and Bluemel, G., "A Ten Year Survey of Skiing Injuries," in *Ski Trauma and Skiing Safety IV*, W. Hauser, J. Karlsson, and M. Magi, Eds., Publication Series of TÜV-Edition, Munich, 1982, pp. 153–163.

Robert J. Johnson,[1] Carl F. Ettlinger,[2] and Jasper E. Shealy[3]

Femoral Shaft Fractures Resulting from Alpine Skiing Injuries

---

REFERENCE: Johnson, R. J., Ettlinger, C. F., and Shealy, J. E., "**Femoral Shaft Fractures Resulting from Alpine Skiing Injuries,**" *Skiing Trauma and Safety: Eighth International Symposium, ASTM STP 1104*, C. D. Mote, Jr. and Robert J. Johnson, Eds., American Society for Testing and Materials, Philadelphia, 1991, pp. 152–157.

ABSTRACT: This study investigates femoral shaft fractures resulting from skiing accidents occurring at a moderate-sized Northern Vermont ski area over a 15-year interval from 1972 through 1987. Twenty-one skiers sustaining femoral fractures were compared to *5240* other injured skiers who sustained *5678* injuries and a control population. The incidence of femoral shaft fractures was approximately 1 for every 80 000 skier days and was unchanged during the study period. Of the 21 fractures, 17 resulted from bending injuries. There was no evidence to suggest that binding dysfunction contributed to these injuries. Skiers sustaining femoral fractures were found to be similar to the control population in age, height, weight, tibial length, skiing ability, and skiing experience and to use similar skiing equipment. They were taller, heavier, more skilled and experienced, involved in fewer falls, skied faster, more frequently injured in collisions, more likely to have a binding release, and more likely to slide or tumble before their injury than skiers sustaining tibial fractures. The age of skiers sustaining tibial and femoral shaft fractures were similar.

KEY WORDS: alpine skiing, injury, femur fracture, epidemiology

Although femoral shaft fractures rarely result from alpine skiing accidents, they have been noted in many studies of ski injuries [*1–15*]. In O'Malley's study, ski patrollers and physicians reported 115 femoral fractures (shaft, 64; hip, 39; supracondylar, 8; and distal femoral epiphysis, 4) resulting from skiing injuries from multiple ski areas largely from the northeastern United States, but the study gives no statistics concerning their causes [*10*]. Although little information exists concerning the incidence of these injuries through the years, O'Malley, Sherry, and Yvars and Kanner stated that a femoral fracture occurred at the rate of 1 to 1.5 per 100 000 skier days [*10,11,13*], and Korbel reported that 7.9% of all the fractures he evaluated near an Australian ski resort involved the femur [*6*]. Femoral fractures ranged from 0.1 to 1.5% of all injuries reported in several studies [*2–7,10–15*]. Moritz and Ellison stated that almost all femoral shaft fractures result from collisions [*8,16*]. Dubravik et al. reported the same high collision rate and suggested that poor snow coverage was an important related factor [*2*]. They noted that temperature, snow conditions, age, skiing ability, and binding function were not related to the occurrence of femoral fractures.

Because femoral shaft fractures represent a severe and debilitating injury and could potentially result from the ski acting as a lever to bend or twist the lower extremity, we

[1]Professor, Department of Orthopaedic Surgery and Rehabilitation, University of Vermont College of Medicine, Green Bldg., Rm. C444A, Burlington, VT 05405.

[2]President, Vermont Ski Safety Equipment, Inc., Box 168, Underhill, VT 05489.

[3]Professor, Department of Industrial Engineering, Rochester Institute of Technology, 1 Lomb Memorial Dr., Rochester, NY 14623.

investigated this injury in some detail. Many investigators in recent years have reported a decrease in the incidence of injuries involving the foot, ankle, and lower leg and, at the same time, have noted an increase in the number of severe injuries to the ligaments of the knee [*17*]. Modern skiing equipment is capable of protecting the lower leg but has not reduced the risk of severe knee injuries. Does this trend also imply that there is a tendency for equipment malfunction to affect adversely the rate of femoral shaft injuries as well? Ascherl noted that there appeared to be an increase in the number of femoral shaft fractures between 1972 and 1981 in his investigation in Germany [*1*]. Yvars and Kanner also noted an increase in the incidence of femoral fractures during 1981 through 1983 [*13*]. However, only three reports of the incidence of femoral shaft fracture relative to the population at risk could be found in the literature [*10,11,13*].

This study will document the incidence of femoral shaft fractures versus the population at risk over a 15-year period, evaluate the characteristics of individuals sustaining fractures of the femur versus those of skiers sustaining tibial fractures and other injuries and a group of uninjured skiers, and ascertain if a relationship exists between equipment malfunction and the generation of femoral shaft fractures in alpine skiers.

Methods

The general method of analysis of the information presented in this paper is the same as that presented elsewhere [*17*]. The study evaluates 39 patients who suffered fractures of the femur at a moderate-sized northern Vermont ski area between 1972 and 1987. Of these fractures, 9 involved the femoral neck or intertrochanteric region, 2 involved the distal femoral epiphysis, and 29 involved the femoral shaft. The 21 femoral shaft fractures that occurred during the 15-year period of analysis at the northern mountain of the ski area are included in the epidemiological analysis presented in this study. The other 8 femoral shaft fractures occurred at the southern mountain of the ski area during the last 6 seasons of the study. They are included only in the roentgenograph analysis of fractures because X-ray film was not available on all the fractures evaluated.

Comparisons of a control group (1817 uninjured skiers), femoral shaft fractures (21), tibia fractures (211), other fractures (649), and all other nonfracture injuries (4798) were used to determine differences between these groups for the various parameters evaluated. The statistics used to determine the significance of observations made included Chi square (Cs), Kolmogorov-Smirnov (KS), student *t*-test (ST), and one-way ANOVA (AN).

Results

Epidemiological Study

During the 15-year epidemiological investigation, we evaluated 5699 ski injuries sustained by 5251 injured skiers resulting from 1 690 000 skiers visits. There was a total of 871 fractures, of which 21 involved the femoral shaft. Thus, femoral shaft fractures accounted for 0.37% of all injuries and 2.4% of all fractures. Of these, 19 were closed injuries; 2 were compound. Ten involved the right leg, and ten involved the left leg. In one instance, the side of the body injured was not recorded. The mean age of these 21 skiers was 22.8 years. Fourteen fractures involved males; seven occurred to females. Males were overrepresented in the femoral fracture group as compared to the control population, but not at a significant level. The incidence of femoral shaft fractures was 1 in 80 295 skier days and was not found to vary significantly during the study. Seasonal totals ranged from 0 (0% of all injuries) to 3 (0.9% of all injuries).

Comparing the age of skiers sustaining femoral fractures (mean 22.8) and tibial fractures (mean 22.9) to those of the control group (mean 25.6) revealed that both fracture groups were significantly younger than the uninjured control skiers (AN $P < 0.0001$). The heights of patients sustaining femoral fractures, fractures other than the tibia and femur, all nonfracture injuries, and controls were not different. Patients sustaining tibial fractures were on average 3.5 in. (9 cm) shorter than the other groups (AN $P < 0.0001$).

Patients sustaining femoral shaft fractures were not lighter than the control population, whereas the tibial fracture group was significantly lighter than the controls (AN $P < 0.0001$). Tibial lengths, measured from the medial joint line to the medial malleolus and tibial head diameters measured transversely just above the fibula head, were recorded for patients in all study groups. The lengths of tibias of the skiers with femoral shaft fractures were not different from those of the control population, while those of skiers who sustained tibial fractures were significantly shorter (mean 3.0 cm, AN $P < 0.0001$). The ratio of tibia length to tibial head diameter was also established. The tibias of patients who sustained femoral shaft fractures were found to be relatively longer and narrower (tibial head diameter) than those who suffered fractures of the shaft of the tibia (AN $P < 0.01$).

The self-determined ability level of skiers suffering femoral shaft fractures was not different from that of the control population but was higher than all other injury groups. Individuals with tibial shaft fractures were found to have the lowest level of ability of all groups examined (femoral fractures, other fractures, and all nonfracture injuries, as well as the control group) (AN $P < 0.0001$).

Skier experience, based on the product of the number of seasons skied and the mean number of days skied each season, revealed that individuals sustaining femoral shaft fractures had 2.3 times more total skiing experience than individuals sustaining tibial shaft fractures and had equal experience to the control population (AN $P < 0.0001$).

Skiers with femoral shaft fractures averaged 3.7 years more seasons skied than those with tibial fractures (ST $P < 0.05$). The total seasons skied for the femoral shaft fracture group was not different from the control population.

All groups of skiers were asked how many times they fell on the last full day they skied before they sustained an injury or were interviewed to be included as a "control" skier in this study. Skiers sustaining femoral fractures had fallen fewer times than any other group, while those suffering tibial fractures had fallen most frequently (AN $P < 0.0001$).

Collisions with trees or other solid objects accounted for 65% of femoral shaft fractures, 15% of tibial shaft fractures, 17% of fractures of bones other than the tibia and femur, and 17% of injuries not including fractures. Thus, femoral shaft fractures involved collisions at a significantly higher rate than the other injury categories (CS $P < 0.0001$).

We observed no differences in the age of boots and bindings of skiers in the fracture groups or the control population. Likewise, no differences in the interval between servicing and adjustment of equipment by a professional shop mechanic or by the skier could be found among the several groups studied. We did find, however, that binding release occurred during the accident more frequently to skiers sustaining femoral fractures (56%) than to those having tibial fractures (34%) (Cs $P < 0.0001$). Skiers suffering fractures to bones other than the tibia and femur and nonfracture injuries had an incidence of release during the accident similar to those sustaining femoral fractures. All skiers were asked if their bindings had released properly in previous falls. Skiers sustaining femoral shaft fractures and control skiers felt that their equipment had functioned properly in over 80% of the cases, while equipment of those sustaining tibial fractures had previously functioned properly in 68% of the instances (Cs $P < 0.0001$).

TABLE 1—*Location of 22 femoral shaft fractures.*

Proximal third	1
Junction	5
Middle third	5
Junction	8
Distal	4
Total	23[a]

[a]One segmental fracture, middle third and junction.

Skier speed at the time of injury tended to be higher for the femoral fracture group than other injury categories (AN $P < 0.01$). Skiers sustaining femoral fractures were more frequently skiing in the fall line than those in the other injury groups who were more frequently traversing at the time of their injury (Cs $P < 0.05$). Seventy percent of skiers with femoral fractures slid or tumbled some distance before sustaining their injury, whereas those in other groups did so less frequently (tibia, 57%; nonfracture injuries, 36%; and fractures other than tibia or femur, 35%; Cs $P < 0.001$).

Roentgenograph Investigation

Original roentgenographs were available for 22 of the 29 patients who sustained femoral shaft fractures at either the north or the south mountain of the ski area. The analysis of these films revealed that the majority of the fractures occurred in the distal portion of the bone (Table 1) and that 17 of 22 skiers had fracture patterns that were consistent with bending rather than torque injuries (Table 2). The relatively low incidence of communication (7 of 22 fractures) suggests that the majority of these injuries resulted from relatively low energy trauma.

Discussion

Our investigation demonstrated that femoral shaft fractures are not increasing in incidence with respect to the population at risk at the ski area we studied. The incidence of femoral shaft fractures of one for every 80 000 skier days was similar to the estimates of O'Malley and Yvars and Kanner [*10,13*].

Binet and Ascherl reported that the incidence of these injuries in Europe has risen [*1*].[4] While this may be true, these authors are reporting results from statistics gathered at medical facilities rather than from the entire population at risk, and their information may simply result from changes in the percentage of femoral shaft fractures in a population of injured skiers they are testing. There would appear to be an increase in the number of femoral shaft fractures they treated if the number of other lower extremity fractures decreased. If, at the same time, the skiing population at risk increased, one would then see an increase in the number of femoral shaft fractures even if the injury rate (based on the population at risk) remained the same or even decreased.

Our analysis also demonstrated that the characteristics of skiers suffering femoral shaft fractures differ dramatically from those sustaining tibial fractures. Although they were similar in age, patients sustaining femoral fractures were taller, heavier, more experienced, more often involved in collisions, more often had a binding release, and more often had properly functioning equipment.

[4]M.-H. Binet, personal communication, presented at the International Society for Skiing Safety meeting, Riksgränsen, Sweden, May 1989.

TABLE 2—*Fracture type of 22 femoral shaft fractures.*

Oblique	10
Transverse	6
Spiral	5
Segmental	1
Total	22

Investigation of the type of fracture pattern revealed that the majority of femoral shaft fractures result from bending rather than torsion. This, coupled with the high incidence of collision involved in the production of these injuries, strongly suggests that torques passed from the ski to the femur are not frequently a contributing factor. Evaluation and functional testing of the equipment associated with the four spiral fractures in the epidemiological portion of this study suggested that in only two cases was there even the potential for binding dysfunction to be a causative factor. Yamada showed that the torsional strength of the femoral shaft is approximately 1.4 times that of the tibia [*18*]. Because the torsional strength of the femur is 40% greater than the tibia (1400 versus 1000 kg/cm), it is logically not possible for a torsional load to pass axially through the boot–binding interface to the boot, to the foot, to the tibia, the knee, and ultimately the femur in sufficient magnitude to cause femur failure in torsion without first experiencing a torsional failure of the tibia. This may explain why no improvement has been seen in the incidence of femur fractures over time and why there is no reason to expect a relationship between the skiing equipment and torsional injuries to the femur. In view of these observations and the vast differences in characteristics of skiers sustaining femoral and tibia fractures, it is safe to conclude that these injuries rarely, if ever, are binding related.

Implantation of the flexed knee into soft snow with the tibia acting as a torque wrench to pass loads through the fixed knee joint could result in a spiral fracture of the femur. Likewise, rotation of the trunk above a femur fixed in the snow could produce a spiral fracture of the femur in a skiing accident. These latter two observations would, however, not implicate binding dysfunction.

Conclusions

1. The incidence of femoral shaft fractures was 1 per 80 000 skier days.
2. The incidence based on the population at risk did not change during the 15 years of the study.
3. Femoral shaft fractures do not appear to be related to ski binding dysfunction.
4. Skiers sustaining femoral fractures were found to be similar to the control population in age, height, weight, tibial length, skiing ability, skiing experience, and skiing equipment used.
5. Skiers sustaining femoral fractures were taller, heavier, more skilled and experienced, involved in fewer falls, skiing faster, more frequently injured in collisions, more likely to have a binding release, and more likely to slide or tumble before their injury than skiers sustaining tibial fractures.

References

[*1*] Ascherl, R., Schlemmer, H., Lechner, F., and Bluemel, G., "A Ten Year Survey of Skiing Injuries," in *Ski Trauma and Skiing Safety IV*, W. Hauser, J. Karlsson, and M. Magi, Eds., TÜEV-Edition, Munich, 1982, pp. 153–163.

[2] Dubravik, P., Szpilberg, M., and Maistrelli, G., "Pattern of Skiing Injuries at Mount Tremblant—A Changing Dimension," in *A Ten Year Survey of Skiing Injuries, Ski Trauma and Skiing Safety IV*, W. Hauser, J. Karlsson, and M. Magi, Eds., TÜEV-Edition, Munich, 1982, pp. 171–177.
[3] Ellison, A. E., Carroll, R. E., Haddon, W., and Wolf, M., "Skiing Injuries: Clinical Study," *Public Health Reports*, Vol. 77, No. 11, 1962, pp. 11–17.
[4] Eriksson, E., "Ski Injuries in Sweden—A One Year Study," *Orthopedic Clinics of North America*, Vol. 7, No. 1, 1976, pp. 3–9.
[5] Jaffin, B., "An Epidemiologic Study of Ski Injuries: Vail, Colorado." *Mount Sinai Journal of Medicine*, Vol. 48, 1981, pp. 353–359.
[6] Korbel, P. J. and Zelcer, J., "A Controlled Study of Skiing Injuries in Australia," in *A Ten Year Survey of Skiing Injuries, Ski Trauma and Skiing Safety IV*, W. Hauser, J. Karlsson, and M. Magi, Eds., TÜEV-Edition, Munich, 1982, pp. 178–183.
[7] Matter, P., Miller, W., and Ott, C., "Frequency of Ski Injuries in the Davos Region," *Orthopedic Clinics of North America*, Vol. 7, No. 1, 1976, pp. 31–35.
[8] Mortiz, J. R., "Ski Injuries," *Journal of the American Medical Association*, Vol. 121, 1943, pp. 97–99.
[9] Nilssen, A., Tuveng, A., Paus, A., and Holter, I., "Skiing Injuries, Alpine Sports," in *A Ten Year Survey of Skiing Injuries, Ski Trauma and Skiing Safety IV*, W. Hauser, J. Karlsson, and M. Magi, Eds., TÜEV-Edition, Munich, 1982, pp. 187–194.
[10] O'Malley, R. D., "Trends in Skiing Injuries," *Physician and Sports Medicine*, Vol. 6, No. 12, 1978, pp. 68–76.
[11] Sherry, E., "Trends in Injuries: Perisher Valley, 1962–1986, Skiing Trauma in Australia," Thesis, University of New South Wales, 1988, p. 104.
[12] Tapper, E. M., "Ski Injuries from 1939 to 1976: The Sun Valley Experience," *American Journal of Sports Medicine*, Vol. 6, 1978, pp. 114–121.
[13] Yvars, M. F. and Kanner, H. R. "Ski Fractures of the Femur," *American Journal of Sports Medicine*, Vol. 12, 1984, pp. 286–390.
[14] Shealy, J. E., "Two Year Statistical Analysis of Skiing Injuries at 13 selected areas in the USA," in *Ski Trauma and Skiing Safety IV*, W. Hauser, J. Karlsson, and M. Magi, Eds., TÜEV-Edition, Munich, 1982, pp. 207–216.
[15] Tapper, E. M. and Moritz, J. R. "Changing Patterns in Ski Injuries," *Physician and Sports Medicine*, Vol. 2, 1974, pp. 39–47.
[16] Ellison, A. E., "Skiing Injuries," *Cibia Clinical Symposium*, Vol. 29, No. 1, 1977, pp. 1–40.
[17] Johnson, R. J., Ettlinger, C. F., and Shealy, J. E., "Skier Injury Trends," in *Ski Trauma and Safety: Seventh International Symposium, ASTM STP 1022*, R. J. Johnson, C. D. Mote, Jr., and M.-H. Binet, Eds., American Society for Testing and Materials, Philadelphia, 1989, pp. 25–31.
[18] Yamada, H., in *Strength of Biological Materials*, F. G. Evans, Ed., Williams & Williams, Baltimore, 1970, pp. 59–69.

Michael K. Lamont[1]

Ski Injury Statistics—What Changes?

REFERENCE: Lamont, M. K., "**Ski Injury Statistics—What Changes?**" *Skiing Trauma and Safety: Eighth International Symposium, ASTM STP 1104*, C. D. Mote, Jr. and Robert J. Johnson, Eds., American Society for Testing and Materials, Philadelphia, 1991, pp. 158–163.

ABSTRACT: Since 1939, reports on the severity of ski injuries have claimed that downhill skiing is dangerous. The reported injury rate varies from 0.8 to 9.1 per 1000 skier days. Two studies at the same ski field, 28 years apart, gave injury rates of 2.7 and 2.4. This was over the period of greatest development for skiing and ski safety equipment. The reported injury rate in 1939 in Norway was 2.7 injuries per 1000 skier days and in 1988 in New Zealand was 4.7 injuries per 1000 skier days. The mean for that 49-year period was 3.5 injuries per 1000 skier days. The mix of injuries has clearly changed, but the actual rate of injury as measured in injuries per skier day has hardly altered. Is skiing safer now than in 1939, or are the comparisons not equal? Well-designed epidemiological studies are needed to measure true incidence accurately; only then can the effectiveness of safety measures be determined.

KEY WORDS: skiing injuries, injury rate (per 1000 skier days), international comparisons (of rate), injury mix, muscle strength, incidence, safety precautions

The return of the Skiing Safety and Ski Trauma Conferences to Riksgransen, Sweden, where it was first held in 1974, allows a review of the past 15 years to determine what impact there has been on skiing safety or, more importantly, what has changed. As a result of the increasing number of skiing injuries and the increasingly popular notion that skiing is excessively dangerous, these conferences were initiated to bring together concerned people from throughout the world to discuss ski trauma. The topics discussed were the incidence of injury, the type of injuries and treatment, but, more importantly, the programs capable of preventing or at least reducing the risk of ski injuries.

In 1939, Bernhardt reported a study of all ski injuries at one Swedish ski area and found a ski injury rate of 2.7 per 1000 skier days [*1*]. Westlin reported a similar study from the same ski area in 1967 and found an incidence of 2.4 per 1000 skier days [*2*]. During the 1960s, a number of papers were published that dealt with ski trauma statistics [*1,3*]. In the early 1970s, a few papers clearly indicated the size of the problem [*4–6*]. In the literature of the 1960s and 1970s, the injury rate varied between 3 and 7 injuries per 1000 skier days [*2,7–9*]. In the 1972/73 ski season, Johnson et al., observed an injury rate at the Glen Ellen (now Sugarbush) ski area in Northern Vermont of approximately 5 per 1000 skier days [*10*]. At Waterfall Valley, New Hampshire, the ski injury rates have declined steadily from 4.2 in 1966 to 2.8 per 1000 skier days for the 1973/74 season [*5*].

In other countries, the ski injury rate has been expressed in different terms. This makes direct comparison impossible.

Campbell et al. reviewed the ski injury statistics for the period December 1972 to April 1978 at the Sugarbush North Skifield in Vermont [*11*]. They reported an overall injury rate

[1]Private physiotherapist, Mangere Health Centre, Waddon Place Mangere, Auckland, New Zealand.

of 4.2 per 1000 skier days, which had declined from 5.3 to 3.3 per 1000 skier days during the 6-year period. Similarly, Crane et al., in updating their Waterville study, confirmed that the accident rate remains stready at slightly less than 3.5 per 1000 skier days [*12*]. In Seattle, Washington, Requa and Garrick reported an injury rate of 9.1 per 1000 skier days for 1971/72 and 1972/73 winters among participants of five major ski schools in that area [*13*]. The highest incident rate was 10.89 per 1000 skier days on a slope classified as "easy."

In a 10-year study in Europe completed in 1981, Ascherl et al. reported an accident rate between 1.1 and 2.8 injuries for every 1000 skier days [*14*]. However, within the last two winters of the study, they noticed an increase in the incidence. In the Laurentian Mountains north of Montreal, Dubravick reported an injury rate of 2.7 per 1000 skier days for the 1979/81 ski seasons [*15*]. In Australia, Korbel and Zeker recorded an injury rate of 1.42 for the 1978 season, 1.31 for the 1979 season, and 1.4 for the 1980 season [*16*]. They also note a 30% increase in the numbers of skiers during that period.

In reviewing the 1979/80 ski injuries in 13 selected ski areas across the United States, Shealy noted an overall injury rate of 2.16 injuries per 1000 skier days, and that this was the same injury rate for the previous year [*17*]. But he commented that it was a 50% reduction over injury rates from 10 to 15 years before, as was documented in the Sugarbush North studies. Shealy, in a review of statistics, has accurately commented that in some studies the overall injury rates decreased from 5.9 injuries per 1000 skier days in the 1960/61 winter season in Austria to 3.4 injuries per 1000 skier days in 1972/73, thus giving a 42% decrease [*18*].

There has clearly been a drop in the lower extremity injuries and an increase in the upper extremity injuries [*19,20*]. Shealy's finding that modern equipment is reducing the lower extremity injury rate while having little or no effect on the upper extremity rate is consistent with findings of many researchers during the past 10 years. Note, however, that these relationships compare studies from the early 1960s to the early 1970s, and that was the time when there was the greatest development in ski binding research and, thus, a significant reduction in tibial fractures. Shealy has continued his overall analysis of skiing data, and, when reporting on ski injuries in the United States during the period of 1978 through 1981, noted that the weighted overall average was 3.2 injuries per 1000 skier days [*21*]. He observed that the earlier downward trend had become somewhat level for the previous 5 years (1972–1977) and attributed that to the high quality of design and manufacture of the boot/binding systems. He postulated that there should not be a dramatic decline in the future.

In a large study in Japan spanning 28 years from December 1956 to April 1984, Kuriyama and Fujimaki reviewed almost 50 000 injuries [22]. They report that the injury rate in the 1960s was between 0.7 and 1%, while the injury rate in the 1984 season was 0.8%. Clearly, there has been very little change in that ski area over that 28-year period, however, they correctly report that the mix of injury within the rate has changed. This has been reported in many instances elsewhere.

The most recent statistics are those from the Cardrona Ski Field in the South Island of New Zealand where the injury rate was 3.8 per 1000 skier days in the winter of 1987, and 4.7 per 1000 skier days in the winter of 1988.[2]

The literature is divided on whether to use the term *skier days* or *skier visits*. There is a subtle difference between the two, and it is likely that various researchers have used the same definition to describe both those events. A skier day could be assumed to be the quantitative measure of skiing done, whereas skier visit simply denotes that x number of

[2]Cardrona Ski Area Medical Report, 1988, p. 1, personal communication, Dr. G. Carpenter, Ski Patrol Director.

people visited the ski field. That does not necessarily mean that they all skied. An international agreement on accepted terminology would be useful so that future studies can be compared equally.

Perhaps the term *injury ratio* (injured skiers [%]/uninjured skiers [%]) would be more appropriate. The "standardization" of the ratio—the numerator and the denominator of the ratio standardized to the same population distribution—would further assist in comparative analyses among ski fields and countries. Ekeland et al. [*23*] has demonstrated that the use of injury ratio is appropriate and effective.

Table 1 depicts the incident rates ranging from the first reported in 1939 to the most recently reported in 1988. The collection of information about the original population has been varied. Some statisticians use ski patrol-based reports, others use clinic or base hospital reports, and still others survey the skiing population to determine the incidence. An unknown number of skiers leave the ski field without reporting their injuries. The underreporting of skier's thumb is a good example. In determining the total population (skiers at risk), researchers have used various measures, but, in the end, they have been satisfied that they have, as well as could be expected, calculated a finite population. At least 22 studies (as herein reported) have used the injury rate calculated on skier days. Accepting that there are variations in the definition of an injury, variations in the definition of the injured population, and variations in the total population, it is nevertheless interesting to observe the changes.

The mean injury rate per 1000 skier days is 3.65 with a standard deviation of 2.088. The 95% confidence limit is between 3.45 and 3.86 injuries per 1000 skier days. In spite of the variations as mentioned above, the 95% confidence level is close, and, thus, the injury rate of 3.65 can be relied on with some certainty. It should be a "benchmark." Those rates have

TABLE 1—*Frequency (per 1000 skier days) of downhill skiing injuries.*

Author	Year(s) of Study		Country
Bernhard [*24*]	1939	2.7	Sweden
Haddon et al. [*25*]	1962	5.9	USA
McAlister et al. [*26*]	1965	7.3	USA
Sponsel [*27*]	1967	4.0	USA
Westlin [*2*]	1967	2.4	Sweden
Johnson et al. [*20*]	1972	5.0	USA
Ellison [*4*]	1973	4.5	USA
Requa et al. [*13*]	1971–73	9.1	USA
Gutman et al. [*28*]	1974	3.4	USA
Young et al. [*17*]	1976	2.8	USA
Campbell et al. [*11*]	1972–78	4.2	USA
Gelehrter et al. [*29*]	1978	5.7	Austria
Ekeland [*30*]	1979	1.13	Norway
Korbel et al. [*16*]	1980	1.4	Australia
Arscherl et al. [*14*]	1971–81	2.4	Germany
Dubravick [*15*]	1979–81	2.7	Canada
Shealy [*17*]	1979–80	2.16	USA
Shealy [*21*]	1979–81	2.16	USA
Kuriyama et al. [*22*]	1956–83	0.9	Japan
Kuriyama et al. [*22*]	1984	0.8	Japan
Personal communication[a]	1987	3.8	New Zealand
Personal communication[b]	1988	4.7	New Zealand

[a]Cardrona Ski Area Ltd., Medical Report 1987, Dr. G. Carpenter.
[b]Whakapapa Skifield Statistics 1988, M. Wood.

TABLE 2—*Sites of injury.*

	Eriksson [*19*] 1974, %	Lystad [*31*] 1981, %
Lower leg	72	43
Upper limbs	20	29 (10% shoulder)
Head	3.1	14

been bettered in 1939 (2.7), 1967 (2.4), and 1976 (2.8), and equalled in 1987 (3.8). In 50 years, the rates have not changed that much, but the injuries themselves have changed.

The Changed Relationships

The site of injury has shifted away from the leg and toward the upper limb, shoulder, and head. Eriksson [*19*] reported at the last Riksgransen meeting in 1974 that, based on information gathered from throughout Sweden 72% of injuries were to the lower leg (29% were to the ankle, 32% were to the tibia, and 16% were to the knee). The upper limb (including the shoulder) accounted for 20% of all injuries, while the head accounted for only 3.1%.

In 1981 in Norway, Lystad recorded 43% of injuries to the lower leg, 29% to the upper limb, 10% to the shoulders, and 14% to the head [*31*]. The Eriksson and Lystad studies are compared in Table 2.

The 1974 Swedish study [*19*] noted 15% knee injuries and 23.6% tibial fractures. At the Cardrona Ski Field in the South Island of New Zealand in the 1988 season, knee injuries accounted for 27% of all injuries and tibial fractures accounted for 6%.[2] At the Whakapapa Ski Field in the North Island of New Zealand, tibial fractures have decreased to 3% of total injuries while knee injuries are 14% of the total.[3] There were as many fractures of the forearm as there were tibial fractures (Table 3)!

Once again, the statistics are variable. With respect to knee trauma, there has been an increase, and this has led to "a sports medicine dilemma" as discussed by Johnson as related to anterior cruciate ligament injuries [*32*].

The population at risk is still the beginner to intermediate skier, the younger skier, and the lighter skier. Collisions with other skiers and ski field obstacles such as lift pylons, rocks, and trees continue to be a problem. High-density skiing, in Japan particularly, produces an alarmingly high risk of collisions. Ski field management has a role to play in minimizing accidents by eliminating known danger areas, protecting on-slope obstacles, and controlling the skiers themselves. The pressure of the skiing public for more skiing and less queuing forces competing ski fields to install greater capacity uphill transport systems, and thereby doubling or tripling the skier density. Recommended skier density standards would guide ski field designers and would minimize the problem of overcrowding.

Because most research has been related to equipment there have been rapid design changes in equipment. All equipment problems are not yet solved.

But research has neglected, to some degree, the skiing environment and the skier. The ski slope can be modified to minimize dangers, as already described. Skiers must become more assertive and patronize those fields that provide the best prepared slope and the "best" injury statistics.

The skier is subjected to a great deal of "propoganda" related to the sport. Skiing safety needs to be part of that. Louie and Mote have advocated joint protection from strong muscles [*33*]. Their timely research clearly shows the influence of muscle activity on joint

[3]Whakapapa Skifield Statistics, 1988, personal communication, M. Woods, Ski Patrol Director.

TABLE 3—*Sites of injury.*

	Sweden 1974, %	Cardrona 1988, %[a]	Whakapapa 1988, %[b]
Knee	15	27	14
Tibia	23.6	6	3
Forearm	?	?	3

[a]Cardrona—Ski Area Ltd., Medical Report 1988, Ski Patrol Director, Dr. G. Carpenter.
[b]Whakapapa—Skifield Statistics 1988, Ski Patrol Director, M. Woods.

stiffness. Skiing revolves around the ability to control momentum precisely. Muscular strength and coordination are vital in that control. The skier cannot rely on bone or ligamentous strength alone. The skier must have muscular strength. Proper preseason ski training is obviously necessary. That, however, is a difficult message to convey to the casual weekend skier who has fashion-oriented ski images and daring "high flyer" ski posters firmly implanted in his or her brain. A serious image showing people sweating, working out at the local gymnasium, and injured skiers being "realigned" in operating theatres needs to compete with the more glamorous image of skiing.

As participants in the Eighth International Skiing Trauma and Safety Symposium and as members of the International Society for Skiing Safety, we need to be committed to reducing the incidence of ski injuries at our own ski areas. We must tackle the problem in three ways—the skier, environment, and equipment. Keep accurate injury statistics (and comparative population information) and systematically analyze that information. Identify the problem areas, the problem skiers, and the problems associated with the equipment; then address those specific issues. The injury rate to better is 3.65 injuries per 1000 skier days. In 2 years' time, at the next conference in Australia, there may be some evidence demonstrating the lowered injury rate. Please accept that challenge and make the sport of skiing safer for everybody.

References

[*1*] Clayton, M. L., "Ski Injuries," *Clinical Orthopedics and Related Research*, Vol. 23, 1962, p. 56.

[*2*] Westlin, N., "Natur Och Frekvens Av Skador Vid Skidakning (Nature and Frequency of Ski Injuries)," *Lakartidningen*, Vol. 64, 1967, pp. 1113–1118.

[*3*] Baumgartner, W., "Sicherheit der Skiabfahrt. (Safety During Downhill Skiing)," *Munchen Med. Wochenschrift*, Vol. 102, 1960, p. 2220.

[*4*] Ellison, A. E., "Ski Injuries," *JAMA*, Vol. 223, 1973, pp. 917–919.

[*5*] Garrick, J. C., "The Epidemiology of Ski Injuries," *Minnesota Medicine*, Vol. 54, 1971, pp. 17, 18.

[*6*] Garrick, J. C., "The Mythology of Ski Injuries," *Sports Medicine*, November, 1973, pp. 35–38.

[*7*] Spademan, R., "Lower Extremity Injuries as Related to the Use of Ski Safety Bindings," *JAMA* Vol. 203, 1968, pp. 103–108.

[*8*] Truchet, P., "Nature et Frequence des Accidents de Ski," *Revue Pratique*, (Paris), Vol. 11, 1961, p. 3259.

[*9*] Westlin, N., "Skidsportskador—Orsak, Uppkomstmekanism, Profylax (Ski Injuries—Their Cause, Origin and Prophylaxis)," *Lakartidningen*, Vol. 66, 1969, pp. 1435–1445.

[*10*] Johnson, R. J., Pope, M. H., and Ettlinger, C., "The Interrelationship Between Ski Accidents, the Resultant Injury, the Skiers' Characteristics and the Ski-Binding-Boot System," *Journal of Sports Medicine*, Dec. 1974.

[*11*] Campbell, R. J., Ettlinger, C. H., Johnson, R. J., and Pope, M. H., "High Risk Injury Groups in Downhill Skiing," in *Ski Trauma and Skiing Safety III*, TUV Publication Series, Munich, 1982, pp. 126–133.

[*12*] Crane, H. D., Young, L., and Cushing, W., "The Influence of Equipment and Ski Factors on Ski Injuries With an Update—13 Year Study," in *Ski Trauma and Skiing Safety III*, TUV Publication Series, Munich, 1982, pp. 134–138.

[*13*] Requa, R. K. and Garrick, J. G., "Skiing Injuries in Children and Adolescents," in *Skiing Safety III*, University Park Press, 1978, pp. 5–10.
[*14*] Ascherl, R., Schlemmer, H., Lechuer, F., and Bluemel, G., "A Ten Year Survey of Skiing Injuries," in *Ski Trauma and Skiing Safety IV*, TUV Publication, Munich, 1982, pp. 153–163.
[*15*] Dubravick, P., Szpilberg, M., and Maistrelli, G., "Pattern of Skiing Injuries at Mount Tremblant: A Changing Dimension," in *Ski Trauma and Skiing Safety IV*, TUV Publication, Munich, 1982, pp. 171–177.
[*16*] Korbel, P. J. and Zeker, J., "A Controlled Study of Skiing Injuries in Australia," in *Ski Trauma and Skiing Safety IV*, TUV Publication, Munich, 1982, pp. 178–183.
[*17*] Shealy, J. E., "Two Year Statistical Analysis of Skiing Injuries at 13 Selected Areas in the USA," in *Ski Trauma and Skiing Safety IV*, TUV Publication, Munich, 1982, pp. 207–216.
[*18*] Shealy, J. E., "Use of Statistics in Identifying Problems in Ski Injury Research," in *Skiing Trauma and Safety: Fifth International Symposium, ASTM STP 860*, R. J. Johnson and C. D. Mote, Jr., Eds., American Society for Testing and Materials, Philadelphia, 1985, pp. 285–292.
[*19*] Eriksson, E., "Ski Injuries in Sweden—A One Year Survey," *Orthopaedic Clinics of North America*, Vol. 7, No. 1, Jan. 1976, pp. 3-9.
[*20*] Johnson, R. J., Ettlinger, C. F., and Shealy, J. E., "Skier Injury Trends," in *Skiing Trauma and Safety: Seventh International Symposium, ASTM STP 1022*, R. J. Johnson, C. D. Mote, Jr., and M.-H. Binet, Eds., American Society for Testing Materials, Philadelphia, 1989, pp. 25–31.
[*21*] Shealy, J. E., "Overall Analysis of NSAA/ASTM Data on Skiing Injuries for 1978 through 1981," in *Skiing Trauma and Safety: Fifth International Symposium, ASTM STP 860*, R. J. Johnson and C. D. Mote, Jr., Eds., American Society for Testing and Materials, Philadelphia, 1985, pp. 302–313.
[*22*] Kuriyama, S. and Fujimaki, E., "Current Trends in Ski Injuries and Their Relationship to Recent Changes in Ski Equipment," in *Skiing Trauma and Safety: Sixth International Symposium, ASTM STP 938*, C. D. Mote, Jr. and R. J. Johnson, Eds., American Society for Testing and Materials, Philadelphia, 1987, pp. 263–270.
[*23*] Ekeland, A., Holtmoen, A., and Lystad, H., "Skiing Injuries in Alpine Recreational Skiers," in *Skiing Trauma and Safety: Seventh International Symposium, ASTM STP 1022*, R. J. Johnson, C. D. Mote, Jr., and M.-H. Binet, Eds., American Society for Testing Materials, Philadelphia, 1989, pp. 41–50.
[*24*] Bernhard, C., "Skiskador i statistik," *Nordisk Medicin*, Vol. 1, 1939, pp. 386–388.
[*25*] Haddon, W., Jr., Ellison, A. E., and Carrol, R. E., "Skiing Injuries: Epidemiologic Study," *Public Health Reports*, Vol. 77, 1962, pp. 975–985.
[*26*] McAlister, R., Brody, J. A., Hammes, L. M., Feltz, E. T., Duncan, D. L., and Williams, M. L., "Epidemiology of Ski Injuries in the Anchorage Area," *Archives of Environmental Health* Vol. 10, 1965, pp. 910–914.
[*27*] Sponsel, K. H., "Weekend Ski Injuries at Mt Telemark, Cable, Wisconsin 1965-1966 Season," *Industrial Medicine and Surgery*, Vol. 36, 1967, pp. 35–40.
[*28*] Gutman, J., Weisbuch, 3., and Wolf, M., "Ski Injuries in 1972–1978. A Repeat Analysis of a Major Health Problem" *JAMA*, Vol. 230, No. 10, 1974, pp. 1423–1425.
[*29*] Gelehrter, R. and Zoth, K., "Zur Epidemiologie des alpinen Skiunfalls in Oesterreich," *Monatsschrift Fuer Unfallheilkunde, H Unfallheilkunde*, Vol. 130, 1978, pp. 35–39.
[*30*] Ekeland, A., "Injuries to Advanced and Expert Skiers During Summer Skiing," in *Ski Trauma and Skiing Safety III*, TUV Publications, Munich, 1982, p. 120.
[*31*] Lystad, H., "A One Year Study of Alpine Ski Injuries in Hemsedal, Norway," in *Skiing Trauma and Safety: Fifth International Symposium, ASTM STP 860*, American Society for Testing and Materials, Philadelphia, 1985, pp. 314–325.
[*32*] Johnson, R. J., "The Anterior Cruciate: A Dilemma in Sports Medicine," *International Journal of Sports Medicine*, Vol. 3, 1982, pp. 71–79.
[*33*] Louie, J. K. and Mote, C. D., "Contribution of the Musculature to Rotary Laxity and Torsional Stiffness at the Knee," in *Skiing Trauma and Safety: Sixth International Symposium, ASTM STP 938*, C. D. Mote, Jr. and R. J. Johnson, Eds., American Society for Testing and Materials, Philadelphia, 1987, pp. 26–52.

Brian C. Oliver[1] *and Fred L. Allman*[2]

Alpine Skiing Injuries: An Epidemiological Study

REFERENCE: Oliver, B. C. and Allman, F. L., "**Alpine Skiing Injuries: An Epidemiological Study,**" *Skiing Trauma and Safety: Eighth International Symposium, ASTM STP 1104*, C. D. Mote, Jr., and Robert J. Johnson, Eds., American Society for Testing and Materials, Philadelphia, 1991, pp. 164–169.

ABSTRACT: To ensure the maximum level of safety for alpine skiers, conditions and factors that predispose to injury need to be identified. This study surveyed potential risk factors for injury in a closed population of skiers using well-defined criteria for injury. Thirteen percent of those skiers answering the survey sustained an injury. The injury rate was 24 per 1000 skier days. Most injuries occurred on the first day of skiing. Icy conditions and fatigue appeared to predispose skiers to injury. The shoulder and knee were the most common anatomical sites of injury. Factors such as age, sex, level of ability, and conditioning, which have been implicated in previous studies as risk factors for injury in alpine skiing, did not appear to predispose the skier to injury in this controlled study.

KEY WORDS: alpine skiing injuries, epidemiology, injury risk, injury rate

Previous epidemiological studies have relied on statistics based on those skiers who reported injuries to the ski patrol or who requested medical evaluation at the ski injury clinic usually located at the base lodge [*1*]. The control populations in these studies were randomly selected individuals at the ski area, uninjured at the time of evaluation and questioning. Injured skiers who are in need of medical attention but who do not present themselves to the ski patrol and injured skiers who see physicians after returning home from their ski vacations are lost to this injury-reporting system.

Established injury rates for alpine skiing in the international literature vary from 3 to 7 injuries per 1000 skier days. Injury rates are usually reported per 1000 skier days with the number of skier days determined by the number of lift tickets sold on a given day [*2,3*].

The ability to ensure the maximum level of safety for alpine skiers rests on recognition of conditions that either increase their risk for injury or protect them from injury. Data concerning the incidence and risk of injury during alpine skiing are only as meaningful as the injury definition used in the study. One solution to the problem of defining a skiing injury, regardless of the perceived severity or medical diagnosis, is to describe the injury in terms of the region of the body involved and the functional consequence to the skier's performance, that is, lost skiing time. This study used a definition of injury based on these criteria.

No particular injury is unique to skiing alone. Sprains, contusions, dislocations, and fractures can occur with any sport. But, because of the nature of skiing and frequency of

[1]Orthropedic surgeon, Sports Medicine Center at Mease Clinic, 3251 McMullen-Booth Rd., Safety Harbor, FL 34695.

[2]Orthropedic surgeon, Atlanta Sports Medicine, 600 W. Peachtree St., N.W., Atlanta, GA 30308.

falls, injury occurs in a fairly predictable fashion. Because of the nature of equipment used in this sport, certain injuries can be anticipated. The ski can act as a lever arm attached to the foot, and, therefore, specific lower extremity injuries would be expected to occur with increased frequency when the bindings fail to release [*4*]. Another mechanism of ski injury is collision [*5*]. These can be caused by an unlimited number of factors and can produce a wide variety of injuries to any part of the body [*6*].

The trends in skiing injuries and their relationship to new ski equipment, improved skiing techniques, and slope grooming have all been well documented [*1*].

Atlanta, Georgia, is an unlikely area to be involved in an epidemiological study of ski injuries because of its geographic location. However, Atlanta has one of the largest ski clubs in the United States with over 5000 members participating in over 50 organized ski trips per year. The purpose of this study was to evaluate the injury rate in this closed population and to determine if factors such as age, sex, level of ability, experience, physical conditioning, skiing equipment, and slope condition contributed to injury.

Method

Members of the Atlanta Ski Club who participated in four one-week-long ski trips were asked to fill out an injury survey after the trip. The survey consisted of two parts. All skiers were asked to fill out Part I, which dealt with questions on age, sex, level of ability, skiing experience, physical conditioning, amount of skiing during the trip, type of equipment, and maintenance of bindings. If a skier sustained an injury that prevented them from skiing at least one day or caused pain in the injured area for two days, they were asked to fill out Part II of the survey. Part II questioned the time of injury, hours skied before injury, day of injury, mechanism of injury, anatomical area injured, classification of injury, and whether medical attention was obtained.

Surveys were distributed to 232 skiers; 167 skiers responded, accounting for a 72% response rate. The respondents were divided into two populations, the injured skiers and the uninjured skiers (control group). The data were then compiled and reviewed (Table 1).

Results

The features of the injured population and the control group were similar with respect to age, sex, level of ability, years of experience, frequency of skiing over the past five years, participation in regular exercise, adjustments of bindings, and hours per day skiing. No statistical difference was found between these groups using Chi-square and *t*-test analysis. Multiple regression analyses/discriminate analyses determined that the only predictor or variable significant between the injured and noninjured group was the number of half days skied.

A higher percentage of skiers used rental equipment in the injured population (43%) than in the control population (34%), but this was not statistically significant using Chi-square analysis.

The majority of injuries occurred during conditions described as icy. The most frequent injuries were strains and sprains involving the shoulder and knee (Table 2). More injuries occurred on the first day of skiing than any other single day (Fig. 1).

Of those skiers responding to the survey, 13% suffered injuries that met the criteria described in this study. Of those skiers injured, only 14% sought medical care or were seen by the ski patrol (Table 3).

TABLE 1—*Results of ski injury survey.*

		Uninjured population (Control)	Injured population
Age	average	37 years	39 years
	range	17–74 years	30–53 years
Sex	male	47% (68)	48% (10)
	female	53% (78)	52% (11)
Level of ability	beginner	14% (20)	14% (3)
	intermediate	66% (96)	62% (13)
	advanced	20% (30)	24% (5)
Years of experience	average	9 years	8 years
	range	0–30 years	0–20 years
No. of ski trips over last five years	average	5 trips	5 trips
	range	0–25 trips	0–10 trips
"Regular" exercise		65% (95/146)	71% (15/21)
hours/week		6.2 h	5.5 h
aerobic		3.4 h	3.0 h
strength		1.9 h	1.4 h
flexibility		1.1 h	0.9 h
Skiing equipment	rental	34% (54/146)	43% (9/21)
	own	66% (96/146)	57% (12/21)
Bindings adjusted		70% (102/146)	71% (9/21)
Hours of skiing per day	average	5.2 h	5.1 h
	range	2–8 h	3–8 h

Discussion

Investigating the epidemiology of ski injuries can be a difficult task. Injuries can be caused by an unlimited number of factors. Central to injury reporting, however, is the definition of injury. This study uses a broad definition of injury, determined by the duration of pain and lost skiing time. Whether the skier was seen by medical personnel or ski patrol was not a parameter for determining injury.

Several factors contribute to alpine skiing injuries [*3*]. Previous reports have noted ski injuries to be more common on weekends [*3*] with a higher injury rate among females than among males and with first-year skiers and beginners more injury prone [*2,3*]. Although

TABLE 2—*Description of injury.*

	Injuries	Percent
Contusion	11	44
Sprain	5	20
Laceration	1	4
Fracture	1	4
Dislocation	1	4
Strain	6	24

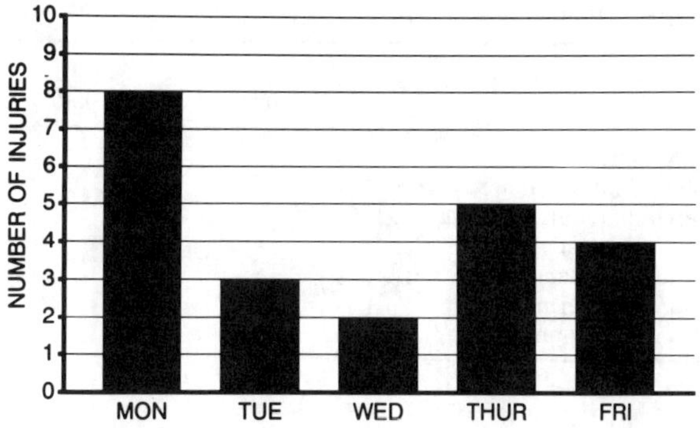

FIG. 1—*Day of week that injury occurred.*

others have found that the likelihood of a skier being injured is a function of ability more than any other single factor [*3*], we did not find this to be the case.

In this study, characteristics of the injured skiing population and uninjured population were similar with respect to age, sex, level of ability, years of experience, frequency of skiing over the past five years, participation in regular exercise, adjustment of bindings, and hours per day of skiing.

Equipment-related factors are also noted to play a role in ski injury. The results of this study reveal that there was no statistical difference in injury rate for those skiers using rental equipment.

Skiing conditions contribute to injury. In this study, the majority of injuries occurred on ice patches or during icy conditions.

Voluntary risk factors have also been described as a possible factor contributing to injury [*3*]. Voluntary risk factors denote an individual skiing on terrain above their level of ability, for example, a beginner skier skiing on an expert level trail. The results of this study reveal that most individuals skied within their described ability (Table 4). Those skiers that were injured were on ski slopes graded at or below their described ability level.

Fatigue may also be a factor contributing to injury. The average amount of time skied before injury has been noted in prior studies to be 2 to 3 h [*3,7*]. In this study, the average number of hours skied before injury was 3 h (Table 5) with most injuries occurring before the lunch break or toward the end of the skiing day. For most recreational skiers, a 3-h period of continuous skiing is probably too long. We agree with recommendations of Westlin that skiers should take short intermissions in their activity to avoid fatigue [*7*].

Established injury rates for alpine skiing vary from 3 to 7 per 1000 skier days [*2,3,8*]. The injury rate from this survey is 24 per 1000 skier days. This injury rate is higher, at least in part, because of documentation of less severe injuries that usually would go unreported in most surveys. If this injury rate is adjusted for only those people who were seen by the ski patrol or physician, the rate becomes 3.6 per 1000 skier days, a value consistent with previous

TABLE 3—*Injury rate.*

Percentage of injured skiers seen by physician or ski patrol	14%
Percentage of skiers injured	13% (21/167)
Injury rate	24/1000 skier days
Adjusted injury rate (skiers seen by physician or ski patrol)	3.6/1000 skier days
Established injury rate	3–7/1000 skier days

TABLE 4—*Voluntary risk factors in skiing injuries.*

Ability level/ski trail rating at time of injury	Number of injured skiers
Beginner/beginner	1
Beginner/intermediate	1
Intermediate/intermediate	9
Intermediate/advanced	2
Advanced/advanced	4
Advanced/intermediate	1
Advanced/beginner	1

TABLE 5—*Time factors in skiing injuries.*

	Hours skiied before injury
Average	3 h
Range	0.5–12 h
	Time of day that injury occurred
A.M.	9 injuries (11 A.M.)
P.M.	11 injuries (2–3 P.M.)

epidemiological reports. Previous prospective evaluations of skiing injuries have been performed [*9,10*]. These studies had the potential of reviewing all injuries sustained by the at-risk population. Hauser's experimental prospective study reported an injury rate of 17.3 per 1000 skier days.

Of those skiers answering the survey questions, 13% sustained an injury that prevented them from skiing at least one day or caused pain in the injured area for two days. The most common injury was a shoulder contusion or strain. The second most common injury was a knee sprain. Of those individuals injured, only 14% saw a physician or ski patrol personnel for care. Injuries that are unreported to the ski patrol or ski injury clinic at the base lodge would be lost to epidemiological surveys based on this type of reporting. Although these injuries may be considered minor in many cases, they do represent morbidity, and, if their etiology can be determined, steps can be taken to prevent their occurrence.

References

[*1*] Johnson, R. J., Ettlinger, C. F., Campbell, R. J., and Pope, M. H., "Trends in Skiing Injuries," *American Journal of Sports Medicine*, Vol. 8, No. 2, 1980, pp. 106–113.

[*2*] Johnson, R. J., Pope, M. H., and Ettlinger, C. F., "The Interrelationship Between Ski Accidents, the Resultant Injury, the Skier Characteristics and Ski Boot Binding Systems," *Orthopedic Clinics of North America*, Vol. 7, No. 1, 1976, pp. 11–12.

[*3*] Young, L. R., Omen, C. M., Crane, H., et al, "The Etiology of Ski Injuries: An Eight Year Study of the Skier and His Equipment," *Orthopedic Clinics of North America*, Vol. 7, No. 1, 1976, pp. 13–29.

[*4*] Ellison, A. E., "Skiing Injuries," *Clinical Symposia*, Vol. 1, 1977, p. 29.

[*5*] Jenkins, R., Johnson, R., Pope, M. H., "Collision Injuries in Downhill Skiing," *Skiing Trauma and Safety: Fifth International Symposium, ASTM STP 860*, R. J. Johnson and C. D. Mote, Jr., Eds., American Society for Testing and Materials, Philadelphia, 1985, pp. 358–366.

[*6*] Johnson, R. J. and Ettlinger, C. F., "Alpine Skiing Injuries: Changes Through the Years," *Clinics in Sports Medicine*, Vol. 1, No. 2, 1982, pp. 181–207.

[7] Westlin, N. E., "Factors Contributing to the Production of Skiing Injuries," *Orthopedic Clinics of North America*, Vol. 7, No. 1, 1976, pp. 45–49.

[8] Eriksson, E., "Ski Injuries in Sweden: A One Year Survey," *Orthopedic Clinics of North America*, Vol. 7, No. 1, 1976, pp. 3–9.

[9] Hauser, W., "Experimental Prospective Skiing Injury Study," in *Skiing Trauma and Safety: Seventh International Symposium, ASTM, STP 1022*, R. J. Johnson, C. D. Mote, Jr., and Marc-Hervé Binet, Eds., American Society for Testing and Materials, Philadelphia, 1989, pp. 18–24.

[10] Shealy, J. E., Geyer, L. H., and Hayden, R., "Epidemiology of Ski Injuries: An Investigation of the Effect of Method of Skill Acquisition and Release Bindings Used on Accident Rates," Industrial Engineering Research Report, State University of New York at Buffalo, 1973.

Jan Sandegård,[1] Börje Eriksson,[2] and Stig Lundkvist[3]

Nationwide Registration of Ski Injuries in Sweden

REFERENCE: Sandegård, J., Eriksson, B., and Lundkvist, S., "**Nationwide Registration of Ski Injuries in Sweden,**" *Skiing Trauma and Safety: Eighth International Symposium, ASTM STP 1104*, C. D. Mote, Jr. and Robert J. Johnson, Eds., American Society for Testing and Materials, Philadelphia, 1991, pp. 170–176.

ABSTRACT: The founding of a nationwide organization of ski areas in Sweden enabled annual collection of data from first aid services about skiing injuries and medical emergencies. The results show that, during the study period (1981 to 1988), the distribution of injuries changed very little.

Wearing a helmet has become more popular. The percentage of head injuries among those injured skiers wearing a helmet is half the percentage of head injuries among those skiing without a helmet. This may be because a helmet has a true head-protecting function, although other factors such as changing the way of falling or skiing should be considered.

Lack of background statistics makes the comparison of relative figures for various injuries presented in our investigation difficult.

KEY WORDS: ski injury, ski trauma

Few studies have been published concerning the frequency of skiing injuries throughout a whole country. One study by Ejnar Eriksson, presented at the 1974 symposium on ski trauma at Riksgränsen [*1*], was based on reports from Swedish doctors treating ski injuries. The doctors were paid for every reported ski injury.

A nationwide organization of ski areas in Sweden, the Swedish Ski Lift and Ski Areas' Organization (SLAO), was founded in 1978. This organization developed a standardized registration card to be filled out with data about injured skiers. The aims of registration are to trace injury pattern trends and to achieve a basis for skiing safety propaganda. About 90% of the ski lifts in Sweden are members of SLAO.

Method

Registration was carried out by ski area staff or ski patrollers who had assisted an injured skier who required evacuation from the area. Less severe injuries, such as skiers' thumb, arm injuries, or other minor injuries, were not included in the registration. The first registration card was used during the 1981/1982 season, with slight modification during the following seasons. The same registration card has been used from 1984 to 1990.

During the 1983/1984 and 1984/1985 seasons, measures were taken to improve the accuracy of reporting the injury.

[1]Associate professor, Department of Orthopaedic Surgery, Östersund Hospital, S-831 83, Östersund, Sweden.

[2]Research coordinator, Folksam, P.O. Box 2520, 104 60, Stockholm, Sweden.

[3]Director of Swedish Ski Lift and Ski Areas' Association, P.O. Box 582, 831 27, Östersund, Sweden.

TABLE 1—*Total ski injuries registered, 1981 to 1988.*

Ski Season	Ski Injuries
1981/1982	663
1982/1983	511
1983/1984	680
1984/1985	1592
1985/1986	2218
1986/1987	1557
1987/1988	1400
TOTAL	8621

First, SLAO, together with the Folksam Insurance Company, developed an insurance policy that was sold to the skier when he or she bought a lift ticket. This policy was bought voluntarily by the skier and was valid during the whole skiing season. The number of downhill skier insurance policies sold covers a small percentage of all Swedish skiers. However, along with the marketing of the insurance, there was a significant ski safety propaganda program consisting of posters, video films, and pamphlets shown at the lift stations.

The back of the registration form was used by the doctor to certify the medical care and diagnosis of the injury.

To encourage participation in the study, ski area staff and ski patrollers took part in a lottery carried out at the end of the season. Two of the completely filled in registration cards from all over the country were drawn, picking one ski area staff member and one ski patroller who won traveling expenses amounting to $1000.

The changing of the registration form during the first three seasons does not make a uniform report of seven seasons possible.

Furthermore, the assumption is made that nonreported ski injuries drop out randomly rather than by a systematic exclusion of certain ski injuries. The acceptance of this assumption gives us the basis to present figures as relative changes in percentage calculated from an average from these four seasons.

Results

A total of 8621 ski injuries were registered during the 1981 to 1988 seasons (Table 1).

The weekly distribution of injuries (Fig. 1) shows that the rate of injury was higher during the first three days of the week. Injury related to the hour of occurrence (Fig. 2) showed fairly even distribution, with more people injured after noon.

Fig. 3 shows that those having attended ski school during the season were in a minority of those injured.

Most injuries occurred while free skiing (Fig. 4). Very few injuries happened during ski school or racing. Accidents in lifts were responsible for less than 2% of the reported injuries. More than 80% of all injuries happened while skiing on the piste. Slightly more than 10% of the injuries occurred off piste (Fig. 5). These injuries, however, especially those in the prohibited areas, were generally more severe than those occurring on piste. The impression that very young skiers are in the majority among those skiing off piste, however, has not resulted in a corresponding domination of the number of accidents occurring off piste.

Weather did not seem to affect ski injury risk (Fig. 6).

Wearing a helmet has been the subject of propaganda since 1982–1983. Even among those injured, the wearing of a helmet is apparent (Fig. 7). The majority of people wearing

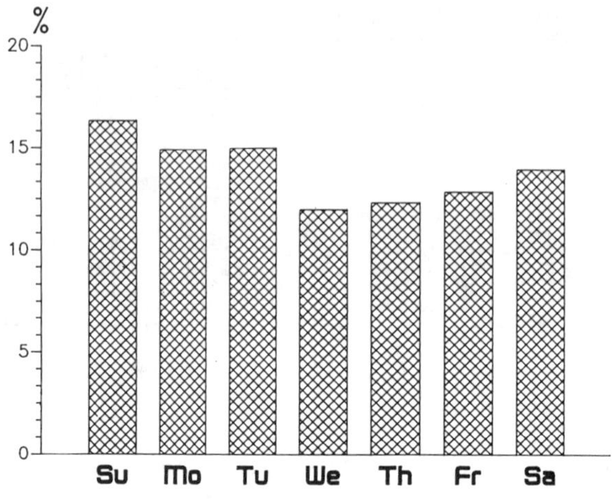

FIG. 1—*Weekly distribution of injuries.*

helmets are under 18 years of age. During the 1985/1986 season, there was a statistically significant lower rate of head injuries among those wearing a helmet. Nine percent of the skiers wearing a helmet registered as injured sustained a head injury. Among those injured and wearing no helmet, 18.6% had a head injury.

A constant finding during the investigated seasons was that four main groups of injuries dominated the statistics. Lower leg fractures, knee injuries, injuries of the arm and shoulder, and head injuries were responsible for more than 80% of the injuries.

Lower leg injuries were more frequent among young skiers; knee injuries were more common among women age 20 to 30; and men sustained injuries to the arm and shoulder more than women did (Fig. 8).

The total number of collisions was constantly between 20 and 25% of all the injuries. It appeared that the risk of acquiring a head injury was greater when colliding; almost half of

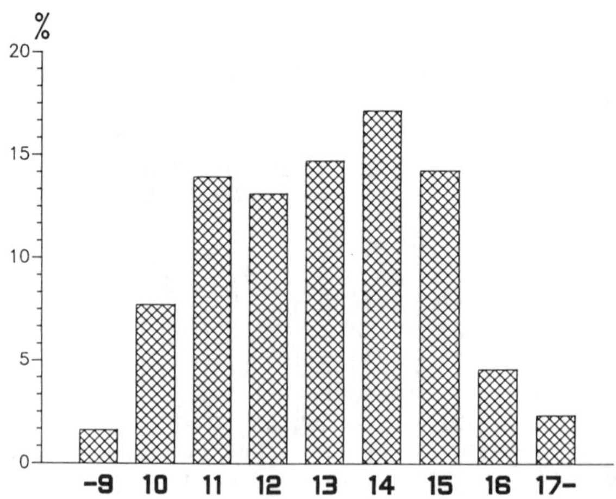

FIG. 2—*Injuries in relation to the hour of occurrence.*

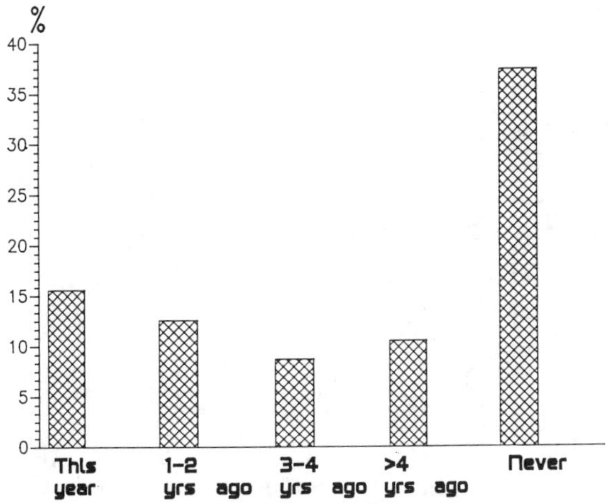

FIG. 3—*Injuries in relation to attendance of skischool.*

the head injuries were the result of a collision (Fig. 9). Two thirds of the collisions were due to colliding with an obstacle; one third involved another skier.

Approximately 5% of all registered persons assisted by ski area staff or ski patrollers were diagnosed as medical emergencies. The most common medical emergency was unconsciousness; respiratory problems were less frequent (Fig. 10).

Discussion

An attempt was made to register as many ski injuries and acute medical emergencies as possible in SLAO ski areas during seven seasons. In one of the largest ski areas in Sweden,

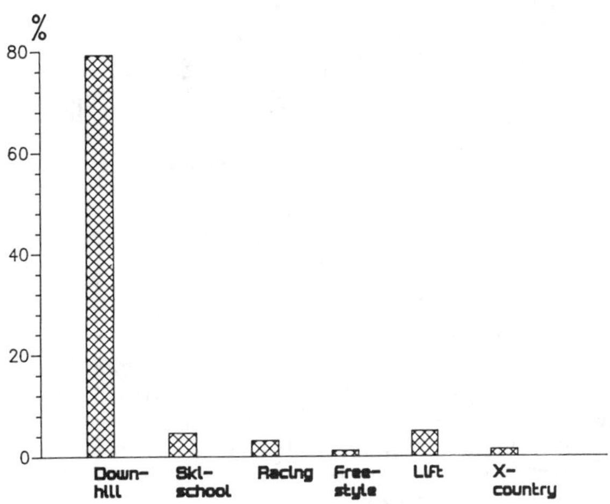

FIG. 4—*Injuries in relation to the type of skiing.*

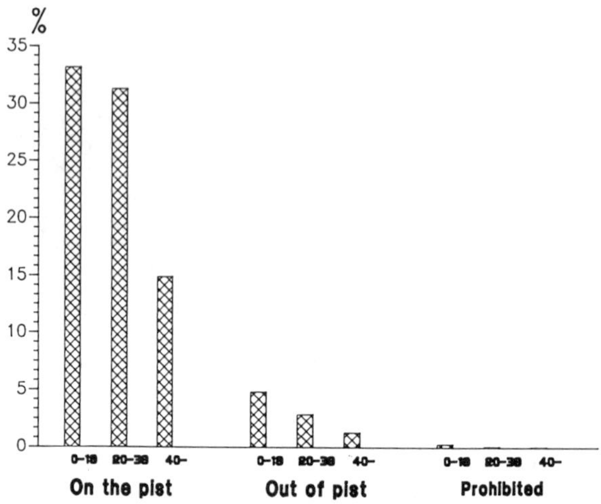

FIG. 5—*Injuries in relation to the piste.*

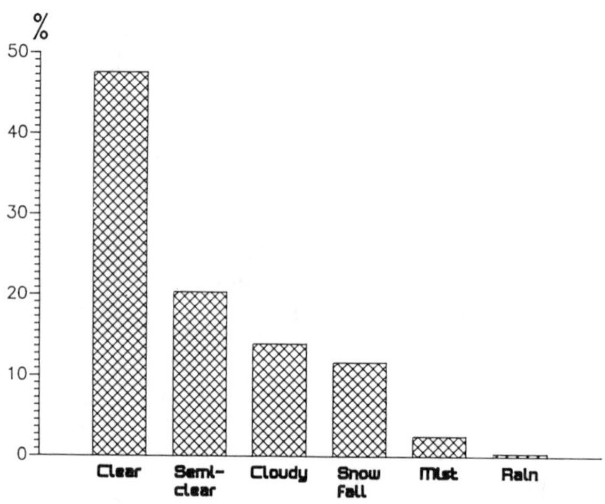

FIG. 6—*Injuries in relation to the weather.*

Åre, the number of injuries taken care of by ski patrollers corresponds to about one fourth of all the ski injuries treated in the one and only local county hospital.[4] Calculating an average number of ski injuries, covering 90% of the ski lift capacity of Sweden, a possible number of all ski injuries in Sweden, per season, is around 6000.[5]

[4]Ann-Sofie Gumaelius, M.D., personal communication, Åre Hospital, 83013 Åre, Sweden, 1986.

[5]For the 1986–1987 season, the registered number of ski injuries was 1557 taken care of by ski patroller or ski area staff corresponds to a total of 4 × 1557 = 6228. For the season 1987–1988, the registered number of 1400 injuries would represent a total of 5600, if the Åre conditions are valid for the rest of the country. Adding 10% to arrive at a figure for the total of ski injuries in Sweden, since the SLAO covers 90% of the Swedish ski lift capacity, must still be done. To give a sum, which is estimated by the above means, I naturally do not claim a strict number. A rough figure could therefore be at 6000 to 7000 injuries for the last two seasons.

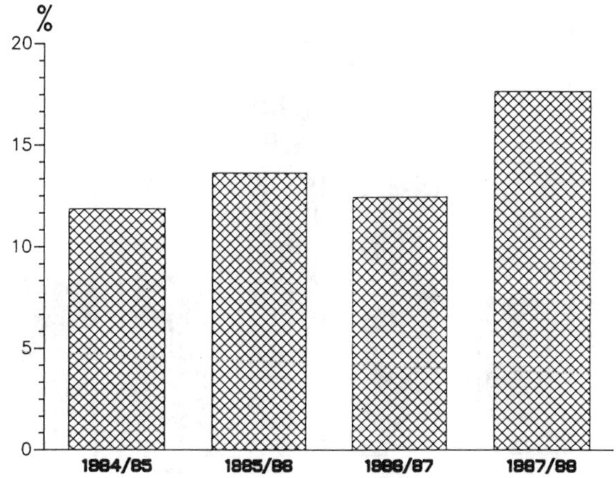

FIG. 7—*Injuries in relation to skiers wearing helmets.*

An interesting finding in the present material is that among skiers younger than 14 years who wear a helmet the risk of head injury seems to have decreased by 50%. To be valid, this conclusion needs to be supported by background data concerning the frequency of wearing a helmet among those not injured. However, we have no reason to suppose that helmets are chosen mainly by more careful skiers, because the wearing of a helmet is mandatory by those participating in racing. One positive effect of wearing a helmet may be that it changes the way of falling or it may protect the head, saving it from a bad blow and resulting in a less severe injury.

The constant number of collisions resulting in an injury during the investigated period is a serious problem. The continuous propaganda to make skiers aware of the risk of collisions and the importance of following safety rules seems to have had no influence.

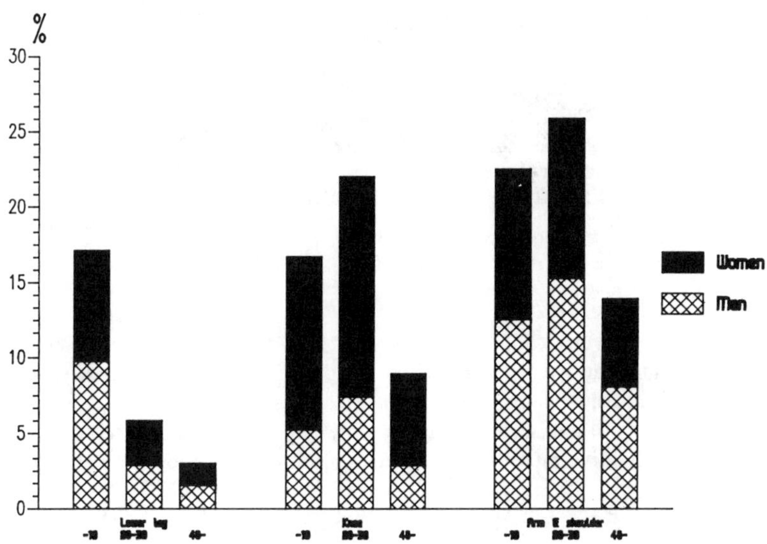

FIG. 8—*Injuries in relation to age and sex.*

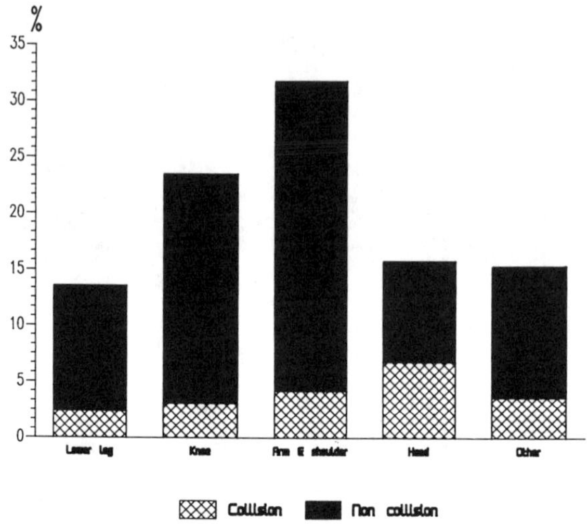

FIG. 9—*Injuries following collision versus noncollision.*

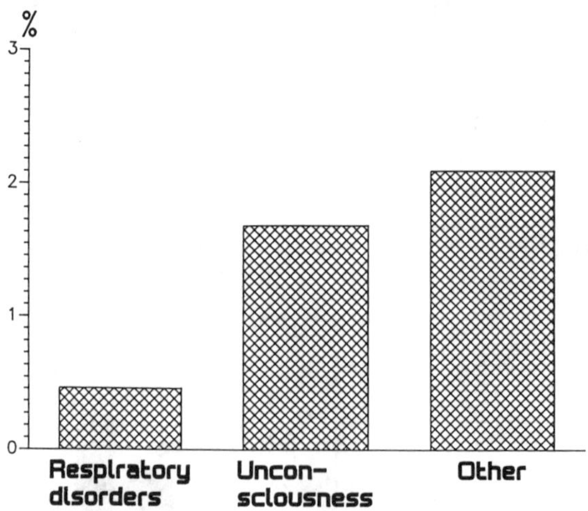

FIG. 10—*Percentages of acute medical illnesses.*

Conclusions

During the studied seven skiing seasons, the pattern of injuries has not changed. Statistically, there is a significantly lower number of head injuries among skiers wearing a helmet than those injured and not wearing a helmet. Despite continuous propaganda, there was an unaltered frequency of collisions during the time of investigation, which thus has focused the need for more effective measures to reduce the number of these most serious injuries.

Reference

[*1*] Eriksson, E., *Orthopaedic Clinics of North America*, Vol. 7, No. 1, Jan. 1976, pp. 3–9.

The Ski Boot

Peter S. Schaff,[1] *P. Ruckdeschl,*[2] *Wolfhart Hauser,*[3] *and B. Rosemeyer*[4]

Pain Threshold Along the Lower Leg in Alpine Ski Boots

REFERENCE: Schaff, P. S., Ruckdeschl, P., Hauser, W., and Rosemeyer, B., "**Pain Threshold Along the Lower Leg in Alpine Ski Boots,**" *Skiing Trauma and Safety: Eighth International Symposium, ASTM STP 1104*, C. D. Mote, Jr. and Robert J. Johnson, Eds., American Society for Testing and Materials, Philadelphia, 1991, pp. 179–185.

ABSTRACT: The pain threshold (PT) along the lower leg was analyzed in both female and male skiers to better understand current sex-related requirements for alpine ski boots. PT was found to be at an average of 32 N/cm^2 for the male group and 23 N/cm^2 for the female group. The difference between groups was significant ($p = 0.05$). We found no significant difference in PT distribution along the lower leg within the groups. Lowering the skin temperature more than 10°C resulted in a significantly higher PT. A 40% higher PT was found with twice as large an area used to apply the pressure ($p = 0.05$). The variation of PT to each subject is comparable to other psycho-physical methods, for example, vibration measurements. Because of a great variation among subjects, a definition of a maximum value to be tolerated in ski boots could not be given within a sufficient confidence interval.

Based on our findings, the following requirements are given: Ski boots must be classified according to sex, because women have a significantly lower PT that may lead to a restriction of motion in a stiff boot designed for male athletes. Temperature isolation for ski boots is very important, not only for comfort but also for safety reasons. Constant sensation feedback, necessary for accurate skiing, is only granted at constant temperature. To avoid pain at low pressure, the force along the lower leg should be distributed homogeneously over a large area. The area of most pressure should not be along the tibialis anterior tendon, because even pressure below the pain level over a long time may lead to a tendovaginitis in that area.

KEY WORDS: skiing, pain threshold, ski boots, ski boot classification, skiing safety

By means of new technologies the interactions between ski boot and lower leg have been examined during recent years [*1–9*]. Pressure measurements revealed different pressure distributions depending on the construction of the boot, with maximum pressure peaks over 30 N/cm^2 at different locations along the lower leg [*10*]. Almost no difference in maximum pressure was found between boots designed for female or male athletes.

To allow maximum dorsiflexion, the pressure may not exceed the 95th percentile of the individual pain threshold (PT) within a range of motion from 0 to 35° forward flexion. If there is a difference in PT between male and female, it should be considered in designing

[1]Head of the Institute for Biomechanical Analysis in Sports and interdisciplinary Studies (BASiS), TÜV Product Service GmbH, Ridlerstr.31, D8000 Munich 2, West Germany.

[2]Physician, Orthopaedics Department University Munich, Harlachingerstr. 51, 8000 Munich 90, West Germany.

[3]Head of TÜV Product Service GmbH, Ridlerstr.31, 8000 Munich 2, West Germany.

[4]Professor and Head of the Orthopaedics Department University of Munich, Harlachingerstr. 51, 8000 Munich 90, West Germany.

and classifying the boot. Therefore, it was necessary to examine the PT along the lower leg and to explore the influence factors on the PT.

Methods

Medoff et al analyzed the PT at six different locations of the lower leg using a hand-held plunger [*11*]. They found the tibia to be the most sensitive area and the heel to be the least sensitive area.

To correlate our pressure data along the lower leg with the PT at that most sensitive area, our goal was to analyze that area in more detail using a special designed machine to apply pressure accurately. The new design should eliminate some disadvantages of a hand-held device:

- Using a machine, it is possible to apply the pressure at a constant velocity.
- The reaction time of the examiner, necessary to stop the application of pressure once the threshold is reached, influences the result. This can be eliminated by letting the subject himself or herself stop the machine as soon as the pain level has been reached.
- On-line data recording with an electrical force ring allows accurate recording versus time.
- The exact vertical application can be achieved easily by a machine.

The new device was built around a universal test machine (Zwick) (Fig. 1). A plastic shell in the shape of the lower leg was placed underneath the tip and padded with a soft cushion to stabilize comfortably the lower leg. The 12- by 17-mm tip was flat with a thin, soft rubber pad on top. The subject sat in a chair. The lower leg was horizontally fixed in the plastic shell. The subject had a remote control to stop the downward movement of the tip once the applied pressure exceeded the pain level. A second safety knob for the examiner and a built-in safety shut-off guaranteed that no damage to the lower leg could happen.

All subjects were healthy with no history of foot problems. There were two groups: 15 males between the ages of 21 and 34, average of 26.5, and 15 females between the ages of 20 and 27, average of 23.2 years.

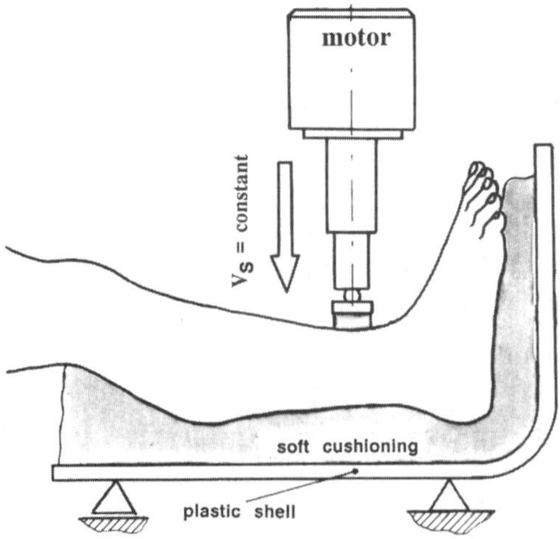

FIG. 1—*Test device with subject. The lower leg is fixed in a plastic shell. The tip with exchangeable tip areas is lowered by means of an electric engine at defined speed.*

The determination of differences along the lower leg required the use of 14 different areas of interest. Areas 1, 5, and 9 were related to anatomical structures. Area 1 was between the malleola, Area 5 reflects the distal 1/6 point of the tibia, and Area 9 was the middle of the tibia. The distance between 1 and 5 was divided by the Areas 2 to 4 in four equal distances as was the distance from 5 to 9 by Areas 6 to 8. Areas 10 to 14 were chosen to be the pretibial muscle tissue. The areas were at the same height, corresponding to the areas along the tibia with rising numbers from proximal to distal. In other words, Area 10 was lateral to Area 9, Area 11 was lateral to Area 8, and so on. All measurements were performed with the downward movement of the tip rectangular to the lower leg at room temperature.

The starting velocity of the machine was set to 60 mm/min. The subjects were told to push the button as soon as they felt pain that was unpleasant. On an affective scale of unpleasant, distressing, and excruciating, this would reflect the first step. Because our main interest was to determine the level at which discomfort occurs, we did no fine scaling of the sensation.

The subjects got an in-depth explanation of the whole procedure, especially the safety features, to avoid false results out of fear of injury.

The test design included the variation of the area of the tip, different skin temperatures, a comparison between manual force ring measurements (where an examiner applied a defined pressure by means of a manual force ring that was placed on the skin) and machine measurements, and a follow-up study within 5 min and another at four months.

Results

We found a sex-related difference of almost 10 N/cm^2. The pain threshold (PT) for males was 31.3 N/cm^2 (SD 10.8) and for females was 22.7 N/cm^2 (SD 7.9). The difference was significant at $p = 0.05$ (t-test; Fig. 2).

The influence of skin temperature was found to be an increased pain threshold at lower temperature. Whereas at normal skin temperature (28°C) the PT was at 30 N/cm^2, a temperature drop at 14°C caused the PT to be at 56 N/cm^2. The difference was significant at $p = 0.01$ for the matched pair test (Wilcoxon test; Fig. 3).

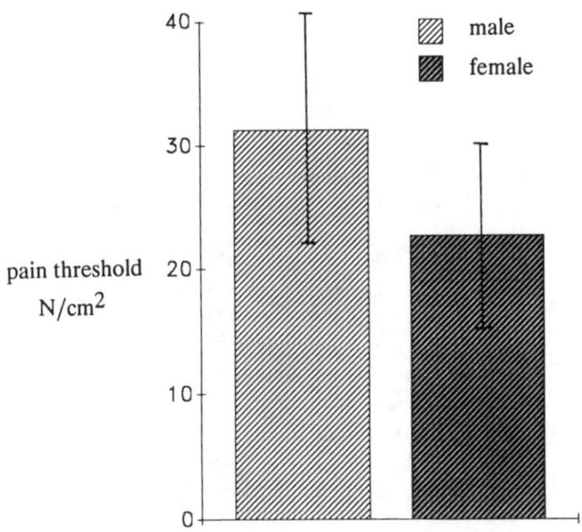

FIG. 2—*Pain threshold along the lower leg for male and female subjects. Differences are significant at* p = *0.01* (t-*test*).

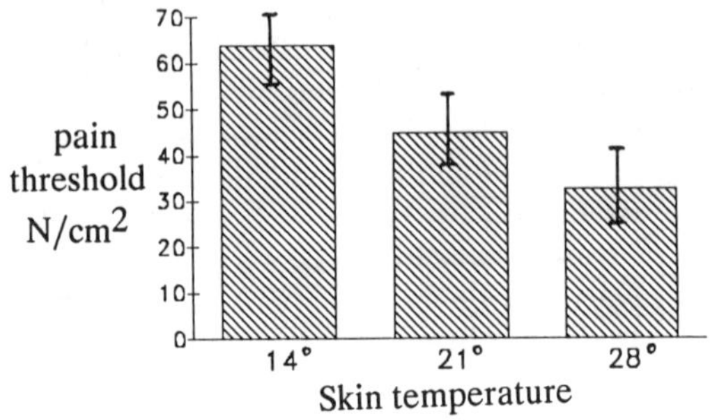

FIG. 3—*Influence of skin temperature on pain threshold.*

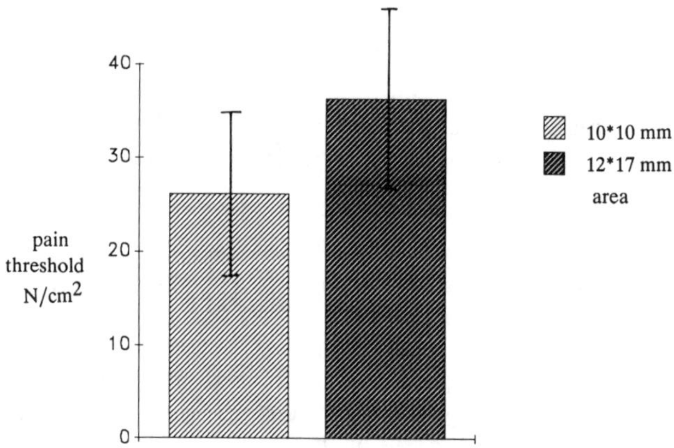

FIG. 4—*Influence of pressure transmitting area on pain threshold.*

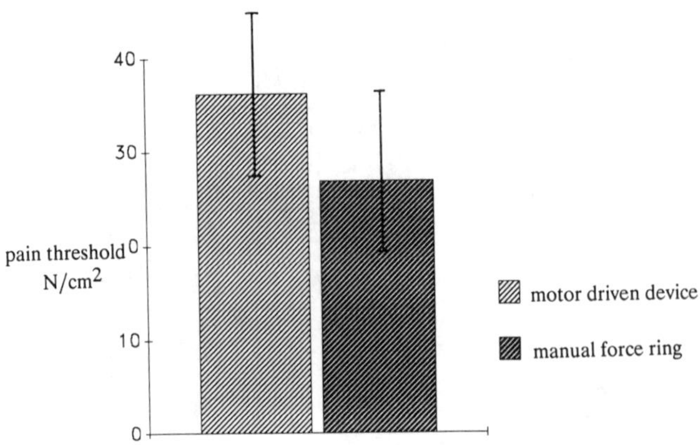

FIG. 5—*Comparison between manual measurements with a hand-held plunger and measurements with a test machine. The differences are significant at* p = *0.01.*

The influence of the pressure distributing area showed a higher PT for the larger area. PT of 26.2 N/cm² was measured with an area of 10 by 10 mm and 36.4 N/cm² with 12 by 17 mm. Again, the difference was significant at $p = 0.01$ for the t-test for paired samples (Fig. 4).

The values obtained with a hand-held device were about 10 N/cm² lower than with the machine (PT = 26.9 versus 36.3 N/cm², respectively; $p = 0.01$; Fig. 5).

We found only small differences for various test locations (Fig. 6). The average values were:

	Male	Female
Tendon	35.4 N/cm²	22.2 N/cm²
Tibia	28.4 N/cm²	21.8 N/cm²
Muscle	31.0 N/cm²	23.7 N/cm²

According to the Fridman rank test, there was no significant difference.

No difference in PT could be found with the follow-up study after four months. Follow-up studies within 5 min showed a short-term variability of 15 to 18% at the areas of interest (maximum deviation to the initial value of up to 59%). No signs of adapting could be found. The long-term variability was up to 53%.

Discussion

The corresponding values for the intraindividual variability in the literature vary. The smallest variability in PT was found if heat or electricity were used to induce pain. Hardy, Wolff, and Goodell [*12*] report variabilities of up to 12% for the PT using heat. Vibration measurements are in the range of 10 to 15% [*13*] with long-term variability up to 90% [*14*]. Our results are well within the range of comparable measuring techniques [*15*].

The interindividual variability was around 35%. Merskey and Spear [*16*] found 22% for males and 33% for females when they measured PT on the subject's head. With electricity as stimulus, variability is recorded to be around 50% [*15,17*], whereas with heat waves,

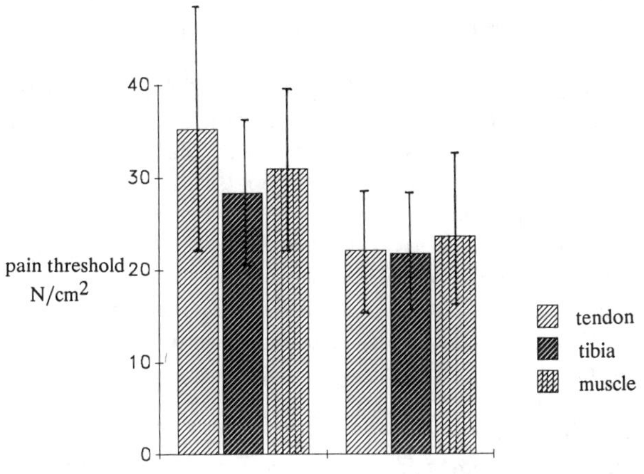

FIG. 6—*Pain threshold along the lower leg for different areas of interest. No significant differences could be observed.*

variability was between 5 and 55% [*12,18,19*]. Thus, the results of our study do not show higher values in variability than was to be expected from the literature.

The reported variabilities of PT measurements are rarely below 15%. One reason for this is that the central cerebral processing of the afferent impulses is influenced more by psychological than by physiological factors. For the alpine skier this would mean that deep powder on a sunny day may raise the PT to higher values, whereas gusty winds or bad luck may cause the PT to be lowered, therefore limiting the range of motion within the boot. This shows the importance of an adjustable boot. For a short time, for the benefit of nice turns on a perfect day, the skier may be willing to be above the pain level along the lower leg.

There is no problem with excessively tight boots, as long as the maximum pressure does not affect anatomical structures in the long run. A ski boot that has maximum pressure over 32 N/cm^2 along the tibialis anterior tendon is critical, whereas the same values along the shin may hurt, but not damage the foot. Some skiers even need a "painful" feedback to get the optimal feeling. For instance, ski racers are often willing to undergo pain in their struggle for milliseconds.

However, recreational skiers must have a boot that allows painless skiing over the full range of forward flexion. To transmit moment to the ski easily, a boot with low values near the instep is preferable to a boot with high values near the instep.

The significant sex-related differences corresponded well with Sherman's results [*20*]. He found by analyzing pressure-induced pain to the frontal head that the PT of female subjects was about 30% below the value for male subjects. Della Corte [*16*], using heat waves, and Merskey and Spear [*18*] found a reduction around 18%. This leads to the conclusion that ski boots designed for female athletes have to have lower pressure values at comparable forward position. Thus, only changing the color of the boot does not meet the requirements for a women's model.

The International Association for Safety in Skiing (IAS) has developed guidelines for ski binding (IAS 100) and ski boot (IAS 150) testing [*21*]. The revised version of the IAS 150 guideline for ski boot testing will consider sex-related differences. To help the consumer choose the right boot, such test routines will reveal improperly classified boots.

Such tests have to include temperature behavior, also. The significant rise of the PT at lower temperature may influence the performance of a poorly temperature-isolated boot. "Cold feet do not feel as good as warm feet!" Therefore, temperature isolation is an important topic for ski boots and will be included in the new IAS 150.

The results of using different areas to apply the pressure show that the same pressure applied over a greater area results in a lower PT. This leads to the conclusion that there is probably no spatial summation for pain. Hardy et al. [*12*] found the same result in 1940 for pain but, however, a clear summation for the temperature sensation. There may be a spatial summation that determines pain but how it works is not known and is not accessible by our test design. Consequently, the construction of ski boots should not include any high localized pressure. Even distribution of pressure over the full range of forward flexion is necessary. Bending of the shaft against a sharp edge, such as we found over the instep in some traditional models [*8*], is critical and should be avoided.

Choosing the right ski boot is still not an easy task! Passive safety in skiing, however, may be influenced by the performance of the ski boot. Individual adaptations are necessary. The skier is sometimes not able to adapt the boot to his or her needs because a detailed description of "how to" and "what if" is not provided. Test routines that can be developed out of these findings together with other results to classify the boot [*22*] should lead to objective statements on performance features. A general description of all features of a boot will help the skiing athlete choose the right and safe equipment in the future.

References

[*1*] Albert, H., Baumann, C., and Lorke, W., "Computergestützte Untersuchung des Biegeverhaltens von Skischuhen," *Qualitätstednik*, Vol. 33, Heft 8, 1988, pp. 413–416.

[*2*] Bahniuk, E. and Strunk, J., "The Use of an Anthropometric Dummy for Testing a New Ski Binding-Boot System," in *Skiing Trauma and Safety: Sixth International Symposium, ASTM STP 938*, C. D. Mote, Jr. and R. J. Johnson, Eds., American Society for Testing and Materials, Philadelphia, 1987, pp. 225–232.

[*3*] Bodem, F., Menke, W., and Casel, J., "A Laboratory for Biomechanical Analysis of the Traumatology of Ski Falls," in *Skiing Trauma and Safety: Fifth International Symposium, ASTM STP 860*, R. J. Johnson and C. D. Mote, Jr., Eds., American Society for Testing and Materials, Philadelphia, 1985, pp. 76–90.

[*4*] Danner, F., Mösch, S., and Müller, J., "Determination of Ski Boot Stiffness Using the Human Leg," presented at the Eighth International Symposium on Ski Trauma and Safety, Rîksgräsen, Sweden, 15-21 May 1989.

[*5*] Hauser, W., Asang, E., and Schaff, P., "Influence of Ski Boot Design on Skiing Safety and Skiing Performance," in *Skiing Trauma and Safety: Fifth International Symposium, ASTM STP 860*, R. J. Johnson and C. D. Mote, Jr., Eds., American Society for Testing and Materials, Philadelphia, 1985, pp. 159–194.

[*6*] Schattner, R., Hauser, W., and Asang, E., "Basic Mechanics of Boot/Skier Interaction," in *Skiing Trauma and Safety: Fifth International Symposium, ASTM STP 860*, R. J. Johnson and C. D. Mote, Jr., Eds., American Society for Testing and Materials, Philadelphia, 1985, pp. 151–158.

[*7*] Schaff P. and Hauser, W., "Druckverteilungsmessungen am menschlichen Unterschenkel in Skischuhen," *Sportverletzung-Sportschaden*, Vol. 3, 1987, pp. 118–129.

[*8*] Schaff, P., Schattner, R., and Hauser, W., "Biomechanical Inquiries on Ski Boots and Resulting Practical Requirements," in *Skiing Trauma and Safety: Sixth International Symposium, ASTM STP 938*, C. D. Mote, Jr. and R. J. Johnson, Eds., American Society for Testing and Materials, Philadelphia, 1987, pp. 154–165.

[*9*] Schaff, P., Kulot, M., Hauser, W., Rosemeyer, B., "Einflußfaktoren auf die Druckverteilung unter der Fußsohle in Skischuhen," *Sportverletzungen-Sportschaden*, Vol. 4, No. 2, Jahrgang, 1988, pp. 164–171.

[*10*] Schaff, P. and Hauser, W., "Dynamische Druckverteilungsmessung mit flexiblen Meßmatten—ein innovatives Meßverfahren in der Sportorthopädie und Traumatologie," *Sportverletzung-Sportschaden*, Vol. 4, 1987, pp. 185–222.

[*11*] Medoff, H., Rosen, J., Pope, M., and Johnson, R. J., "Pressure Induced Pain in the Foot and Leg," in *Skiing Trauma and Safety: Fifth International Symposium, ASTM STP 860*, R. J. Johnson and C. D. Mote, Jr., Eds., American Society for Testing and Materials, Philadelphia, 1985, pp. 110–116.

[*12*] Hardy, J. P., Wolff, H. G., and Goodell, H., "Studies on Pain," *Journal of Clinical Investigation*, Vol. 19, 1940.

[*13*] Goldberg, J. M., "Standardised Method of Determining Vibratory Perception Thresholds for Diagnosis and Screening in Neurological Investigation," *Journal of Neurosurg. Psych.*, Vol. 42, 1979.

[*14*] Fagius, J. and Wahren, L. K., "Variability of Sensory Threshold Determination in Clinical Use," *Journal of Neurological Sciences*, Vol. 51, 1981.

[*15*] Notermans, S. L. H., "Measurement of Pain Threshold Determined by Electrical Stimulation and Its Clinical Application," *Neurology*, Vol. 16, 1966.

[*16*] Merskey, H. and Spear, F. G., "The Reliability of the Pressure Alpometer," *British Journal of Social and Clinical Psychology*, Vol. 3, 1964.

[*17*] Lanier, L. H., "Variability in Pain Threshold," *Science*, Vol. 97, 1943.

[*18*] Della Corte, M., "A Study on the Cutaneous Pricking Pain Threshold in Normal Man," *Archivio di Fisiologia*, Vol. 64, 1965.

[*19*] Chapman, W. P. and Jones, C. M., "Variations in Cutaneus and Visceral Pain Sensitivity in Normal Subjects," *Journal of Clinical Investigation*, Vol. 23, 1944.

[*20*] Sherman, E. D., "Sensitivity to Pain," *Canadian Medical Association Journal*, Vol. 48, 1943.

[*21*] Asang, E., "The Work of the IAS in Skiing Safety," in *Skiing Trauma and Safety: Fifth International Symposium, ASTM STP 860*, R. J. Johnson and C. D. Mote, Jr., Eds., American Society for Testing and Materials, Philadelphia, 1985, pp. 17–26.

[*22*] Hall, B. L., Schaff, P., and Nelson, R., "Dynamic Displacement and Pressure Distribution in Alpine Ski Boots," in this volume, pp. 186–199.

Barbara L. Hall,[1] *Peter S. Schaff,*[2] *and Richard C. Nelson*[3]

Dynamic Displacement and Pressure Distribution in Alpine Ski Boots

REFERENCE: Hall, B. L., Schaff, P. S., and Nelson, R. C., "**Dynamic Displacement and Pressure Distribution in Alpine Ski Boots,**" *Skiing Trauma and Safety: Eighth International Symposium, ASTM STP 1104,* C. D. Mote, Jr. and Robert J. Johnson, Eds., American Society for Testing and Materials, Philadelphia, 1991, pp. 186–199.

ABSTRACT: The motion of the lower leg and the pressure at the interface between boot and lower leg were analyzed in both skiers and nonskiers to better understand current requirements of alpine ski boots for varying levels of skiing experience. Sixteen subjects, eight skiers and eight nonskiers, were tested. Five boots, including traditional, rear entry, and mid-entry designs, were studied. In each of the pairs of boots, subjects performed a series of rapid downward movements ("unweighting") on skis that were rigidly attached to a platform. Pressure data were collected using a capacitance measuring mat with six measuring points located 4 through 17 cm above the ankle along the anterior surface of the right lower leg; displacement of the leg and boot was determined from two-dimensional video analysis. Results indicate that the pressure generated on the lower leg by experienced skiers was larger than pressure generated by nonskiers. The range of motion (flexion) of the boots was also greater for the skiers. The ratio of pressure to angular displacement was consistent across groups within each boot, indicating that flexion characteristics are governed by material properties of the individual boots. This pressure-to-displacement ratio did vary among boot designs. With this in mind, it is recommended that, to achieve the range of motion necessary for proper performance of an alpine ski boot, beginning skiers should use a boot with a greater angular deflection for a given applied pressure. Information of this nature could be included in commercial specifications.

KEY WORDS: skiing safety, skiing performance, ski boots, pressure distribution, boot testing, displacement

Skiing techniques are improving, and ski equipment is changing to fit new consumer demands and help skiers avoid injury. Recent research done in alpine skiing focuses more and more on the boot. Some studies of pressure on the front of the leg have been conducted using static pressure measurements on artificial and human legs [*1–5*]. In addition to measurements with artificial legs, measuring along the human leg inside a ski boot can add some valuable information to our knowledge of the interaction between skier and ski boot. Eventually, on-slope data collection can help improve the design and performance of alpine ski boots and will help to develop recommendations that can be used by alpine ski boot manufacturers and by the commercial sales force to ensure that a pair of alpine ski boots meets the needs of the user.

[1]Master's student, Penn State University, Biomechanics Lab; currently, Institute for Biomechanical Analysis in Sports and interdisciplinary Studies (BASiS), TÜV-PS, Ridlerstr. 31, 8000 Munich 2, West Germany.

[2]Head of the Institute for Biomechanical Analysis in Sports and interdisciplinary Studies (BASiS), TÜV-PS, Ridlerstr. 31, 8000 Munich 2, West Germany.

[3]Professor and Head of Penn State Biomechanics Lab, Penn State University, University Park, PA 16802.

The purpose of this investigation was to develop a method for determining the displacement of parts of a ski boot and the pressure distribution at the interface of the boot with the skier during skiing. The method was used to determine differences in displacement and pressure distribution between experienced skiers and nonskiers and among several boot models.

Material and Methods

The work of Schaff et al. was continued in this study. During a motion mimicking a movement made frequently during alpine skiing, pressure distribution on the lower leg was recorded and the motion of the subject was videotaped and analyzed so that information on the relative movement of parts of the ski boot and lower leg was obtained. All data were collected at the Penn State University Biomechanics Lab during the summer of 1988.

Subjects

Sixteen male subjects, two groups of eight, aged 20 to 38 years, with U.S. shoe size 8½ to 9½ were recruited for the study. Each member of one group, skiers (S), had many years of alpine skiing experience (mean + standard deviation, 15.88 + 9.79), while members of the second group, nonskiers (N), had never skied in alpine ski boots. The skiers were recruited primarily from the ski school and racing team at Tussey Mountain Ski Resort near State College, Pennsylvania. Nonskiers were recruited from the student population at Penn State University.

Preparation of Subjects

Each subject was informed about the experiment and signed a consent form. Results from a thorough examination, including measurement of the contour of the foot and lower leg, of the right foot of each subject indicated no foot abnormalities for any of the subjects. A capacitive pressure mat containing seven pressure measuring points was attached to the right leg so that the center of the lowest point was located 4 cm above the medial malleolus. The mat was aligned on the leg such that the line of the measuring points followed the bony spine on the front of the tibia. The mat was taped onto a sock so that all edges of the mat were secured.

Critical landmarks were marked on the right leg and boot using black adhesive dots. Locations marked included: top of fibula, top of mat, top of front and back of boot shell, front of binding, ankle joint. The center of the ankle joint of the subject was marked externally to the boot. The horizontal and vertical locations of the ankle joint were determined from the height of each subject's ankle, the thickness of each boot sole, and the location of padding to secure the ankle in each boot. It was assumed that the ankle joint did not move within the ski boot during motion and that the ankle joint was the pivot point of both the lower leg on the foot and the upper boot on the lower boot (Fig. 1).

Equipment

Four brands of ski boots were used (Table 1) to create five boot conditions. Each subject was tested in each boot condition.

The mat used to determine the pressure distribution on the front of the leg was constructed of seven capacitive measuring points embedded in rubber and coated with plastic foil. For

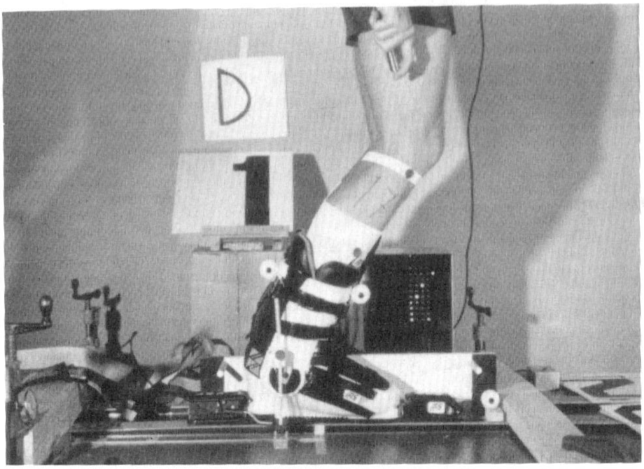

FIG. 1—*Position of the reflective markers.*

a complete description of the mat see References *2*, *3*, and *5–7*. Before data collection, the pressure mat was calibrated using an in-house calibration device designed and built at the Center for Locomotion Studies at Penn State University.

Two cameras were used to record pressure and motion. One, a Panasonic AG 170 high-speed shuttered camcorder set at 1/500 second exposure and 30 frames (60 fields) per second, recorded subject motion. The second, a Panasonic AG 500 unshuttered video camera, recorded pressure data shown on a video screen. Timing lights were used to synchronize the cameras.

The same pair of 200-cm-long skis with ESS Var bindings was used for all trials. This binding allows for simple adjustment to the correct position for any boot on the ski. The skis were spaced parallel to each other at a distance equivalent to "shoulder width" and rigidly fastened to a work bench.

Data Collection

Instructions to Subjects—Because the skiing backgrounds of the two groups of subjects were different, all instructions were given without the use of skiing jargon that might be unfamiliar to the nonskiers. The required motion was described to each subject in two ways. First, the idea of dropping body weight as quickly as possible was explained. Subjects were told to "drop into the ski boot" by letting the body drop straight down rather than by "leaning forward or backward." Second, subjects were encouraged to bend ("flex") the

TABLE 1—*Letter designations for five boot conditions.*

Boot Name	Letter Designation
Salomon SX 92 (soft)—rear entry boot	A
Salomon SX 92 (stiff)—rear entry boot	B
Koflach Comp 512—front entry (traditional boot)	C
Dachstein VC6R—mid entry boot	D
Dynafit ETS—rear entry boot	E

front of the ski boot as much and as quickly as possible. Initial practice attempts were monitored, and the subject was instructed to repeat the motion until repetitions were similar. After hearing the description of the motion, many of the subjects with skiing experience asked if they should perform an "unweighting motion."

Data Analysis

Analysis of the data collected during the described procedure was conducted in four phases. First, preliminary evaluations were made to determine if one trial was a good descriptor of the five trials performed by each subject. Second, the pressure data were evaluated to select a good indication of pressure for a complete trial to be used for statistical evaluation. Third, the motion of thc subjects was digitized to determine changes in ankle angles. Fourth, two-way analyses of variance were conducted to evaluate differences between the skiers and nonskiers and among the five boot conditions [*8*].

Pilot Analysis of Pressure Data

A pilot analysis was conducted to determine if one trial was a good descriptor of the five trials performed by each subject. Analysis of the data was performed beginning with the last two frames of data that were at "zero" pressure values before the pressure spike started in any measuring point and up to the decay in pressure readings after the peak. The portion of motion after peak pressure and compression were achieved was not controlled, and, therefore, no attempt was made to analyze this portion of the data.

For the pilot analysis, the raw pressure data for the middle three of five trials for one nonskier and one skier were examined for consistency. Using a chi-square test for comparison, calculations were done to analyze differences among the three trials. The data sets for the three trials were aligned so that the times of maximum pressure were simultaneous for each of the six measuring points (MPs). Alignment was conducted for each of the six MPs separately. Samples of three data points (one from each trial) were selected from this group of synchronized data through time, and the variance of each sample was compared to the overall variance among the three trials over time. The initial rise portion of trials was consistent for both subjects. The results of this analysis supported the decision to analyze only one trial per boot per subject. The middle trial (C) was selected unless there was some problem with the data from that trial for a given subject or boot.

Calibration of Pressure Data and Selection of Pressure Indicant

The pressure data for each of the 80 trials were read off the videotapes, reviewed for specific events, used to determine the time sequences to be analyzed, entered into a database, calibrated, and smoothed. Mathematical combinations of the smoothed pressure data were examined to determine the best single number to describe changes in pressure distribution through a full trial. A buffer zone of two frames was established at either end of the data for smoothing purposes. In this format, the data were smoothed using a five-item moving average, which proved a satisfactory method for eliminating fluctuations from the data.

The pressure data, in the smoothed form, were a time sequence of pressure readings (a pressure matrix) for the period of interest during the forward flexion of the ski boot. For analysis purposes, it was necessary to select a standardized (nontime dependent) indicant of pressure that could be used for statistical evaluation. Five possible indicants (Table 2) were investigated. A correlation matrix (Table 4) was developed for these five indicants, and, on the basis of careful review of the correlation matrix, P_{max} was selected for all pressure analysis.

TABLE 2—*Five indicants of pressure.*

Indicant	Description
P_{max}	maximum pressure reading occurring during the trial
F_E	weighted combination of the pressure readings for each MP at the time when maximum pressure occurred
P_{Pmax}	mean of all pressure measurements at the time when the maximum pressure occurred
P	mean of all pressure measurements for time before and including the time when maximum pressure occurred
Max of P_1	the average pressure across all MPs at the time when that average is a maximum

Displacement Data

Retrieval of data from the videotape of the subject motion was done using a digitizing system developed by Peak Performance Technologies (1987). For digitizing, a stick figure was developed such that the angle made by the tibia-ankle-front of binding was determined. All digitized data were filtered using a Butterworth second-order, double-pass digital filter with a cut-off frequency of 2 Hz. Angles were calculated from the filtered data, and the data were transferred to a spreadsheet program for analysis.

Data Analysis

For statistical analysis of ankle angles, eight parameters were compared among boots and between subject groups (Table 3). All significance tests were based on a Type I error probability of 0.05.

Results

Pilot Pressure Analysis

Figure 2 illustrates the method by which three trials from one subject were aligned so that the maximum pressure for each trial occurred at the same time. The pilot pressure analysis was done with uncalibrated, unsmoothed data. The initial portion of the trial (compression) is shown for Subject 6 in Boot A, Trials 2, 3, and 4. Only the results for measuring Point 4 are shown (Fig. 2).

For each increment of time (1/30th of a second), the variance of the three data points was compared to the overall variance among the three trials. Results indicate that among

TABLE 3—*Parameters investigated.*

Parameter	Description
P_{max}	maximum pressure
Angle_{Pmax}	angle at P_{max}
Angle_0	angle at time 0
Angle	(angle at P_{max}) − (angle at time 0)
Angle_{min}	minimum angle (that is, maximum compression)
m	slope of compressive portion of pressure versus angle curve
t_{Pmax}	time to P_{max}
$t_{anglemin}$	time to minimum angle

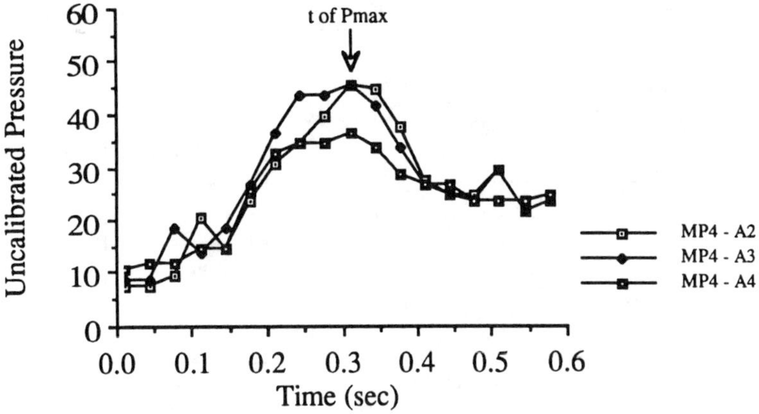

FIG. 2—*Uncalibrated pressure versus time for selected trials.*

the three trials, during the time when pressure was increasing, the differences were not significant. The main differences occurred after maximum pressure was achieved. These post-maximum differences were not considered, however, because only the compressive phase of the movement was analyzed. Analysis of the data led to the decision to analyze only one trial per subject and to use only measuring Points 1 through 6 for analysis. Problems with measuring Point 7, because of its location (in many cases above the top of the ski boot), caused inconsistent data even within single trials.

The correlation matrix for the five mathematical combinations of the pressure data (Table 3) is presented in Table 4. The correlation coefficient between any two of the five values is very high ($r > 0.80$). Because P_{max} is a reasonably good predictor (accounts for 64% of variation) of each of the other four indicants, it was used for statistical analysis purposes [7]. Empirical importance and simplicity of calculation are additional reasons to select P_{max} as the indicant of pressure.

For all analyses requiring one numerical value representing pressure for each trial, P_{max} was used. For all analyses requiring a time sequence of values to represent changes in pressure through time, pressure data from the measuring point at which maximum pressure occurred were used.

Pressure and Displacement Analysis

The results of a two-factor analysis of variance for groups (abilities) and boots are shown in Table 5. The table shows which parameter was investigated and whether there were significant differences between skiing abilities or among the five boots. The right side in-

TABLE 4—*Correlation matrix for five indicants of pressure.*

	P_{max}	F_E	P_{Pmax}	P	Max of P_1
P_{max}	1				
F_E	0.83	1			
P_{Pmax}	0.82	0.97	1		
P	0.82	0.80	0.82	1	
Max of P_1	0.83	0.99	0.99	0.81	1

TABLE 5—*Results of ANOVA's investigating differences between groups (abilities) and among boots.*

PARAMETER	ABILITY p	BOOT A	B	C	D	E	p
P_{max}	NS < S (0.0001)	1	2	5	3	4	(0.70)
$\angle P_{max}$*	NS > S (0.0003)	3	4	2	1	5	(0.12)
$\angle_0$*	NS > S (0.59)	4	3	1	2	5	(0.24)
$\angle_0 - \angle P_{max} = \Delta\angle$	NS < S (0.018)	5	1	3	4	2	(0.49)
$\angle_{min}$*	NS > S (0.0001)	1	5	3	2	4	(0.15)
$\lvert m \rvert$	NS > S (0.85)	1	4	5	3	2	(0.0006)
t to P_{max}	NS < S (0.43)	4	5	3	2	1	(0.64)
t to $\angle_{min}$	NS > S (0.55)	4	2	5	3	1	(0.24)

NS = Non-Skier
S = Skier
* Bigger $\angle$ = less flexion
[shaded box] = Statistically significant ($p < 0.05$)

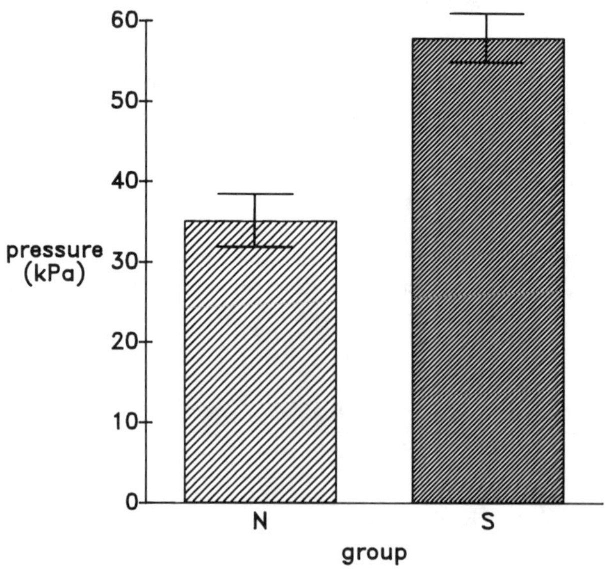

FIG. 3—*Comparison of maximum pressure between groups.*

dicates the order of boot performance (considering data for both skiers and nonskiers) with 1 representing the smallest mean value and 5 representing the largest value for each parameter. On the left side of Table 5, the comparison between the mean values for each group is indicated for each parameter. Significant values are in parentheses. The interactions between abilities and boots were not significant for any of the eight parameters.

Pressure—Figure 3 (representing data from all 80 trials) shows the maximum pressure (P_{max}) values for both groups. The skiers were able to generate a larger P_{max} than the nonskiers (mean + standard error: 57.96 + 3.08 kPa versus 35.14 + 2.24 kPa). There were no differences in the maximum pressures generated among the five boots (Fig. 3).

Angular Displacements

$Angle_{P_{max}}$—Skiers generated a greater absolute flexion (at P_{max}) than nonskiers, as indicated by a smaller $angle_{P_{max}}$ (65.23 ± 1.00°) than nonskiers (70.40 ± 0.92°). Figure 4 illustrates the $angle_{P_{max}}$ for both groups. There were no significant differences in $angle_{P_{max}}$ among the five boots.

$Angle_O$—There was not a significant difference in the initial angle between the two groups of subjects (N: 82.26 ± 0.46°, S: 81.88 ± 0.54°). Furthermore, there were no differences among the boots.

Angle—A comparison of the change of angle of flexion indicates that the skiers traveled through a wider range of motion than the nonskiers (16.64 ± 1.15° versus 11.86 ± 0.93°; Fig. 5). As with other parameters, there were no significant differences in angle among the five boots.

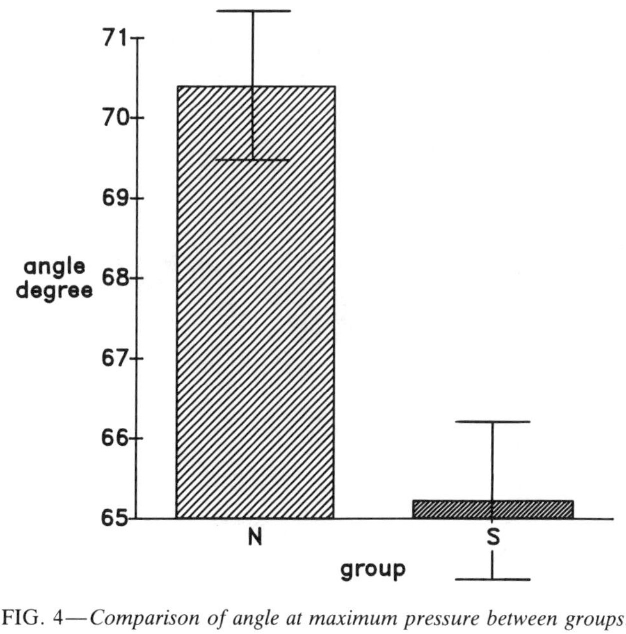

FIG. 4—*Comparison of angle at maximum pressure between groups.*

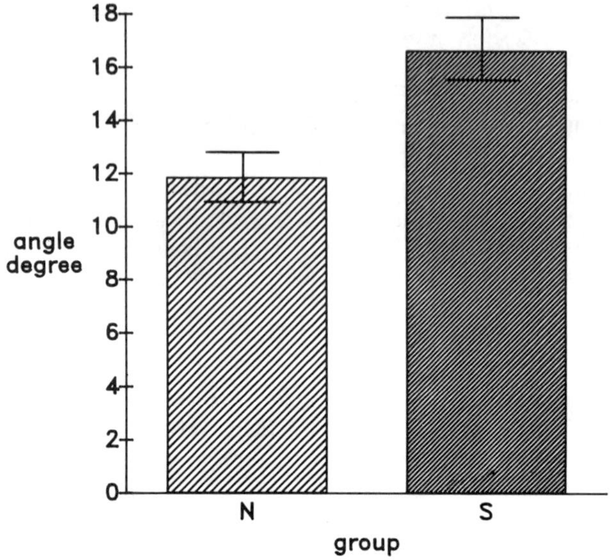

FIG. 5—*Comparison of change in angle between groups.*

Angle$_{min}$—Because in many cases the minimum ankle angle achieved by most subjects was nearly equal to the angle at P_{max}, it is not surprising that the results for angle$_{min}$ are similar to those for angle$_{P_{max}}$. Skiers generated a greater absolute flexion than nonskiers (N: 69.87 ± 0.94°, S: 64.31 ± 1.00°). (Note: Smaller angle$_{P_{max}}$ = greater flexion.)

Slope of Pressure versus Ankle Angle Curve

m—A slope was determined for the best fit line representing the compressive phase of the pressure versus ankle angle curve for each trial. Figure 6 is an example of determination

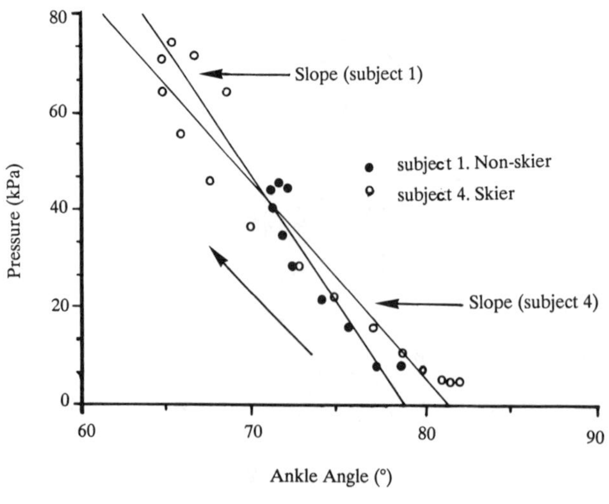

FIG. 6—*Typical pressure versus angle curves for a skier and a nonskier (Trial D3, MP4).*

of the slope for a skier and a nonskier. The slope of the best fit line is calculated using only the data points before maximum pressure. In contrast to most of the other parameters tested, the difference between the two groups was *not* significant overall (N: −3.35 + 0.28 kPa°; S: −3.29 + 0.20 kPa°; Fig. 7), and there *was* a significant difference among the boots (see Table 5). More specifically, the slope for Boot A was different from the slopes for the other four boots (see Figs. 6 and 7).

Temporal Relationships

$t_{P_{max}}$—The time to P_{max} was not different between groups (N: 0.40 ± 0.02 s, S: 0.42 ± 0.02 s) or among boots.

t_{min}—The time to $angle_{min}$ was not different between groups (N: 0.38 ± 0.05 s, S: 0.35 ± 0.01 s) or among boots.

Discussion

The major purpose of this study was to develop methods for collecting motion and pressure data in a controlled laboratory environment. Once developed, the method was used to characterize the differences among several boot designs. In addition, the response of the five different boot conditions to the movement of subjects with varying amounts of skiing experience was investigated. Significant differences were observed between the pressure and displacement responses of skiers and nonskiers.

The research of Schaff et al. [*1–6*] was aimed primarily at developing a pressure mat and making static measurements of pressure with the leg at several fixed angles of forward flexion. As an extension of the research of Schaff et al., the present study used video analysis in conjunction with the mat to study the dynamic motion of the lower leg and ski boot and the pressure distribution at the interface between the boot and the skier.

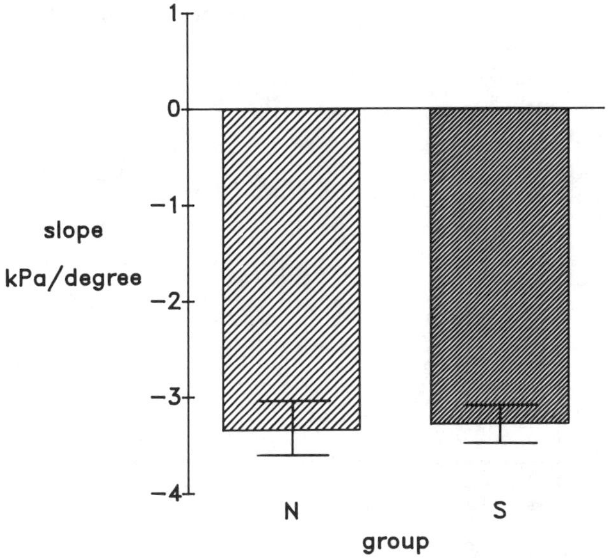

FIG. 7—*Mean slopes of pressure versus angle curves for both groups.*

As a methodological development, it has been shown that use of the maximum pressure created by a subject performing the motion described in the present study is a good indicant of the pressure changes throughout the complete compressive motion.

The interface between the skier and ski boot is important for transferring the actions of the skier down through the boots and into the skis. It is critical that the motion of the leg be transmitted to the boot successfully, but without injury to the lower leg and ankle. For this to happen, the boots must flex enough to allow forces from the lower leg to control the ski, but not so far that the ankle joint is allowed to flex beyond a safe region. This upper limit of the safe region is influenced by sex and age. Shealy [9] points out that the average value for males is 35° and for females 49°. The 5th to 95th percentile range for males is 23 to 45°, and for females it is 36 to 63°. According to IAS 150, it is stated to be 40 to 45°. That might be an oversimplification but may serve as an orientation [7]. Further studies should address that topic to come up with a proper definition that can serve as a guideline.

Perhaps the most important results from the present study are those regarding the pressure versus angle slopes for the 80 trials. The slope analyzed was a combination of maximum pressure data and ankle angle displacement data. By calculating the slope of the best fit line in the compressive phase of the unweighting motion, one obtains the response of the ski boots to changes in pressure. Results indicate that there was not a significant difference between the slope values for skiers and nonskiers. Conversely, there was a difference in the slope values between Boot A and each of the other four boots. This indicates that the design of the boot itself governs the rate of flexion with the application of a pressure. In other words, a boot flexes a given amount with the application of 40 kPa of pressure regardless of whether the skier is experienced or not, or, biomechanically spoken: the boot flexes in response to a torque, which depends on pressure distribution.

Therefore, for a skier to obtain the range of motion required for proper skiing technique, he or she must use boots with flexion characteristics that allow near maximum flexion of the boot with the application of maximum pressure by the skier (Fig. 8). There is a potential risk to the ankle joint if an alpine ski boot allows forward flexion much past 50° from horizontal. However, it is beneficial to performance for the skier to be able to use most of the 25° available between the set initial flex and the mechanical stop at around 40° of forward flexion that should be built into most boots [7]. This range is presented as the "ideal range

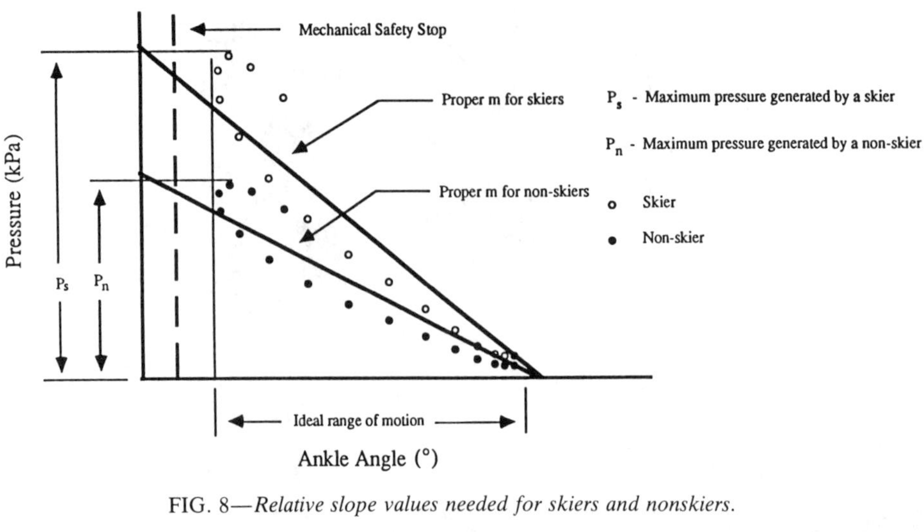

FIG. 8—*Relative slope values needed for skiers and nonskiers.*

TABLE 6—*Results of ANOVA's investigating differences in change of angle between groups within each boot condition.*

	Boot				
Parameter	A	B	C	D	E
Angle	N<S	N<S	N<S	N<S	N<S
p	(0.21)	(0.93)	(0.06)	(0.06)	(0.08)

of motion" in Fig. 8. It is advantageous for *all* skiers to have access to the ideal range of motion. The experienced skier can generate a larger maximum pressure than the nonskier. Consequently, the proper boot for an experienced skier should achieve the ideal range of motion at a greater final pressure than the boot of the beginning skier. The absolute value of the slope for the skier's boot should be greater than that for the nonskier. The slope value for Boot A is less than for any of the other boots, and, consequently, it is soft enough to allow nonskiers to cover a displacement close to the ideal range of motion.

Experimental Observations

Evaluation of results using statistical means provides information on the relative similarities and differences present in sets of data. Conclusions from statistical results require predetermined levels of significance, and there is frequently information that is not statistically significant but that is interesting to the researcher. In the present study, the idea of range of motion was of particular interest because this is the premise on which boot evaluation was based. Because of observation of the performance of the subjects as well as comments made by the subjects, there was reason to believe that the change of angle (angle) was different for the two groups in different boots (that is, that interaction between boots and groups was occurring). Therefore, although no significant interaction was present between boots and groups, further analyses of range-of-motion characteristics were carried out within each of the five boot conditions.

Results of a comparison of change of angle between skiers and nonskiers within each boot are interesting (Table 6). Trends in the data indicate that the skiers had a larger relative angular displacement, within each boot, than the nonskiers. For Boots C, D, and E, the p values, although not indicating significance at the $\alpha = 0.05$ level, are low ($p = 0.06, 0.06$, and 0.08, respectively) compared to the p values for Boots A and B. It is reasonable to assume that at the softer flexing setting (A) the boot does not respond differently depending on ability because it is very soft; but, at more stiff settings (B), the boot is too stiff even for advanced skiers, and, therefore, there is no difference in flexion between the two groups of subjects.

It is possible for an alpine ski boot to be too soft and to flex too easily. In fact, it may be that the similarity between Angle values between the two groups in boot A is due to the fact that although the nonskiers were able to flex the boots within the full ideal range, the skiers flexed the boot through and past this ideal deflection to the protective mechanical stops (see Fig. 8). Because the ideal flex range is just less than the controlled stop range, the results for the skier and nonskier are similar. Likewise, at the stiff setting, boot B is *so* stiff that neither the skiers nor the nonskiers were able to cause forward flexion.

Conclusions

Alpine ski boots that fit properly can improve the skiing performance of the skier. Modern skiing techniques require a large forward flex movement [*10*]. Performance is improved by allowing the skier enough forward flexion to control the ski properly. Increased control also may help to improve safety because the skier is better able to control speed and direction on the ski slope.

Specifically, the results of this study led to several conclusions regarding differences between the nonskiers and skiers and among the five boots.

1. Experienced skiers are able to generate a larger maximum pressure than nonskiers when performing the motion required for the present study.
2. Experienced skiers are able to flex (both relatively and absolutely) the front of an alpine ski boot farther than nonskiers when performing the motion requested for the present study.
3. The rate of flexion of an alpine ski boot is the same for experienced skiers as for nonskiers for the motion requested for the present study.

Practical Application

The combined evaluation of the results from the present study suggests the following practical application. The rate of flexion (change of ankle angle with changes in pressure) of an alpine ski boot is a function of the boot and not a function of the strength or experience of the skier. Therefore, because beginning skiers are not able to generate as great a pressure as experienced skiers, beginning skiers should use a ski boot with a flexion rate that allows travel through the complete ideal range of motion required by the skiing technique with the pressure that beginners *are* able to generate. From a performance point of view, the absolute value of the slope of the pressure versus ankle angle curve for the skier's boot should be greater than that for a nonskier.

We hope that our suggestions may lead to a better understanding of the performance aspects of the boot. Future studies have to prove whether there is a close correlation between enhanced performance by properly adapted boots (passive safety) and injury prevention.

References

[*1*] Hauser, W., Asang, E., and Schaff, P., "Influence of Ski Boot Design on Safety and Skiing Performance," in *Skiing Trauma and Safety: Fifth International Symposium, ASTM STP 860*, R. J. Johnson and C. D. Mote, Jr., Eds., American Society for Testing and Materials, Philadelphia, 1985, pp. 159–164.

[*2*] Schaff, P. and Hauser, W., "Measurements of Pressure Distribution in the Human Lower Leg in Ski Boots," *Sportsverletzung Sportschaden*, Vol. 3, 1987, pp. 118–129.

[*3*] Schaff, P. and Hauser, W., "Dynamic Measurement of Pressure Distribution Using a Flexible Mat as Capacitor—an Innovative Measuring Method in Sports Orthopaedics and Traumatology. Development—Application—Informative Value," *Sportsverletzung Sportschaden*, Vol. 4, 1987, pp. 185–222.

[*4*] Schaff, P., Schattner, R., and Hauser, W., "Biomechanical Inquiries in Ski Boots and Resulting Practical Requirements," in *Skiing Trauma and Safety: Sixth International Symposium, ASTM STP 938*, C. D. Mote, Jr. and R. J. Johnson, Eds., American Society for Testing and Materials, Philadelphia, 1987, pp. 154–165.

[*5*] Schattner, R. S., Asang, E., Hauser, W., and Velho, F., "A Degree for Measuring the Influence of Ski Boot Design on the Pressure Distribution in the Lower Leg," in *Skiing Trauma and Safety: Fifth International Symposium, ASTM STP 860*, R. J. Johnson and C. D. Mote, Jr., Eds., American Society for Testing and Materials, Philadelphia, 1985, pp. 182–188.

[*6*] Schaff, P., Hauser, W., Schattner, R., and Kulot, M., "Pressure Measurements Inside Shoes and Application in Alpine Skiing," in *Biomechanics: Basic and Applied Research Selected Proceeding of the Fifth Meeting of the European Society of Biomechanics, September 1986, Berlin, F.R.G.*, G. Bergmann, R. Kolbel, and A. Rohlmann, Eds., Martinus Nijhoff Publishers, Dordrecht, W. Germany, Sept. 1987, pp. 659–666.

[7] International Association for Safety in Skiing, *Adult Ski Boots Greater Than Size 36. Requirements and Tests, (IAS Specification No. 150)*, Author, Munich, W. Germany, 1980.
[8] Glass, G. V. and Hopkins, K. D., *Statistical Methods in Education and Psychology*, 2nd ed., Prentice-Hall, Inc., Englewood Cliffs, NJ, 1984.
[9] Shealy, J. E. and Ettlinger, C. F., "The In-Boot Fracture" in *Skiing Trauma and Safety: Sixth International Symposium, ASTM STP 938*, C. D. Mote, Jr., and R. J. Johnson, Eds., American Society for Testing and Materials, Philadelphia, 1987, pp. 113–126.
[10] Kuchler, W., *Skilehrplan No. 8*, BLV Verlag München, 1987, pp. 48–49.

Veit Senner,[1] Peter Schaff,[1] and Wolfhart Hauser[2]

A New Artificial Leg for Ski Boot Testing

REFERENCE: Senner, V., Schaff, P., and Hauser, W., **"A New Artificial Leg for Ski Boot Testing,"** *Skiing Trauma and Safety: Eighth International Symposium, ASTM STP 1104*, C. D. Mote, Jr. and Robert J. Johnson, Eds., American Society for Testing and Materials, Philadelphia, 1991, pp. 200–207.

ABSTRACT: For years, artificial legs have been used in ski boot testing, mainly for the determination of shaft-stiffness, flexibility range, and pressure distribution. Pressure distribution measurements with the existing standard leg (TUEV prosthesis) showed significant differences from measurements on human legs. This study improves the old prosthesis to get results comparable to a real-life situation. By comparing the individual pressure distribution of 14 male subjects with the group's statistically determined average pressure distribution, the person with the fewest differences from the average distribution curve was found. By rebuilding his lower leg in shape and size, changing the joint position, using a plastic shell to simulate the tibialis anterior, and finally, cushioning it with a flexible material to simulate soft tissue, a new prosthesis was designed that showed a major improvement to the old standard leg.

KEY WORDS: skiing safety, ski boots, shaft design, pressure distribution, artificial leg, prosthesis measurements, standard boot testing

Four years ago at the Sixth International Symposium on Skiing Trauma and Skiing Safety, Walkhoff and Baumann [*1*] showed the great disparity between prosthetic and human test subjects when determining ski boot stiffness and the dissipated energy. They concluded that there is a need for a boot flex machine (for example, as described by Danner [*2*]) and a standardized prosthesis that will give consistent, comparable, and repeatable tests on different boots.

Current Standard

The current standard for adult ski boot stiffness and flexibilty range, the International Organization for Skiing Safety (IAS) standard No. 150, uses a boot flex machine in its testing program. The advantage of this method lies in its high reproducibility and easy applicability. On the other hand, it shows the great influence of the artificial leg that is used on the results. This may not be of much interest if one is only classifying ski boots. But when determined moments, energy dissipation factors, or pressure distributions (Schaff et al. [*3*]) are used in investigations of binding setting or safety aspects in general, prosthesis that is used must simulate as close as possible the given anthropometric situation.

[1]Mechanical engineer and Medical doctor, respectively, Institute for Biomechanical Analysis in Sports and interdisciplinary Studies (BASiS), TUEV Product Service, Ridlerstr. 31, 8000 Munich 2, West Germany.

[2]Medical doctor and head of the TUEV Product Service, Ridlerstr. 31, 8000 Munich 2, West Germany.

Material and Methods

Criterion of Comparison

As a criterion of comparison and a factor that describes the interaction between boot and leg, the pressure distribution inside the boot along the tibia is most suitable. Its pattern and values depend on the type of boot tested and, of course, on the shaft's flexion angle. All changes made to the prosthesis (such as size, shape, material, or position of the joint axis) were aimed at achieving the same pressure pattern as the human leg. The method of determining the pressure distribution inside the ski boot is described by Schaff et al. [*3*], Hauser et al. [*4*], and Schattner et al. [*5*].

We used the so-called average pressure distribution derived from 14 individual distributions that were statistically treated and then approximated by a spline function (see section entitled "Statistical Treatment of the Data").

Figure 1 shows the average pressure distribution inside a ski boot at 35° forward flexion, determined with a human leg, with the old prosthesis, and with our new prosthesis.

Analysis of the Discrepancy

The reasons for the discrepancy between the results determined by the physiologic measurement and those determined by artificial leg tests can be summarized as follows:

(1) measurement-technical reasons,
(2) different joint kinematics,
(3) different shape and size,
(4) different position of the joint axis, and
(5) different material, hardness, flexibility.

To avoid discrepancy caused by measurement technique, it was necessary to conduct both series of tests under exactly the same conditions (instruments, calibration, temperature, and reference points).

Recent investigations of the kinematics of the ankle in ski boots show that with increasing forward flexion, simple rotation around the joint axis is overlaid by a translation movement in the sagittal plane [*6*]. This means that the turning point in the physiologic case (in contrast to the artificial leg) is not constant.

Figure 2 shows this effect, which might cause a reduction of the measured pressure in the lower parts and an increase in the upper parts of the boot shaft. The realization of this effect with an artificial leg would demand the development of an artificial ankle joint that, among other characteristics, exactly models the elasticity and flexibility of the human ankle. The construction of such an artificial ankle might be the last step toward the "perfect" artificial leg.

Constructive Changes of the Old Prosthesis

The recognition of the physiologically correct size and shape of the new prosthesis revealed the problem of identifying and constructing the average lower leg. We solved this problem by comparing the individual pressure distributions of our 14 test persons to the group's average pressure distribution. This comparison was done for 8 different ski boots, so in total we had 8 average pressure curves and 8 times 14 individual pressure curves to compare. In this manner we found the person whose pressure distributions in all boots showed the least

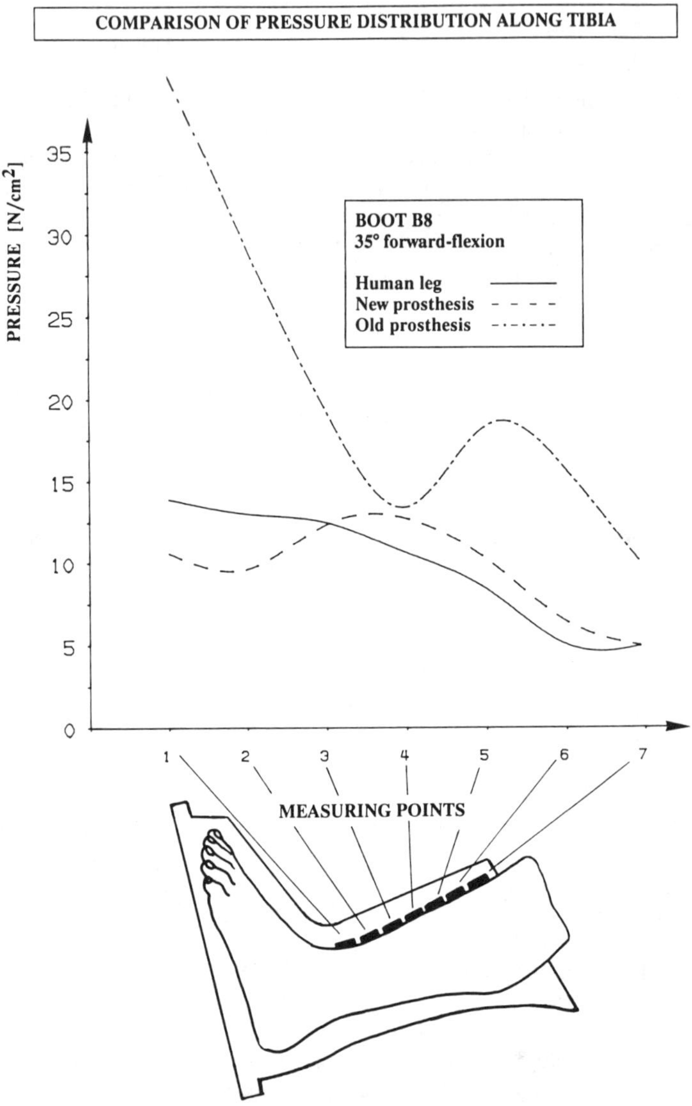

FIG. 1—*Pressure distribution in boot B8 at 35° forward flexion for the human leg, the old prothesis, and the new prosthesis.*

difference to the corresponding average pattern. The lower leg of this "ideal" person was then constructed in exact shape and size.

Figure 3 shows the model of our "ideal" lower leg, with the four horizontal cuts as they are shown in Fig. 4. Cut 1 lies at 140 mm, Cut 2 at 195 mm, Cut 3 at 255 mm, and Cut 4 at 305 mm above standing level. The physiologically correct position of the joint axis was also taken from our "ideal" subject. The difference between the vertical position of the medial malleolus of our "ideal" lower leg and the joint axis of the old prosthesis came to a total of 23 mm. With the new prosthesis, it was possible to reduce this difference to less

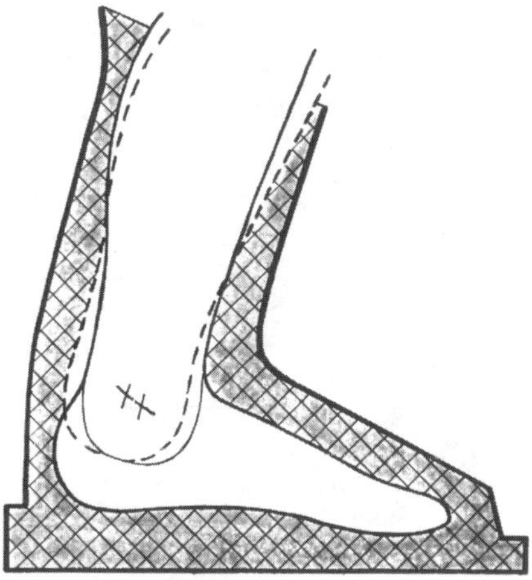

FIG. 2—*Movement of the ankle axis in sagittal plane with increasing forward flexing angle.*

than 7 mm. To realize a higher physiologic flexibility and hardness of the surface of our new prosthesis, we replaced some wooden parts with a special rubber foam. The thickness of this layer varied from 4 mm in the area of the margo anterior tibiae to 22 mm in the area of the musculus triceps surae.

A flexible plastic shell held by two spiral springs was placed on the new prosthesis (see Fig. 3) to simulate the projection of the tibialis anterior in case of dorsal flexion.

Measurements with the New Prosthesis

The first pressure distribution measurements with the new prosthesis were performed in August 1987. To identify how closely the new artificial leg mimicked real-life behavior, we

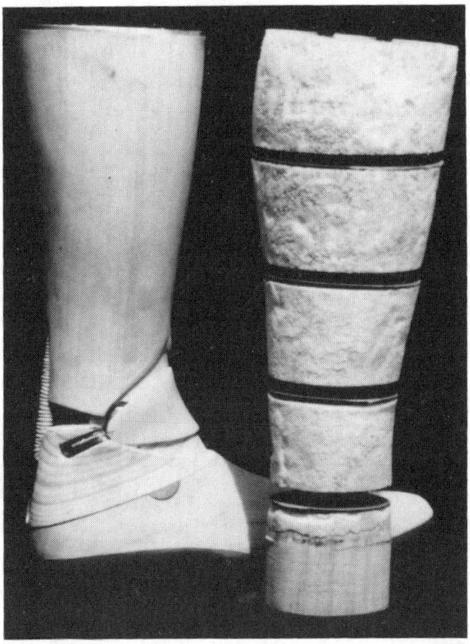

FIG. 3—*The new prosthesis and its model with four horizontal cuts.*

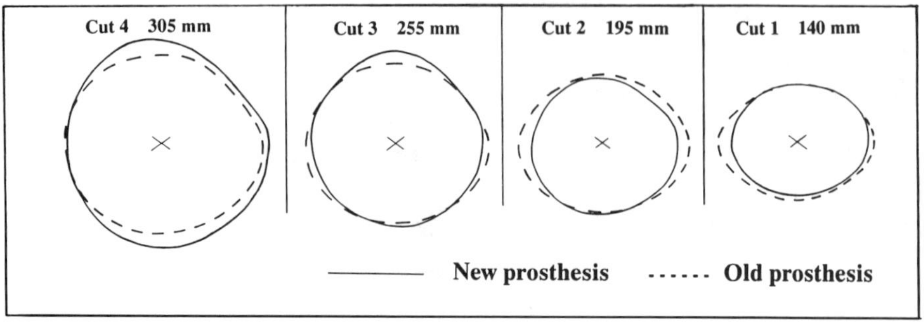

FIG. 4—*Size and shape of the old and the new protheses shown by four horizontal cuts. The given values indicate the distance of the levels above standing plane in millimeters.*

had our "ideal" test person perform the same measuring program on the same day that the new prosthesis was tested. This ensured equal testing conditions and, therefore, comparable pressure data. Two different types of boots were used in the test:

Boot B8—conventional overlap type, Size 7 and
Boot D8—rear entry design, Size 7.

The measuring program was conducted as follows:

(1) installation of the pressure distribution measurement device,
(2) calibration and mounting of the capacitive force-measuring mat on the human lower leg,
(3) physiologic measurement, Boots B8 and D8
(4) control of the testing conditions; comparison of actual and old pressure data,
(5) mounting of the measuring mat on the prosthesis, insertion of the prosthesis into the boot,
(6) installation of boot and prosthesis onto the boot flex machine,
(7) prosthesis measurement, Boots B8 and D8, and
(8) statistical treatment of the data; graphic representation.

To collect the pressure data, we used the device described by Schaff et al. [*3*]. The measuring mat, consisting of eight capacitive transducers, was fixed to the leg as follows (Table 1 below indicates the distance in millimeters of the center of each measuring point above the ankle joint).

TABLE 1—*Distance of the center of each measuring point above the ankle joint.*

Measuring Point	Distance Center of Measuring Plane Above Malleolus Medialis, mm
1	56
2	82
3	108
4	134
5	160
6	186
7	212

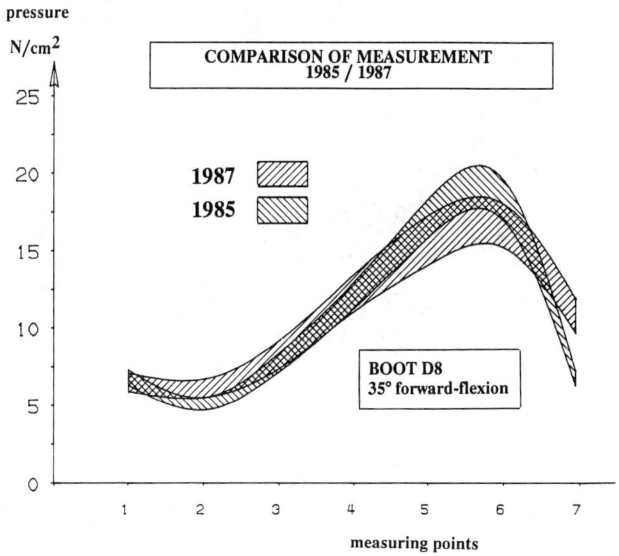

FIG. 5—*Comparison of the pressure data after 2 years: physiologic measuring in 1985 and 1987, Boot D8, 35° forward flexion.*

Both physiologic and prosthesis measurements were repeated ten times with each boot. The analyzed forward-flexion angle was 35°. For the physiologic measurements, our subject was advised to hold the flexion angle by muscular force. For the prosthesis measurements, we used the boot flex machine described by Danner [2] to control flexion angle. To eliminate any dynamic influence on the pressure pattern, the machine was set at a constant 35° angle before the prosthesis measurements were done.

Considering equal testing conditions, the device setting was controlled by comparing the actual pressure data of our subject with his data of 1985 (we had tested him under the same experimental parameters: Boot D8 and 35° forward-flexion angle). Figure 5 shows the results of this comparison of the physiological measurements of 1985 and 1987. The two pressure functions have been replaced by their corresponding deviation ranges. (Further information about the determination of the deviation range can be found in Refs *7* and *8*.)

The good correspondence between the data of 1985 and the data of 1987 mean that we had endured similar testing conditions.

Statistical Treatment[3] of the Data

The determined pressure values were treated as follows:

(1) transformation of the values to N/cm^2-equivalents,
(2) elimination of data out of range based on Nalimoff test criteria,
(3) calculation of the mean value and standard deviation,
(4) for each measuring point: calculation of the maximum statistical error d_{max} and the maximum measuring error u_{max},
(5) approximation of the derived mean values by a smoothing spline,

[3]The entire statistical treatment is described by Senner [7].

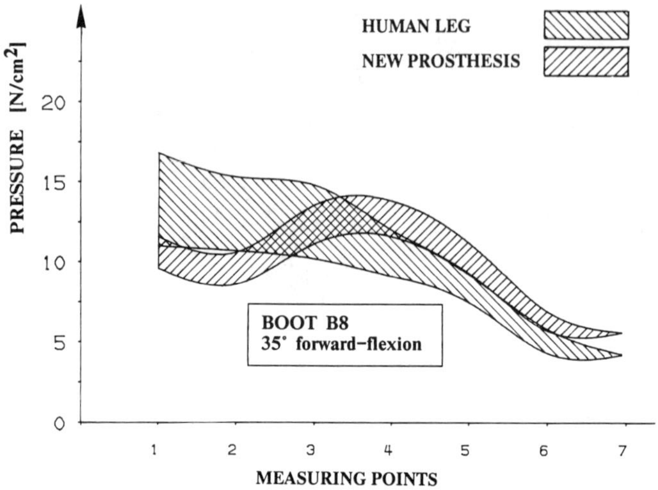

FIG. 6—*Pressure distribution deviation ranges derived from data achieved by physiologic measuring and measuring with the new prosthesis (Boot B8).*

(6) calculation of the deviation range using the mean value and the calculated measuring error, and
(7) storing all the calculated data and plotting the derived spline functions.

Results, Conclusions, and Requirements

Figure 1 shows the results of our first measurements using the new prosthesis and the ones testing the human being, compared to the pressure values determined with the old leg (all Boot B8 at 35° forward flexion). Figure 6 indicates the corresponding deviation ranges calculated for the human leg and the new prosthesis.

It is obvious that the pressure distribution with our new artificial leg is a major improvement to the standard leg used up to now. Especially in the range of measuring Points 1 and 2, where our new prosthesis is not as thick as the old one (see Fig. 4), the reduction of the existing discrepancy (Fig. 1) between the pressure values of the old prosthesis and those of the human leg is significant.

Another look at Fig. 6 shows that at no point of the measuring field does the determined pressure pattern of the new leg differ more than 2.3 N/cm^2 from the physiologic one.

Analyzing the effects on the pressure pattern caused by the different constructive changes, we can say that the change of the size and shape was the most effective one, followed by the change of the joint ankle position. The effect caused by the soft cushioning is comparatively less significant. Future enhancements including a new more anatomic artificial joint might provide a further improvement. To simulate human movement within ski boots, the prosthesis should resemble the human leg as close as possible. The improvements toward real-life behavior that we have achieved with our new artificial leg are so significant that we can no longer recommend the use of the old type leg.

Future test procedures that require an artificial leg should therefore use our enhanced version of the standard TUEV prosthesis.

References

[*1*] Walkhoff, K. and Baumann, C. W., "Alpine Ski Boot Hysteresis Characteristics Interpreted for Skier Target Groups Within the Current Standards," in *Skiing Trauma and Safety: Sixth International*

Symposium, ASTM STP 938, C. D. Mote, Jr. and R. J. Johnson, Eds., American Society for Testing and Materials, Philadelphia, 1987, pp. 127–144.

[2] Danner, F., Die Stellung des Fusses im Skischuh. Diplomarbeit an der Fachhochschule Muenchen zu Erlangung des akademischen Grades eines Diplomingenieurs (FH). Fachbereich Materialpruefung des TUEV-Bayern, Ed., Munich, West Germany, 1989.

[3] Schaff, P., Schattner, R., and Hauser, W., "Biomechanical Inquiries on Ski Boots and Resulting Practical Requirements," in *Skiing Trauma and Safety: Sixth International Symposium, ASTM STP 938*, C. D. Mote, Jr. and R. J. Johnson, Eds., American Society for Testing and Materials, Philadelphia, 1987, pp. 154–175.

[4] Hauser, W., Asang, E., and Schaff, P., "Influence of Ski Boot Design on Skiing Safety and Skiing Performance," in *Skiing Trauma and Skiing Safety: Fifth International Symposium, ASTM STP 860*, R. J. Johnson and C. D. Mote, Jr., Eds., American Society for Testing and Materials, Philadelphia, 1985, pp. 159–164.

[5] Schattner, R., Asang, E., Hauser, W., and Velho, F., "A Device for Measuring the Influence of Ski Boot Design on the Pressure Distribution in the Lower Leg," in *Skiing Trauma and Skiing Safety: Fifth International Symposium, ASTM STP 860*, R. J. Johnson and C. D. Mote, Jr., Eds., American Society for Testing and Materials, Philadelphia, 1985, pp. 182–188.

[6] Shealy, J. E. and Miller, D. A., "Dorsiflexion of the Human Ankle as It Relates to Ski Boot Design in Downhill Skiing," in *Skiing Trauma and Safety: Seventh International Symposium, ASTM STP 1022,* R. J. Johnson, C. D. Mote, Jr., and M.-H. Binet, Eds., American Society for Testing and Materials, Philadelphia, 1989, pp. 146–152.

[7] Senner, V., "Entwicklung eines Programmes zur statistischen Auswertung vorhandener Messwerte im Schaftbereich alpiner Skischuhe," Study at the Technische Universitaet Muenchen. Institut fuer Biomedizin und Ergonomie, TUEV-Bayern, Ed., Munich, West Germany, 1986.

[8] Senner, V., Schaff, P., and Hauser, W., "Entwicklung einer optimierten Prosthese," Institut fuer Biomedizin und Ergonomie, TUEV-Bayern, Ed., Munich, West Germany, 1988.

Paolo Zucco[1]

Ski Boot Thermography Method and Its Significance

REFERENCE: Zucco, P., "**Ski Boot Thermography Method and Its Significance,**" *Skiing Trauma and Safety: Eighth International Symposium, ASTM STP 1104*, C. D. Mote, Jr. and Robert J. Johnson, Eds., American Society for Testing and Materials, Philadelphia, 1991, pp. 208–213.

ABSTRACT: Protection from cold is one of the most important functions considered in designing and manufacturing ski boots. Thermography is used for evaluating cold protection capacity of various kinds of inner shoes and boot shells. We performed thermal analysis of three boot categories using two thermography methods, and the results were compared. We observed that (1) thermography is a valid method for boot cooling studies; (2) both an inner shoe and boot shell aid in thermal insulation; (3) progressive cooling and forced warming of the boot give the same results in identifying heat exchange areas; (4) blood flow, muscle activity during skiing, and boot fit must be considered in designing ski boots; and (5) because of the importance of this boot function, a standardized method of analysis should be adapted by all manufacturers. We concluded that the structure must be analyzed with thermography testing. It is not necessary to use an artificial limb inside the boot to obtain satisfactory data.

KEY WORDS: infrared thermography, ski boot fitness, skiing safety

In the last 15 years, much laboratory and field research has been conducted to find ways to improve ski boots technically. Accurate radiographic and telemetric studies of ski boots [*1*,*2*] have provided much information about the interaction between the human foot and ski boot during skiing. The ski boot must protect the foot from impact with the snow and from the cold environment. If we consider that skiers are exposed for several hours to below-zero temperatures, thermal isolation is necessary for maintenance of comfort and proprioceptive feedback.

Materials used in the construction of ski boots have greatly improved in recent years. When ski boots were made with a single leather shell, thick socks were required to protect the skier's foot from the cold. Today, ski boots have much more practical inner boots. Different materials and shapes have been used to minimize cooling of the foot. The shell itself has undergone several changes to improve permeability and to reduce external-internal conductivity with the ambient environment. To evaluate ski boot efficiency in temperature isolation, infrared thermography has been used [*3*,*4*].

Methods

We used a liquid nitrogen AGA thermovision consisting of an infrared camera and a monitor connected to a computer displaying an image called a thermogram (Fig. 1). A thermogram shows temperature variations by means of different colors that vary according

[1]Assistant professor, Orthopaedic Clinic of the University of Pavia, Policlinico S. Matteo, I.R.C.C.S., Via Taramelli 3, 27100 Pavia, Italy.

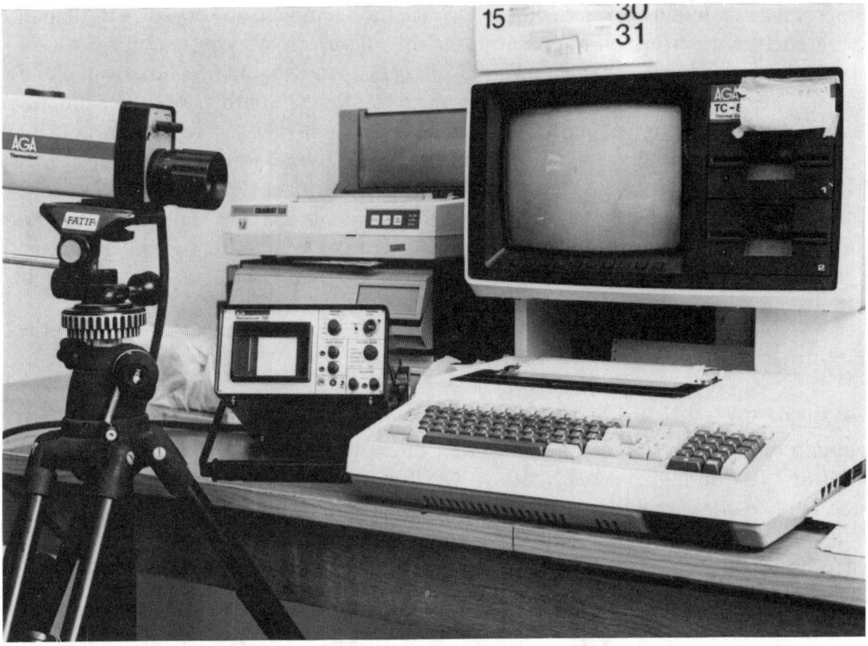

FIG. 1—*AGA Thermovision camera with computer displaying thermograms.*

to thermal patterns indicated by the equipment. A thermal gradient from one color to another can be chosen in relation to the material under examination. In our tests, temperature difference from one color to another ranged from 0.8 to 1.6°C [*5*].

Three different kinds of ski boots were analyzed: high level, medium level, and junior. An old model made about 15 years ago was also analyzed. The boot categories were based on both cost and manufacturers' statements. The main difference in our study's boots was in the shell material (polyurethane for high level and thermoplastic rubber for medium level) and in the inner boot characteristics. In our group of high level boots, we chose both rear entry and front entry models (with four buckles) to evaluate the impact of the ski boot structure on thermal losses. In total, ten boots were analyzed.

In a first test, we analyzed the boot at room temperature to ensure that the temperature distribution was uniform. Then, following the method of Roberts, hot air was introduced at a constant pressure into the boot by a special device that controls air temperature and pressure [*3,4*]. The boot buckles were tightened, and an adapter connected the air pipe to the boot's top to avoid air leakage. We did not measure the temperature within the boot because we were only interested in heat loss through the boot. The first thermogram was taken at the constant ambient temperature. A second thermogram was taken after 2 min, and a third was taken 4 min after the introduction of hot air. For the junior boot, the time was reduced by half to make significant thermograms because the temperature gradient would have otherwise decreased too much and the resulting temperature would have been too uniform.

A second test was carried out simulating real conditions. This time the ski boot was worn by a test subject and introduced for 30 minutes into a container of ice. The subject was required to make some simple movements with his toes and to do some bends and extensions with his ankle to maintain adequate blood flow. He then removed his foot from the container. Thermograms were performed after 5 and 10 min to discover arèas of heating. We used this method and not a cold chamber for two reasons: (1) a cold chamber is not available in our institute. In the future we intend to perform the tests directly on the slopes to simulate real conditions. (2) For testing the junior models, we used an 8-year-old boy who was available for on-slope tests but not for the cold chamber tests of 30 minutes.

Each test was done on two different days. We also performed thermograms of separate parts of the boot, including the inner shoe. In the thermograms, the high temperature areas are light and the low temperature areas are dark. The background appears dark in the first tests because of the heated boot and light in the second one because of the cooled boot, so that the background radiation was higher.

Results

Our results are based on the observation of the thermograms and the variation and distribution of colors in the image at different times.

In the first test on higher level boots, in which hot air was introduced into the ski boot, the rear entry model obtained the best results with a uniform performance and only a low permeability to air at the ankle joint (Fig. 2). The other design (front entry, four buckles) revealed areas of thermal leakage at the articulation and at the buckles where the shell overlapped. One model (high level boot) showed high permeability to air, perhaps due to the characteristics of the inside shoe and to some faults in the assembly of the shell (Fig. 3). The performance of the medium level model was good with only a small area of leakage at the ankle joint.

The old model showed localized leakage at the buckles and at the overlapping at the top of the shell (Fig. 4). The junior model, a rear entry boot, showed remarkable leakage, along the lines of connection between the different parts of the shell (Fig. 5).

The second test allowed evaluation of the areas of progressive heating after cooling in ice. The results were not the same as the first test for the high level models: for both rear entry and front entry designs heat loss occurred primarily along the sole and at the toe (Fig. 6).

The performance of medium level and junior models in this second test was quite similar to the first test results. In particular, the junior model showed very defined areas of heat loss (Fig. 7). The second test was more appropriate for the evaluation of heat conduction

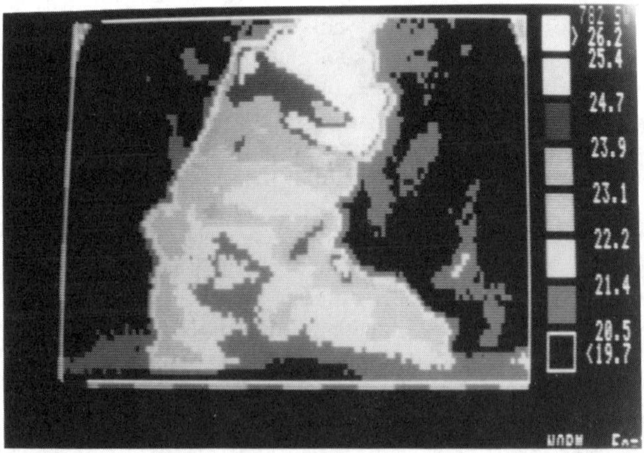

FIG. 2—*Good performance of a modern boot after 4 min of hot air. Only litte heat loss areas.*

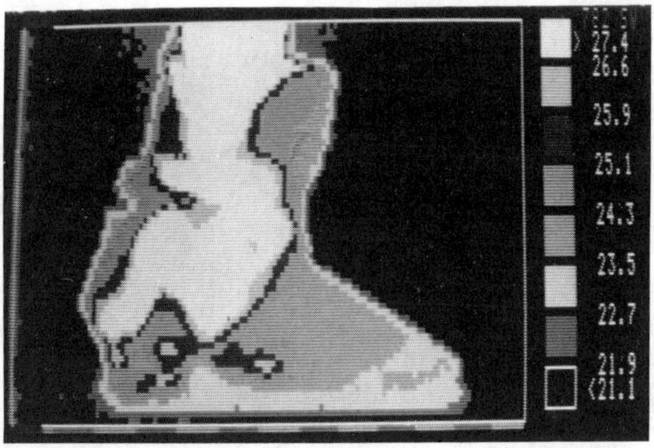

FIG. 3—*Large heat loss area is very evident in the ankle joint and the upper part of the shell of a modern rear entry boot after 4 min.*

of the ski boot because the thermal exchange is more progressive and heating of the structure is produced directly by the foot.

Discussion

Our conclusions are based primarily on the analysis of thermograms and of the boots' structure with the aim of discovering the reason for poor performance. One high level model, the junior boot, and the old boot revealed a high amount of leakage as a result of faults in manufacturing or assembly. For instance, in the old model, leakage was due to poor quality sewing and to poor fit of the various plastic components of the shell. In the junior model, the inside shoe provided uniform heat loss and had a good design, but there was some leakage in the assembly of the rear part of the shell and at the ankle joint.

Our tests revealed that both the inner boot and the outer shell are important for good insulation. Absence of sewing within the inner boot and a tight fit of the components of the

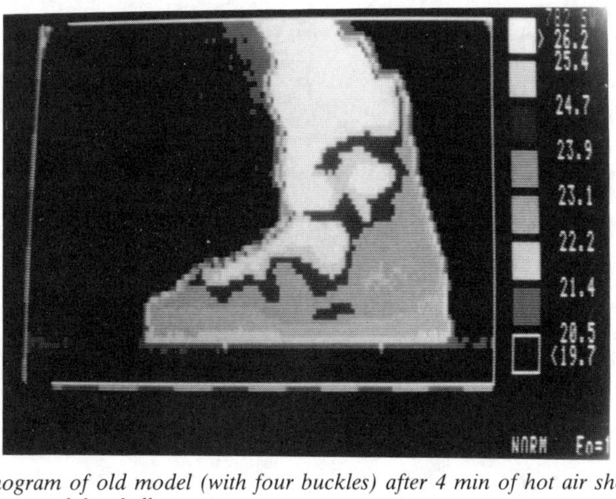

FIG. 4—*Thermogram of old model (with four buckles) after 4 min of hot air shows large heat loss area at the overlapping of the shell.*

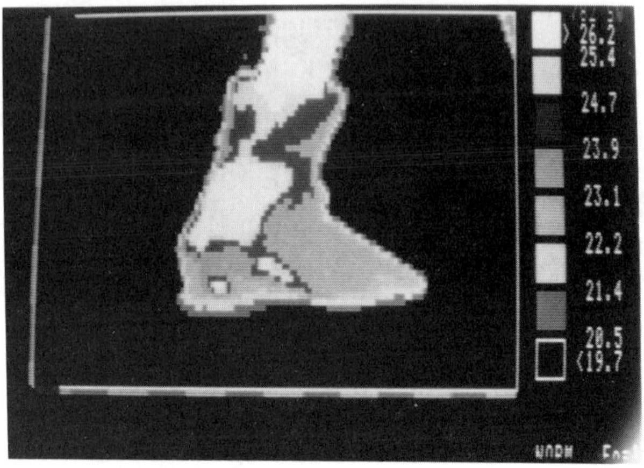

FIG. 5—*Junior rear entry boot shows a large area of heat loss with only 1 min of hot air inside. The heat losses follow the shell assembling lines.*

shell reduce heat loss. The kind of material and distribution of the inner boot padding, as well as its positioning within the shell, are also important.

Foot cooling is due to the physical condition of the skier as well as to the ski boot performance; the characteristics of the blood flow and the muscular activity of the skier are important but cannot affect the thermal resistance of the ski boot. If the latter is inadequate, the foot rapidly chills in the cold skiing environment. On the basis of the tests performed, we think that simulation of real skiing conditions is important but rather difficult to obtain. The cooling in the laboratory of the boot worn by a human foot, with ice or within a cold chamber, is sufficient, in our opinion, to produce reliable and useful data. The hot air test, which is more easily performed, is preferred for its ease of standardization. The results of our hot air tests were useful to demonstrate insulating characteristics of a boot's structure. In conclusion, we think that cold protection has great significance in skiing safety and injury prevention especially for junior skiers [*3*]. Application of infrared thermography in the thermal analysis of ski boots is promising even with its shortcomings.

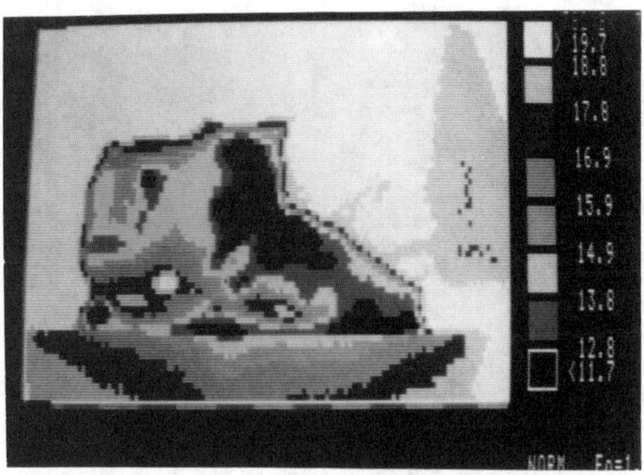

FIG. 6—*Modern boot with four buckles was taken out of the ice worn by the tester. This thermogram taken after 10 min of observation shows the beginning of thermal exchange in the lower part of the shell.*

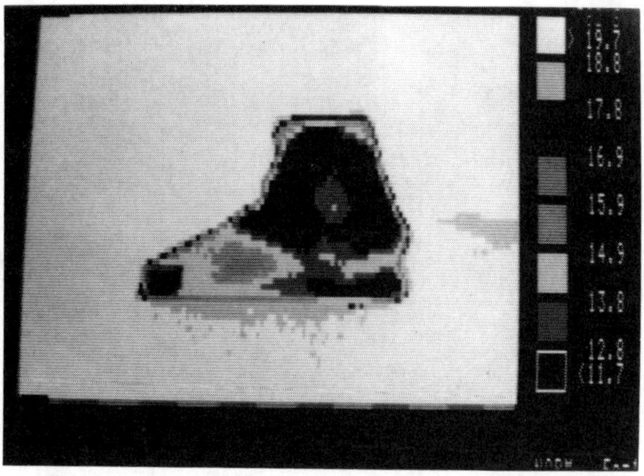

FIG. 7—*The same boot as in Fig. 5 10 min after being taken out of the ice. The tester was still wearing the boot and the thermogram shows thermal exchange in the lower part of the shell.*

We believe it would be well advised to work out a standard test with the hot air method or with a heated artificial limb, which could allow a comparison of ski boot models on the market. The goal of such testing should be better temperature isolation of all ski boots.

References

[*1*] Zucco, P., Moschi, A., and Zingoni, G., "La funzionalità delle calzature da sci dal punto di vista della biomeccanica articolare e della adattabilità del piede. Parte II: le forze agenti sulla pianta del piede; significato e metodo di studio," *Medicina dello Sport*, Vol. 36, No. 3, 1983, pp. 261–271.

[*2*] Medoff, H., Pierce, J., Pope, M., and Johnson, R. J., "On-Slope Testing of an Instrumented Alpine Ski Boot," in *Skiing Trauma and Safety: Fifth International Symposium, ASTM STP 860*, American Society for Testing and Materials, Philadelphia, 1985, pp. 165–172.

[*3*] Roberts, C. C., Jr., "Infrared Thermal Imaging and Skiing Safety," in *Skiing Trauma and Safety: Fifth International Symposium, ASTM STP 860*, American Society for Testing and Materials, Philadelphia, 1985, pp. 445–463.

[*4*] Roberts, C. C. and Reinke, K. L., "Infrared Thermography in the Hands of the Research, Development and Engineering Consultant," Infrared Information Exchange—1978, AGA Corporation, Secaucus, NJ, 1979.

[*5*] Hauser, E. R. and Nelson, G. D., "Thermographic Evaluation and Heat Flow Analysis of Clothing and Garment Design," Infrared Information Exchange—1978, AGA Corporation, Secaucus, NJ, 1979.

The Ski

Anthony A. Renshaw[1] *and C. D. Mote, Jr.*[1]

A Model for the Turning Snow Ski

REFERENCE: Renshaw, A. A. and Mote, C. D., Jr., **"A Model for the Turning Snow Ski,"** *Skiing Trauma and Safety: Eighth International Symposium, ASTM STP 1104*, C. D. Mote, Jr. and Robert J. Johnson, Eds., American Society for Testing and Materials, Philadelphia, 1991, pp. 217–238.

ABSTRACT: A model is developed to investigate the steady-state solutions of a turning snow ski. A rigid body skier executes a constant radius turn on a horizontal snow surface. Two types of forces are assumed along the ski bottom: *skidding forces*, which arise when shearing a new snow surface, and *carving forces*, which maintain the curvature of the ski as part of the running surface of the ski slides along its own track without shearing the snow. Using the equations of conservation of linear and angular momentum, dynamic equilibrium is established for the three forces and accelerations acting on the skier/ski system: the force generated along the flexing ski, gravity, and the centripetal acceleration of the turn. Turn radius and speed are insufficient to specify a unique solution to these equations. To quantify the effects of different ski designs on the model, a range of possible dynamic equilibrium solutions is calculated for each turn radius and speed and compared using two indices, one measuring the mechanical efficiency of the turn resulting from the energy dissipation of shearing the snow surface, and the second measuring the equilibrium solution sensitivity to human control and regulation. When possible solutions are mapped onto the plane of these two indices, a characteristic solution behavior emerges, which has been corroborated with experimental results found using a model ski turning on Astroturf.® This behavior provides a quantitative basis for comparing different ski designs and proposing new design strategies.

KEY WORDS: ski design, skiing mechanics, skiing, snow, sports mechanics, ski, sports equipment, skiing trauma, skiing safety, mechanical modeling, design optimization

Nomenclature

$C(s)$	Angle between $\hat{v}(s)$ and $\hat{n}(s)$, degree; Fig. 2
C_{init}	Angle of carving initiation, degree
$d(s)$	Depth of ski edge in snow, m
$\underline{EI}(s)$	Transverse flexural ski stiffness, N-m^2
$\overline{EI}(s)$	Original $EI(s)$, N-m^2
$F_c(s)$	Force generated during carving, N/m
$F_i(s)$	Force generated by shearing ice, N/m
$F_i'(s)$	Force generated during shearing snow, N/m
F_r	Radial force on experimental ski, N
$F_s(s)$	Snow force along the ski running surface, N/m
$\underline{F}_s(s)$	Vector representation of F_s, N/m
F_t	Thrust force applied at the skier center of mass, N

[1]Graduate student and professor and chairman, respectively, Department of Mechanical Engineering, University of California, Berkeley, Berkeley, CA 94720.

F_t/W Normalized thrust—mechanical efficiency performance index
f_{max} Maximum increase in stiffness for $f[h(-1)]$
$f[h(-1)]$ Proposed nonlinear stiffness increase of $EI(s)$
g Gravitational constant, m/s^2
$GJ(s)$ Torsional ski stiffness, N-m^2
$\overline{GJ}(s)$ Original $GJ(s)$, N-m^2
$h(s)$ Deflection of ski from undeformed state, m
I_x,I_y,I_z Principal moments of inertia of the skier, kg-m^2
K_d Smoothing function for numerical stability
K_f Scaling factor for snow shearing force
L Ski length, m
l Distance from skier center of mass to skier/ski attachment (that is, the boot), m; Fig. 3
M Experimentally measured moment about pivot point corresponding to M_x, N-m
M_X Moment created by $\underline{F}_s(s)$ about an axis through the skier center of mass parallel to the X-axis, N-m
$-\frac{\partial M_X}{\partial \varepsilon_t}\frac{1}{Wl}$ Normalized sensitivity—human control performance index
m Mass of the experimental ski, kg
$\hat{n}(s)$ Unit normal to the bottom of the ski
R Radius of the turn, m
$\hat{r}-\hat{\theta}-\hat{Z}$ Orthogonal unit vectors of cylindrical representation of $X-Y-Z$
s Length coordinate along undeformed ski, m
$X-Y-Z$ Fixed coordinate system (inertial); Fig. 3
$x-y-z$ Coordinate system fixed on the skier at the center of mass; Fig.3
$x'-y'-z'$ Coordinate system fixed on the skier at the boot; Fig. 3
$\hat{x}-\hat{y}-\hat{z}$ Orthogonal unit vectors in $x-y-z$
$\hat{v}(s)$ Ski velocity unit vector
W Skier weight, N
$w(s)$ Half-width of ski, m; Fig. 1
Z Height of skier center of mass above snow, m; Fig. 3
$\alpha_X, \alpha_Y, \alpha_Z$ Rotation angles of the skier, rad; FIg. 3
$\beta(s)$ Angle between cutting surface and snow or ice surface, rad; Fig. 2
$\underline{\Delta}(s)$ Vector from skier center of mass to point of application of $\underline{F}_s(s)$, m
$\delta(s)$ Distance from ski midline to point of application of $\underline{F}_s(s)$, m
ε_r, ε_r Rotation angles of the ski, rad; Fig. 3
$\eta(s)$ Angle of twist of ski due to torsion, rad
$\underline{\omega}$ Angular velocity in $x-y-z$, rad/s
$\omega_x, \omega_y, \omega_z$ Components of $\underline{\omega}$, rad/s
$\rho(s)$ Curvature of the ski, m
θ Angular position of the skier/ski in the turn, rad
$\dot{\theta}$ Angular velocity of the skier/ski in the turn, rad/s

Introduction

Despite the variability of skier ability and skiing conditions, design parameters of skis typically lie within narrow ranges. The search for an optimal ski design within or around these ranges has been retarded by the absence of any model relating the design of the ski and the skiing technique to the efficiency of the skiing process. This paper introduces a theoretical model of a turning ski and examines effects of the ski design variables on two parameters possibly predicting its turning efficiency: the mechanical efficiency associated with energy losses in the turn, and the efficacy of the human control action maintaining the turn. The objective of such research is to understand better the mechanics of the skiing process to be able to compare quantitatively different ski designs and suggest design strategies.

The literature on ski design is descriptive, and based principally on observation. Schultes [*1*] claims that between 88 to 98% of the strain energy of the ski is in bending rather than torsion, depending on the hardness of the snow. He claims that the side cut of the ski shown in Fig. 1 is unnoticeable during the turn itself, although it may have a significant role in turn initiation. Sakata [*2*] examines the relative importance of the bending stiffness compared to the torsional stiffness by surveying the bending and torsion stiffnesses of skis sold between 1975 and 1986. From consistency of the design parameters over time he concludes that the bending stiffness is significantly more important than the torsional stiffness. He also notes that the moment of inertia and natural frequencies of skis changed little between 1975 and 1986, while the mass of skis decreased slightly.

This paper builds on the model of a turning snow ski by Lieu and Mote [*3*]. The model has been recast into a more general formulation, and the results are extended to include a

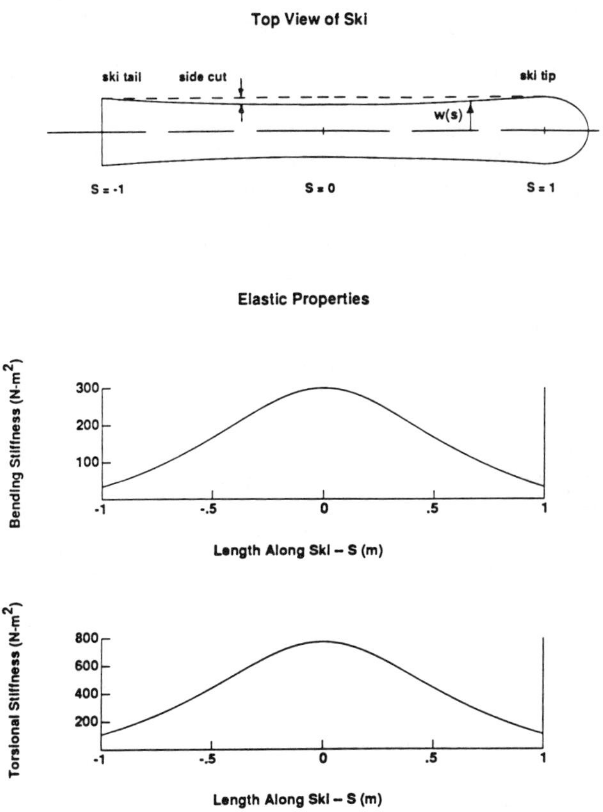

FIG. 1—*Geometric and elastic properties of skis.*

wider variety of turns and skis. More importantly, the presentation format of the results is entirely new and allows a direct comparison of different turns and skis using two performance indices.

The model considers a rigid skier riding a single ski that executes a constant radius, constant speed turn on a horizontal snow surface. The skier is propelled through this turn by a hypothetical thrust force acting at his or her center of mass and tangent to the circular turn trajectory. This force replaces the gravitational gradient normally responsible for overcoming the forces of the snow on the ski. If gravity were used to propel the skier in this model, then several cumbersome definitions and assumptions would have to be made to describe the terrain and location of the skier through the turn. By executing the turn on a horizontal surface and artificially providing an external thrust to propel the skier indefinitely through a circular turn, these complications are avoided. This thrust does not arise as a result of the skier-ski-snow modeling. Instead, it is supplied externally and at whatever magnitude is necessary to maintain the constant speed momentum balance of the turn. Gravity remains in the model only to establish equilibrium with the vertical direction. It acts perpendicularly to the thrust.

The single ski is assigned a length, boot position, and flexural stiffness, torsional stiffness, and side cut distributions. These variables are used to determine the forces between the ski and snow causing an equilibrium (steady-state) deflection of the ski as it executes a turn. These forces are combined with the external thrust and the weight of the skier normal to the plane of the snow to determine steady-state turning configurations. Ski terminology and sample bending and torsional stiffness distributions are shown in Fig. 1.

The forces of interaction between the ski and the snow are assumed to be of two types, each with a different mechanism and magnitude of force generation dependent on the ski orientation and deflection in the snow. *Skidding forces* at points along the bottom ski edge are generated when the trajectory of the ski causes the edge of the ski at those points to shear the snow surface. These skidding forces are assumed proportional to the forces generated in the machining of ice and are estimated from ice-cutting experimental data. As the afterbody of the ski deflects, a configuration can often be reached in which the trajectories of points on the ski edge have no velocity component normal to the bottom edge of the ski. These points, therefore, slide on the snow surface rather than machining a new surface. This phenomenon, termed *carving*, requires forces smaller than the skidding forces. The *carving forces* are only those required to maintain the curvature of the ski without machining the snow surface. A smooth transition between the skidding and carving forces is assumed, and frictional forces are not considered.

For a given turn radius and speed, the model does not lead to a unique solution to the equations of dynamic equilibrium, namely conservation of linear and angular momentum. To understand the model's results adequately, it is necessary to compare quantitatively a range of skidding and carving solutions at each radius and speed. Two parameters are defined to assist this comparison. The mechanical efficiency of the solution is given by the externally supplied thrust directed tangent to the trajectory that is required to maintain the constant speed and constant radius turn on the horizontal surface. The smaller the thrust, the more efficient the turn. The sensitivity of the human control of each solution is quantified by the derivative of the fore–aft moment generated by the snow forces at equilibrium with respect to the tilt of the ski at the location of the boot. This sensitivity parameter measures the gain of the control action generated by the skier when tilting the boot. A small sensitivity is often desirable because it implies that the equilibrium moment is less sensitive to small tilting errors at the boot.

Equilibrium solution maps of these two parameters are computed for ranges of ski designs and modeling assumptions. The results show that the flexural stiffness of the ski, the centripetal acceleration of the skier, and the snow hardness are the most important parameters of the model influencing the steady-state turning efficiency.

The analytical solutions are compared qualitatively with empirical results obtained in a scaled experiment using a small aluminum ski turning on a rotating Astroturf surface. The turning results show similar characteristic behaviors of the skier thrust and sensitivity as functions of the ski orientation.

The Model

Snow/Ski Interaction

The skidding forces are assumed proportional to forces required to machine ice from Lieu and Mote [*4*]. Their experiments show that the force per unit length, F_i, necessary to machine the ice surface is always normal to the cutting edge and that its magnitude is determined by the depth of cut d into the ice and the cutting angle β between the cutting plane and the surface of the ice (Fig. 2). The value F_i is given by the empirical relation:

$$F_i = \left[\frac{16120}{\sin^{3.7}\beta} - 15510\right] [39.37\, d]^{(-0.37\beta + 0.7)} \text{ N/m} \qquad d > 0 \tag{1}$$

At any section along the length of the ski that is skidding, the force F_i can be assigned. The position along the length of the ski is s (Fig. 1). The values d and β are implicit functions of s. Hence, $F_i = F_i(s)$.

This formula is scaled to model the cutting of snow instead of ice by the two coefficients, K_f, and K_d.

$$F_i'(s) = K_f\, K_d(s)\, F_i(s) \tag{2}$$

Coefficient K_f scales the magnitude of F_i to represent snow rather than ice. The cutting force of snow is initially assumed to be 2% of the cutting forces of ice, giving $K_f = 0.02$. K_f respectively decreases or increases for softer or harder snows. The derivative of F_i with respect to d in Eq 1 is large near $d = 0$. Coefficient K_d smooths F_i' near $d = 0$ for numerical stability:

$$K_d = \begin{cases} \dfrac{1}{2}\left[1 - \cos\left(\pi \dfrac{d}{0.002}\right)\right] & 0 < d < 0.002 \text{ m} \\ 1 & 0.002 < d \text{ m} \end{cases} \tag{3}$$

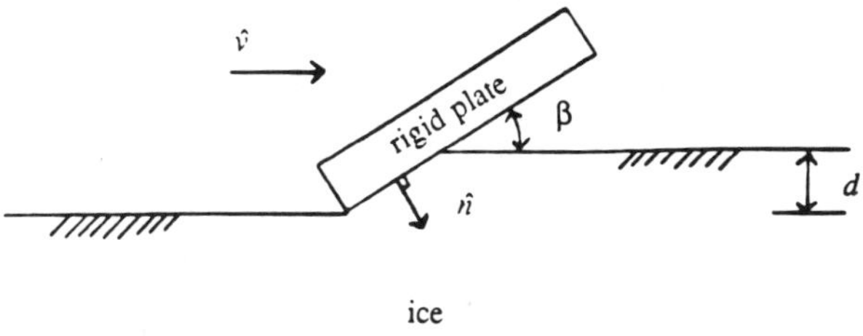

FIG. 2—*Schematic of an ice-cutting experiment used to determine the force per unit length required to machine ice. The angle between velocity $\hat{v}$ and plate normal $\hat{n}$ determines whether the plate is cutting or sliding on the ice.*

Because this only affects the forces on sections of the ski penetrating less than 2 mm into the snow, the form of K_d is not significant to the equilibrium solutions.

Carving

The skidding force $F_i'(s)$ is an upper bound on the ski forces. When a point on the afterbody of the ski slides in the track cut by the edge of the ski, the forces on the ski are necessarily reduced and bounded from below by the equilibrium forces required to maintain the curvature of the ski, denoted $F_c(s)$:

$$F_c(s) = \frac{d^2}{ds^2}\left\{\frac{EI(s)}{\rho(s)}\right\} \tag{4}$$

$EI(s)$ is the transverse flexural stiffness of the ski, and $\rho(s)$ is the radius of curvature of the ski (see Fig. 1).

The transition between skidding forces, F_i', and the carving forces, F_c, is regulated by the velocity decomposition at each point along the ski into a component cutting into new snow and a component sliding along the previously cut snow surface. The angle $C(s) = \cos^{-1}[\hat{v}(s) \cdot \hat{n}(s)]$ between the unit velocity vector $\hat{v}(s)$ and the unit ski normal $\hat{n}(s)$ in Fig. 2 is an indicator of this transition. The transition force between skidding and carving is modeled using a cosine envelope such that carving force transition begins at $C(s) = C_{\text{init}}$ and is fully achieved at $C(s) = 90°$. Combining the three types of forces together, one obtains the modeled ski force $F_s(s)$ at any point s on the ski:

$$F_s(s) = \begin{cases} F_i'(s) & 0 < C(s) \le C_{\text{init}} \\ F_i'(s) + \frac{1}{2}[F_c(s) - F_i'(s)]\left[1 - \cos\left(\pi\frac{C(s) - C_{\text{init}}}{90 - C_{\text{init}}}\right)\right] & C_{\text{init}} < C(s) \le 90° \\ F_c(s) & 90° < C(s) \le 180° \end{cases} \tag{5}$$

C_{init}, the angle of carving initiation, is arbitrarily assigned an initial value of 80° and is independent from K_f. Although $C(s)$ is always less than or equal to 90° in the equilibrium solutions, the solution algorithm uses a continuous force function for angles greater than 90° during intermediate phases of the calculations.

Skier/Ski Geometry and Position

The skier is modeled as a rigid body mounted on a single ski executing a constant radius, constant speed turn in a horizontal plane (Fig. 3). The ski is rigidly attached to the skier, although two of the angles of attachment, the roll side to side and the tilt forward and backward, can be varied. The rigid body has a mass W/g and three principal moments of inertia, I_x, I_y, I_z, where the x–y–z coordinate system is fixed in the body with its origin at the center of mass. The skier position is described by six degrees of freedom. They are the radius of the turn, R, the angle in the turn, θ, the height Z of the center of mass above the snow surface, and three noncommutative, finite rotation angles, α_Z, α_Y, α_X that rotate the

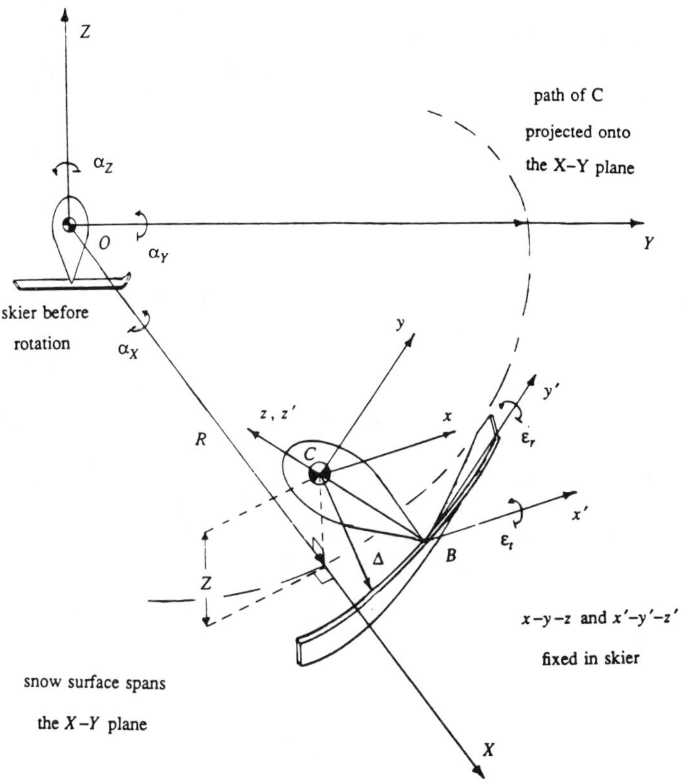

FIG. 3—*Geometry of the modeled turn. Rotations* α_x, α_y, *and* α_z, *are right-handed while* ε_t *and* ε_r *are left-handed.*

x–y–z coordinate system from a reference orientation in the fixed X–Y–Z system (see Appendix A).

The skier and x–y–z system are located in the fixed X–Y–Z coordinate system by a sequence of rotations followed by a translation. The positioning begins with the x–y–z and X–Y–Z systems coincident. The skier faces in the positive y direction with z vertical, and the center of mass lies at the origin, point O, located at the center of the turn and on the snow surface, which is spanned by the X–Y plane. The first rotation α_Z about the Z axis causes the ski tip to twist counterclockwise (to the left). A negative rotation α_Y about the Y axis banks the skier to the left about an axis parallel to the original longitudinal axis of the ski. Finally, the rotation α_X about the X axis rotates the head backward and the feet forward. Descriptive names for the three rotations are: the twist angle (α_Z), the bank angle (α_Y), and the recline angle (α_X). Following these rotations, the skier and the x–y–z system are translated to the point ($X = R$, $Y = 0$, $Z = Z$).

The principal axis of inertia for I_z is the z axis, defined by the line joining the center of mass, C, and the boot position, B. The boot is at a constant distance l from the center of mass. The orientation of the ski at the boot is described by two noncommutative finite rotation angles, the ski roll angle, ε_r, and the ski tilt angle, ε_t, about the y' and x' axes, respectively. The x'–y'–z' axes are fixed in the skier with coincident z and z', and x'–y'

parallel to $x-y$. The origin of the $x'-y'-z'$ is located at the point $(0,0,-l)$ of the $x-y-z$ system. A rotation of the ski about the z' axis is not considered.

The ski is modeled as an Euler-Bernoulli beam of length L with stiffness and geometry varying along the length s. The forebody of the ski is defined by $s > 0$ and the afterbody by $s < 0$ (see Fig. 1). The ski half-width or side cut is $\pm w(s)$, the transverse flexural stiffness is $EI(s)$, and the torsional stiffness is $GJ(s)$. The ski mass is negligible compared to the skier mass.

Steady-State Equations

The snow/ski interaction creates a distributed force on the bottom of the ski, $\underline{F}_s(s)$, whose orientation is assumed normal to the deflected ski surface. The value $\underline{F}_s(s)$ denotes the vector representation of the ski force in the $X-Y-Z$ coordinate system. Two additional forces contribute to the steady-state equilibrium. The weight of the skier, W, is directed perpendicular to the horizontal snow surface and, hence, does not contribute to the propulsion. An externally supplied thrust, F_t, is required at the center of mass directed tangent to the circular trajectory and perpendicular to W to propel the skier through the turn at constant speed.

In the cylindrical coordinate representation of $X-Y-Z$ with unit vectors $\hat{r}$, $\hat{\theta}$, and $\hat{Z}$, the linear momentum balance at equilibrium becomes:

$$\int [\underline{F}_s(s) \cdot \hat{r}]\, ds = -(W/g)R\dot{\theta}^2 \tag{6a}$$

$$F_t + \int [\underline{F}_s(s) \cdot \hat{\theta}]\, ds = 0 \tag{6b}$$

$$-W + \int [\underline{F}_s(s) \cdot \hat{Z}]\, ds = 0 \tag{6c}$$

The angular momentum balance is evaluated in the principal coordinate system, $x-y-z$, where the thrust force and the weight that both act through the center of mass give no contribution. The vector $\underline{\Delta}(s)$ is measured from the center of mass to the point of application of $\underline{F}_s(s)$ (see Fig. 3), and $\underline{\omega}$ is the angular velocity in the $x-y-z$ coordinates, calculated from α_X, α_Y, and α_Z (see Appendix A). The angular momentum balance at equilibrium is:

$$0 = \int [\underline{\Delta} \times \underline{F}_s(s)] \cdot \hat{x}\, ds + (I_y - I_z)\omega_y\omega_z \tag{7a}$$

$$0 = \int [\underline{\Delta} \times \underline{F}_s(s)] \cdot \hat{y}\, ds + (I_z - I_x)\omega_z\omega_x \tag{7b}$$

$$0 = \int [\underline{\Delta} \times \underline{F}_s(s)] \cdot \hat{z}\, ds + (I_x - I_y)\omega_x\omega_y \tag{7c}$$

where $\hat{x}$, $\hat{y}$, and $\hat{z}$ are unit vectors.

The deflection of the ski is calculated using Euler-Bernoulli beam and classical torsion theories. For this calculation, the distributed force $\underline{F}_s$ is assumed to act normal to the undeflected running surface of the ski, which is satisfactory for sufficiently small deflection. The deflection, $h(s)$, is calculated by treating the forebody and the afterbody of the ski as independent cantilever prismatic beams extending from the boot location on the ski. The bending deflection, $h(s)$, is determined from:

$$F_s(s) = \frac{d^2}{ds^2}\left[EI(s)\frac{d^2}{ds^2}h(s)\right] \tag{8a}$$

with boundary conditions

$$h = 0 \quad \text{and} \quad \frac{dh}{ds} = 0 \quad \text{at} \quad s = 0 \tag{8b}$$

$$\frac{d^2h}{ds^2} = 0 \quad \text{and} \quad \frac{d^3h}{ds^3} = 0 \quad \text{at the tip and tail of the ski} \tag{8c}$$

The angle of twist $\eta(s)$ is determined by:

$$F_s(s)\,\delta(s) = -\frac{d}{ds}\left[GJ(s)\frac{d}{ds}\eta(s)\right] \tag{9a}$$

with $\delta(s)$ equal to the distance from ski midline to the point of application of F_s. In this model, it is assumed that F_s is located on the surface half way between the embedded edge of the ski and the undisturbed snow surface at $Z = 0$. If both ski edges are entirely below the X–Y plane, F_s is applied at the ski midline. The boundary conditions are

$$\eta = 0 \quad \text{at} \quad s = 0 \tag{9b}$$

$$\frac{d\eta}{ds} = 0 \quad \text{at both the tip and tail of the ski} \tag{9c}$$

Initial Configuration

The initial ski, skier, and snow properties, hereafter termed the *original ski*, are given below. This ski was analyzed by Lieu and Mote [*3*]. With this choice of speed and turning radius, the bank angle of the turn is about 45°.

Turn:

$$R = 10 \text{ m} \qquad \dot{\theta} = 1 \text{ rad/s}$$

Skier:

$$W = 686 \text{ N} \qquad l = 1 \text{ m}$$

$$I_x = 23.5 \text{ kg} - \text{m}^2 \qquad I_y = 24.0 \text{ kg} - \text{m}^2 \qquad I_z = 0.78 \text{ kg} - \text{m}^2$$

Snow:

$$K_f = 0.02 \qquad C_{\text{init}} = 80°$$

Ski:

$$L = 2\ m, \text{ with the midpoint at } s = 0$$

$$w(s) = \pm(0.035 + 0.010\ s^2)\ \text{m} \qquad -1 \leq s \leq +1\ \text{m} \tag{10a}$$

$$\overline{EI}(s) = \frac{200}{s^2 + 0.5} - 100\ \text{N} - \text{m}^2 \qquad -1 \leq s \leq +1\ \text{m} \tag{10b}$$

$$\overline{GJ}(s) = \frac{500}{s^2 + 0.5} - 225\ \text{N} - \text{m}^2 \qquad -1 \leq s \leq +1\ \text{m} \tag{10c}$$

Solution Technique

The linear and angular momentum balances (Eqs 6 and 7) depend on the four unspecified degrees of freedom of the skier/ski system: Z, α_X, α_Y, α_Z, and the two allowable ski degrees of freedom ε_r, ε_t. The equations describing dynamic equilibrium (Eqs 6 and 7) and the flexure and twist of the ski (Eqs 8 and 9) are nonlinear and cannot be solved analytically. In fact, there is no unique solution if these six variables are unconstrained. Specification of two variables, α_X, the recline angle, and α_Z, the twist angle, leads to a unique solution when a solution can be found. The equilibrium configurations are found using an iterative two-phase modified steepest descent algorithm. First, the ski deflection is predicted by iteratively calculating it from the snow forces generated by the deflection of the previous iteration. Convergence of the ski deflection prediction is achieved when the calculated snow/ski interaction force varies less than 0.4% between iterations. Second, positioning of the skier and ski are varied to satisfy dynamic equilibrium. Convergence of the linear and angular momentum balance relationships is satisfied when the residuals are less than 0.45% of $W(N)$ and $Wl(Nm)$, respectively.

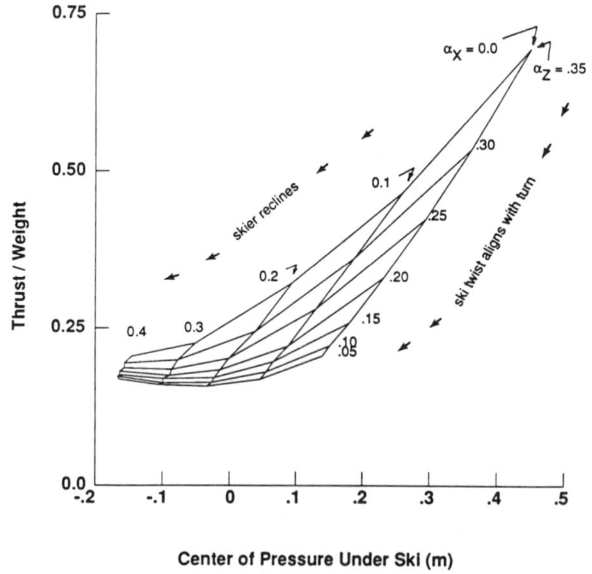

FIG. 4—*Solutions for the original ski mapped onto the location of the center of pressure of the ski forces and the thrust necessary to maintain the constant radius, constant speed turn.*

Analytical Results

Solution Characteristics

Solutions are computed for the original ski for pairs of $\alpha_X - \alpha_Z$ coordinates. α_X assumes values 0.0, 0.1, 0.2, 0.3, and 0.4 rad and α_Z the values 0.05, 0.10, 0.15, 0.20, 0.25, 0.30, and 0.35 rad. At $\alpha_X = 0.0$, the model is erect; the skier leans backward when $\alpha_X > 0$. When $\alpha_Z = 0.0$, the ski at $s = 0$ is tangent to the trajectory, and $\alpha_Z > 0$ rotates the forebody of the ski toward the center of the turn.

Figure 4 shows the external thrust required to maintain the equilibrium velocity of the ski plotted against the location of the center of pressure of the snow forces along the running surface of the ski. Thrust is reduced by moving the center of pressure toward the tail of the ski by either increasing the recline angle α_X or decreasing the twist angle α_Z. The thrust reduction converges to a lower limit. The center of pressure on the ski can lie either behind or ahead of the boot. In all cases, the strain energy of bending is at least ten times greater than the strain energy of torsion, supporting estimates by Schultes [*1*].

Figure 5 shows typical equilibrium force distributions on the running surface of the ski for a skidding solution, a solution in the transition between skidding and carving, and a carving solution. In the skidding solution, the force is nearly symmetrically distributed along

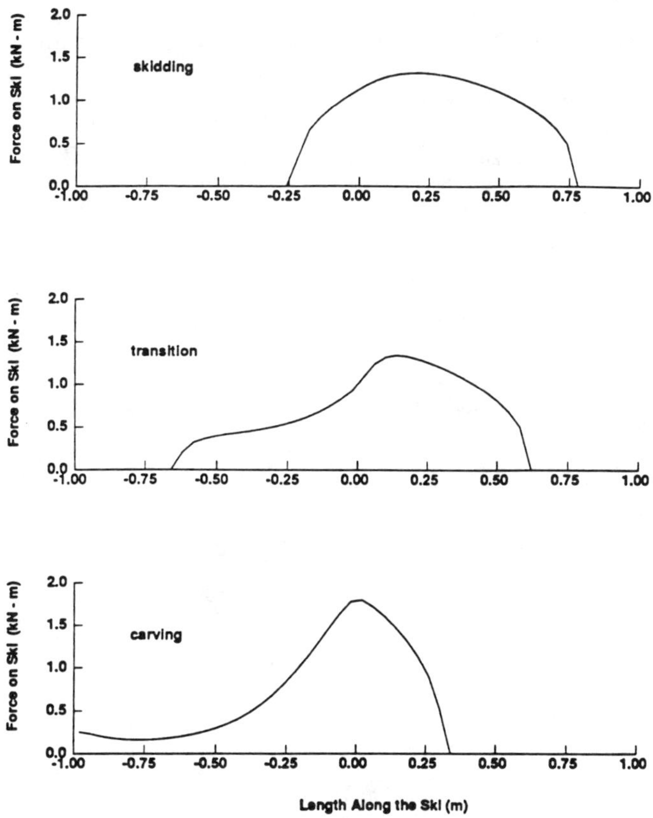

FIG. 5—*The force distribution along the bottom of the ski for three representative solutions: a skidding ski, a ski in transition between skidding and carving, and a fully carving ski.*

the length of the ski about a point on the forebody of the ski. The tip and the tail of the ski both rise out of the snow. At the initiation of carving, the tail of the ski is pushed into the snow, the force distribution shifts back along the ski, and the symmetry is destroyed.

Solution Indices

To compare different ski designs, the equilibrium solutions are presented using two solution indices. The first index is the normalized thrust (F_t/W) required. The thrust balances the energy dissipation in the turn and is used as a measure of the mechanical efficiency of the turning ski. Turn solutions with small dissipation, and therefore small required thrust, are expected to be faster than those of large dissipation. The second solution index, $-(\partial M_X/\partial \varepsilon_t)/(1/Wl)$, is evaluated numerically at each equilibrium solution. M_X represents the moment created by the snow force, $F_s(s)$, about an axis parallel to the X axis at the center of mass computed through static equilibrium with the forces on the ski bottom. This normalized derivative is referred to as the solution *sensitivity*. Solution sensitivity is a measure of the ease of human control of the equilibrium solution. Low sensitivity states that small tilting of the boot at equilibrium produces small changes in the equilibrium moment. Small moment imbalance can probably be more easily regulated than larger imbalances. Thus, a low sensitivity turn should be more easily maintained by the skier.

In Fig. 6, the full range of solutions for the original ski are represented in a map of the two solution indices. The solutions are classified into three separate regions: the skidding region where decreasing thrust accompanies increasing sensitivity, a transition region where sensitivity reaches a maximum value, and a carving region where sensitivity is greatly reduced as thrust reaches a minimum value. Examination of the force distribution and deflection of the ski is used to make this classification.

The solution map summarizes the possible turning solutions for this ski design, skier, and

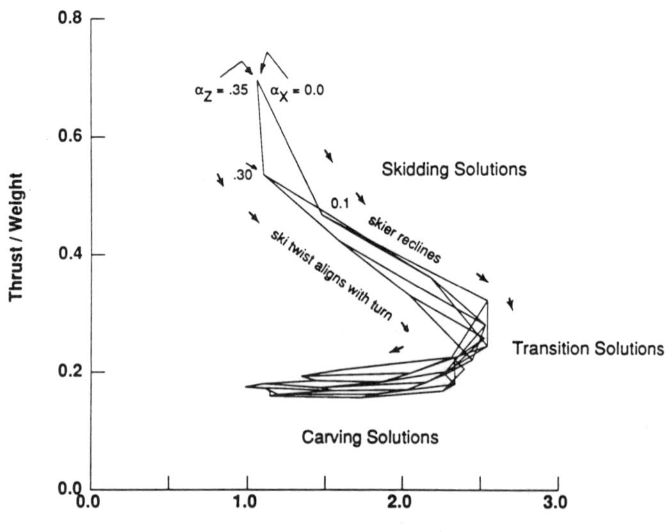

FIG. 6—*The two solution indices for the original ski. Three regions of interest are labeled: skidding, transition between skidding and carving, and carving solutions. This curve is used as a benchmark for comparing different ski designs.*

specified turn. The maximum sensitivity turn and the minimum thrust turn bracket the possible solutions to the specified turn. By allowing the ski design and selected modeling assumptions to change, the contribution to the performance indices and the bracketing solutions can be evaluated. Some results are summarized below.

Snow Hardness

Figure 7 compares the solutions for the original ski on snows of different hardness, characterized by coefficient K_f. Solutions in the softest snow ($K_f = 0.005$) show little differentiation in sensitivity or thrust. As the snow hardness increases, differences between the skidding and carving solutions are identified. The maximum sensitivity is directly proportional to K_f, and the minimum thrust is inversely related to it. Harder snows produce smaller minimum thrusts and, therefore, *faster* solutions. This speed increase is at the expense of increased sensitivity in the transition solutions between the skidding and carving.

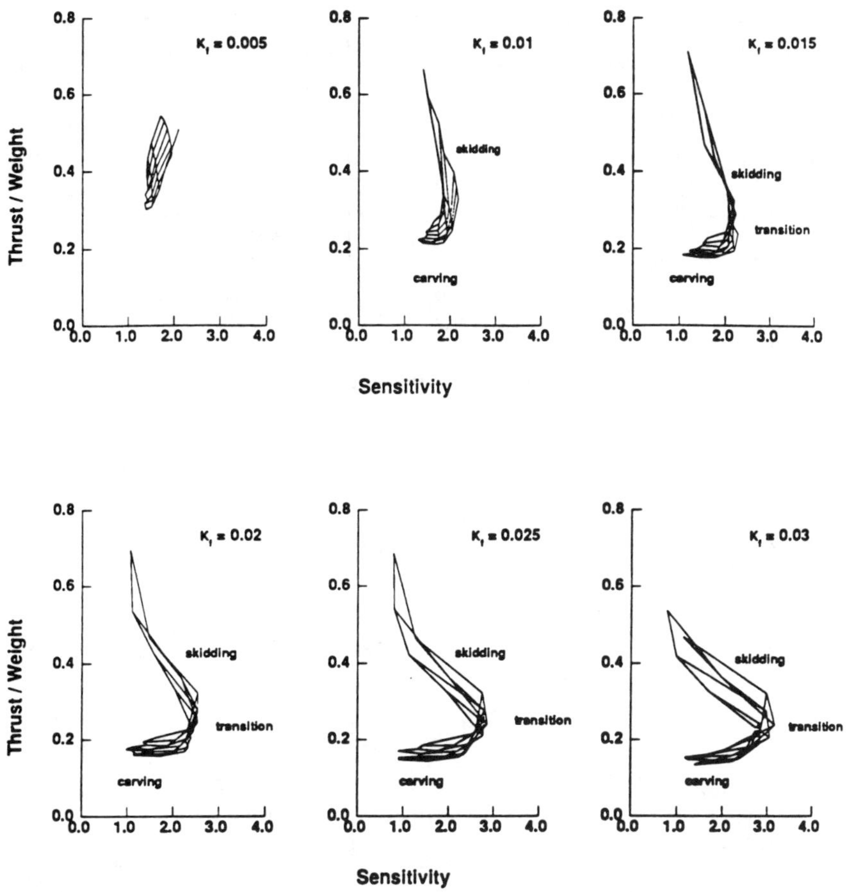

FIG. 7—*Solutions for snows of different hardness* K_f, *the hardness of the snow compared to ice. In the original solution,* $K_f = 0.02$.

Longitudinal Bending Stiffness Distribution

Figure 8 shows the effects of scaling the original stiffness distribution, $\overline{EI}$, by factors of 0.5, 1.0, 1.5, and 2.0. Increasing the stiffness of the ski increases the maximum sensitivity in the transition region proportionally. The minimum thrust needed in the carving solutions is smallest for the highest stiffness. The maximum sensitivity of the lowest stiffness solution is minimized, and the minimum thrust is larger than that of the original ski. These solution behaviors are similar to those found for changing snow hardness.

Other Design Variables

The solution maps for turns with identical centripetal accelerations are indistinguishable. It appears that centripetal acceleration can be used as a parameter of dynamic similarity for

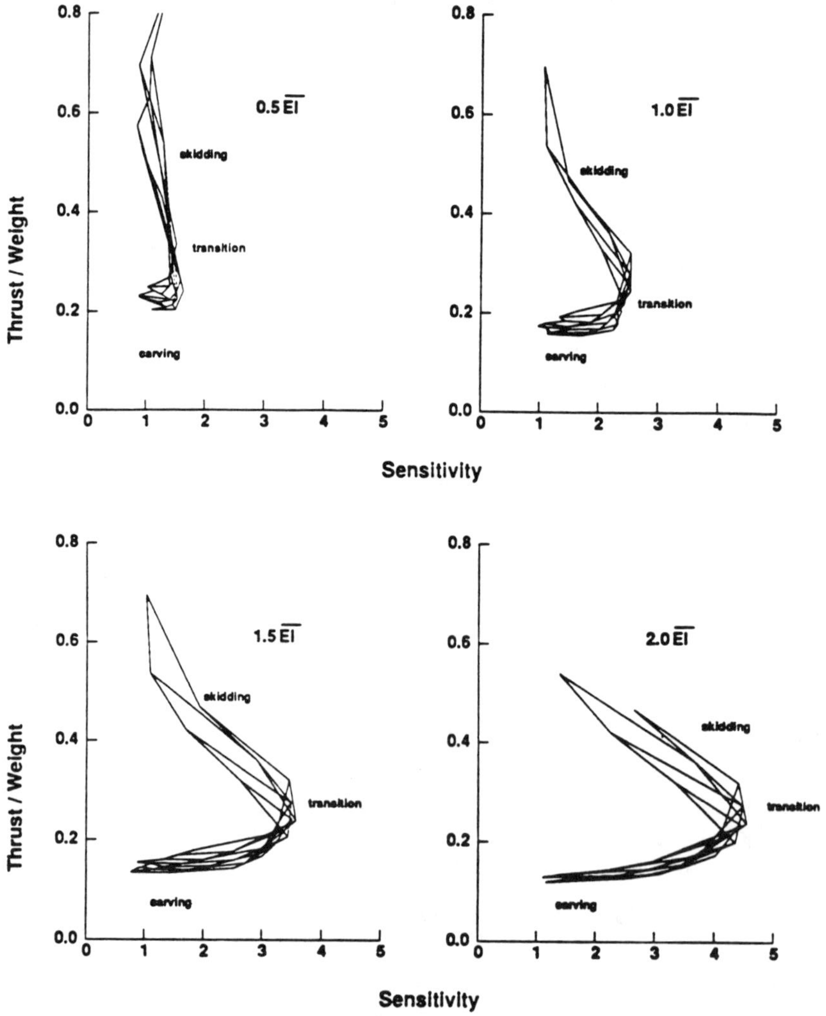

FIG. 8—*The effect of longitudinal stiffness on turn solutions.*

different turns. Changes in torsional stiffness affect only the skidding solutions by reducing the required thrust, but this is significant only for large (> 50%) stiffness changes. Neither the side cut nor the length of the ski afterbody (in the range of 0.5 m to 1.0 m) affects the solution map.

Five Parameter Summary

The effects of five variables on the solution map are summarized in Fig. 9. The five variables are: the snow hardness; the longitudinal bending stiffness of the ski; the centripetal acceleration of the turn; the maximum sensitivity of the transition from skidding to carving; and the minimum thrust achieved when the ski is carving. In general, the harder snow and stiffer ski have smaller minimum thrust at the expense of larger maximum sensitivity. The turns with greater centripetal acceleration have larger minimum thrusts and smaller maximum sensitivities. These variations occur smoothly and provide a basis for predicting the coupled effects of these variables.

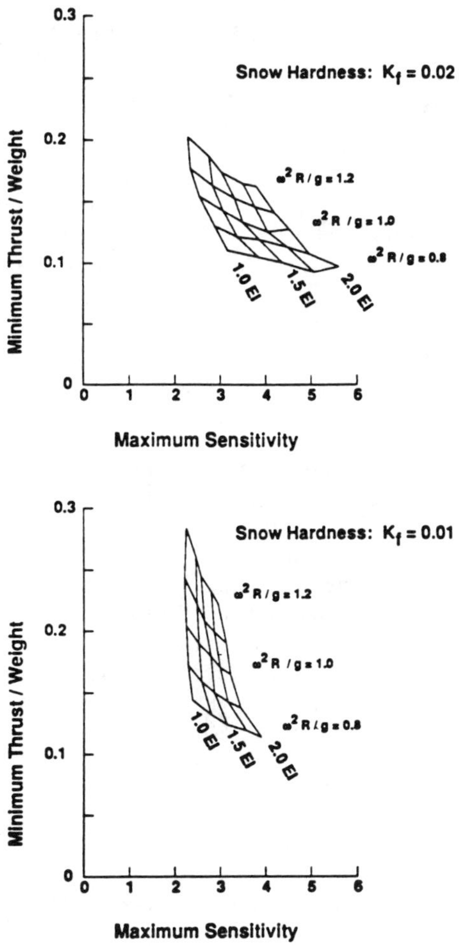

FIG. 9—*Summary of results in terms of five parameters: snow hardness* K_f, *centripetal acceleration, overall longitudinal stiffness, maximum sensitivity, and minimum thrust.*

Adaptive Skis

A ski design strategy is suggested by these results that reduces both the maximum sensitivity and the minimum thrust. During the transition from skidding to carving, a low stiffness is needed to reduce the maximum sensitivity. During the carving state, high stiffness is needed for smaller thrusts. The design problem, then, is recognizing whether the ski is either skidding or carving and modifying the stiffness accordingly.

This problem may be solved by noting that there is a good correlation between the sensitivity of the solution and the deflection of the tail of the ski. High sensitivity solutions are associated with flat skis while the small sensitivity and small thrust carving solutions have large deflections of the tail.

To test whether the maximum sensitivity and minimum thrust can both be reduced by monitoring the tail deflection, an arbitrary, hypothetical stiffness, increasing nonlinearly as a function of the tail deflection up to a maximum increase of f_{max}, is proposed:

$$EI(s) = f[h(-1)]\, \overline{EI}(s) \tag{11}$$

where $h(-1)$ is the deflection of the ski at $s = -1$ and

$$f[h(-1)] = \begin{cases} f_{max} + \frac{1}{2}(1 - f_{max})\left[1 - \cos\left(\pi \frac{0.2 - h(-1)}{0.2}\right)\right] & 0 \le h(-1) \le 0.2 \\ f_{max} & 0.2 < h(-1) \end{cases} \tag{12}$$

The solution maps for this ski are shown in Fig. 10 where f_{max} takes on values 1.0, 1.25, 1.67, and 2.5. The quotation marks on the figure denote the maximum possible increases of stiffness, not a fixed increase. The solution maps show a small maximum sensitivity compared to the sensitivity for a linear, high stiffness ski (see Fig. 8), while the carving solutions have comparable minimum thrusts.

Experimental Corroboration

The following experiment is performed to corroborate predictions from the model. A 1.3-m-diameter plywood disk with Astroturf® bonded to its surface is rotated in the horizontal plane at 50 to 60 rpm. A model aluminum ski 16 cm long located at the end of a pivoting lever arm is lowered onto the Astroturf at a radius of 48 cm and allowed to reach vertical equilibrium in the Astroturf as the ski deflects. A circumferential drag force is created as the Astroturf slides underneath the ski, and the ski is held in specified orientations to capture the different solutions described by the theoretical model.

This experimental system is not a precise representation of the model. Although one can ski on Astroturf treadmills, the forces on the ski from the Astroturf are different from those produced by snow. The absence of a centripetally accelerating mass and the reduction in scale represent substantial changes from the theoretical system. However, the balances of the vertical and circumferential forces as the deformed model ski cuts and carves the surface are major components of the theoretical model that are preserved in the experimental set-up. This similarity provides a limited basis on which to compare the theoretical and experimental systems and solution maps.

The experimental system has three degrees of freedom: (1), the pentration depth of the ski into the Astroturf, regulated by the weight of the ski and the pivoting lever arm (10.2 N); (2), the ski twist about a vertical axis normal to the plane of the snow; and (3), the ski tilt about a horizontal axis perpendicular to the length of the ski located 6 cm above the

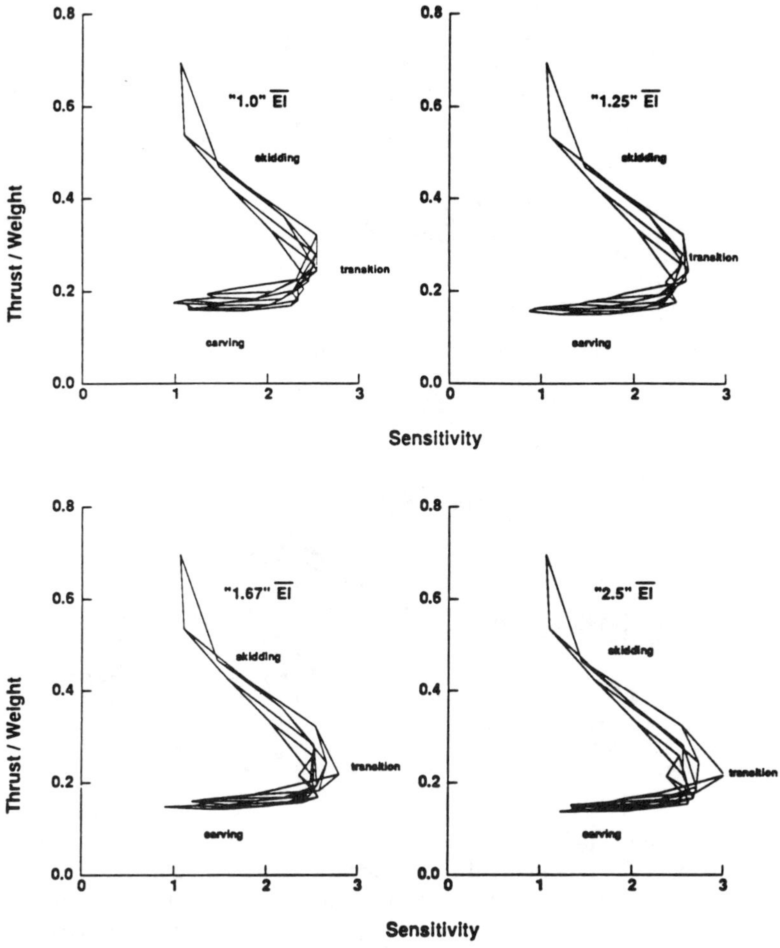

FIG. 10—*Solutions for skis with stiffness shown in Eqs* 11 *and* 12. *Quotation marks identify* f_{max}. *The minimum thrust is reduced by the increased stiffness while the maximum sensitivity remains constant compared with Fig. 8.*

boot (Fig. 11). Variation over the $\alpha_X - \alpha_Z$ grid is simulated by varying the twist and tilt angles. The ski is held at the constant bank angle of 45°.

The experimental skis are made of 16- by 3-cm rectangular strips of aluminum cut from 0.29-mm-thick sheets. Measurements of the stiffness of each individual strip shows an average stiffness of EI = 0.01 N-m^2. To vary the stiffness of the ski, two to four strips are stacked one on top of another, similar to a leaf spring. The location of the boot is 7 cm from the tip. The forebody of the ski is shorter than the afterbody to avoid capture of the tip of the ski by the Astroturf and subsequent rotation of the ski tip under the ski. The ski is not tilted far forward during any experiments for this reason.

Pairs of strain gages are attached on opposite parallel faces of the ski support arm to measure the moment produced by the shear force in the plane of the snow. To measure the location of the center of pressure on the ski, a third pair of strain gages is mounted on the

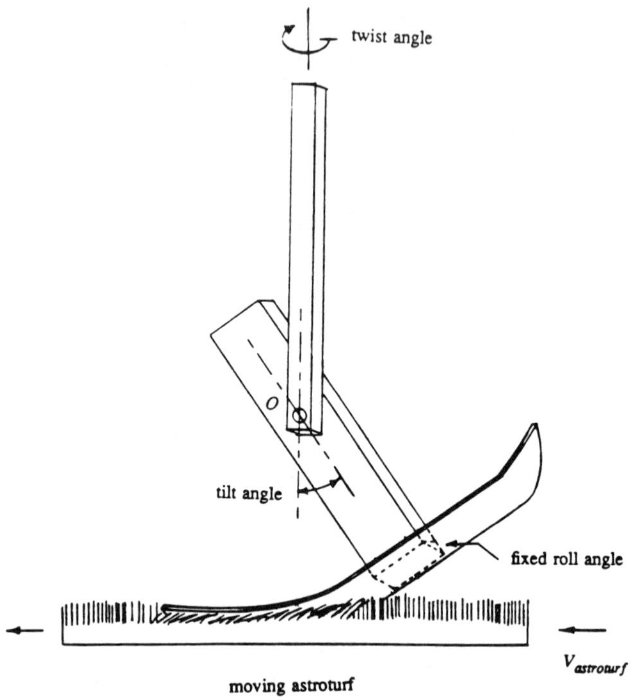

FIG. 11—*An experiment to measure ski solution curves for an aluminum ski resting on a moving Astroturf surface. Forces are measured using a strain gauge dynamometer mounted on the support arm.*

support arm at a different height above the snow. The bending moment caused by the forces in the plane of the snow produces different bending strains in the upper and lower gages while the moment caused by the known vertical force on the ski produces equal strains at both pairs. As a result, the moment produced by the vertical force can be decoupled from that produced by in-plane forces. The in-plane forces are the drag and centripetal forces, and the moment produced by the vertical force is used to determine the sensitivity parameter.

An IBM PC/AT is used to position the ski tilt angle and record the twist angle, forces, and moments on the ski during an experiment. An experimental protocol is followed for two types of Astroturf, one with an average fiber length of 9 mm, and the other, 15 mm. Ski tilt is varied in 2° increments from −6° (the ski tip pushed down into the snow) to 24° (the ski tip out of the snow) where the ski is flat on the table at 0°. The ski twist angle is held at 5, 10, 15, and 20°. At 0°, the ski is tangent to the trajectory, and positive twist rotates the tip toward the center of the rotating Astroturf. Over this range of 64 points (16 tilt angles, 4 twist angles), 3 ski stiffnesses, consisting of 2, 3, or 4 aluminum plys, are tested. The steady-state forces and moments at each distinct set-up are measured 50 times and averaged.

A constant centripetal acceleration is required over the tilt and twist angle configurations for the solution maps to represent a dynamically similar turn. The ratio of F_r/mg, where F_r is the radial force on the ski and mg is the weight of the ski, varies from 0.20 to 0.44. The measured ski turn corresponds to a turn with average blank angle of only 11 to 23°. Typical plots of the drag force and moment about the pivoting point (which serves as the skier location in the experiment) are shown in Fig. 12 for two stiffnesses.

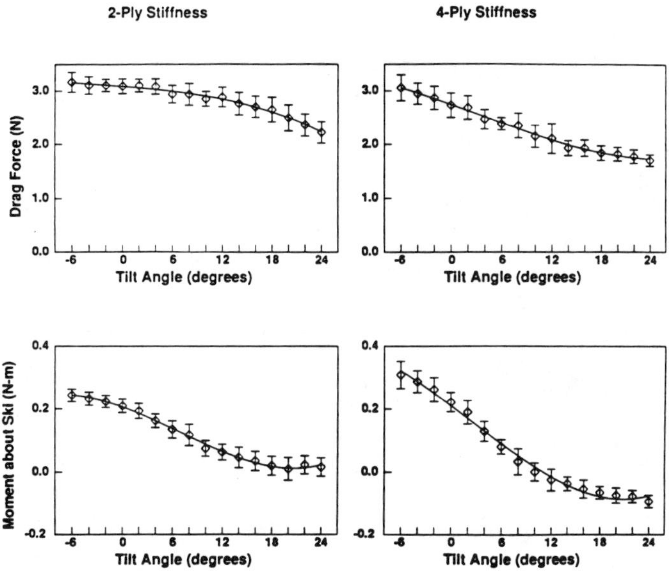

FIG. 12—*Drag and moment measurements for two skis with twist angle = 10°. Error bars show plus and minus one standard deviation.*

The drag (thrust) force and moment caused by the vertical force are plotted against the ski tilt angle and fit by cubic splines. The spline is differentiated to determine the sensitivity $-\ \partial M/\partial \varepsilon_t$. Figure 13 shows the solution maps for the 9-mm Astroturf for the three ski stiffnesses. The 15-mm Astroturf produces similar results. Initially, the drag decreases with increasing sensitivity until a maximum sensitivity is reached. Then, the drag decreases slowly with significant decreases in sensitivity. The maximum sensitivity is approximately proportional to the stiffness of the ski, and the asymptotic drag value decreases as stiffness increases. The drag–sensitivity behavior exhibited by these curves is qualitatively similar to that predicted by the model.

Discussion

Many assumptions are made in defining the model. While most are at least intuitively plausible, it is useful to summarize these assumptions and examine their possible impact on the results.

The model skier skis on a horizontal surface rather than on a downhill course. This assumption allows analysis of a dynamic equilibrium that would not be possible on a terrain that varied during the turn. However, the effects of the unsteady accelerations on the mechanics of the turn cannot be examined [5].

The assumption that ice and snow produce similar shearing forces avoids difficulties associated with experimentally determining a shearing function for snow. These difficulties include manufacturing snow, defining the type of snow, evaluating the manufactured snow, and so forth. Different magnitudes of snow force have been investigated by varying K_f. Dependence of the results on the overall magnitude of the snow force should be greater than variations produced by changes in the particular snow force expression, which do not significantly alter its overall magnitude.

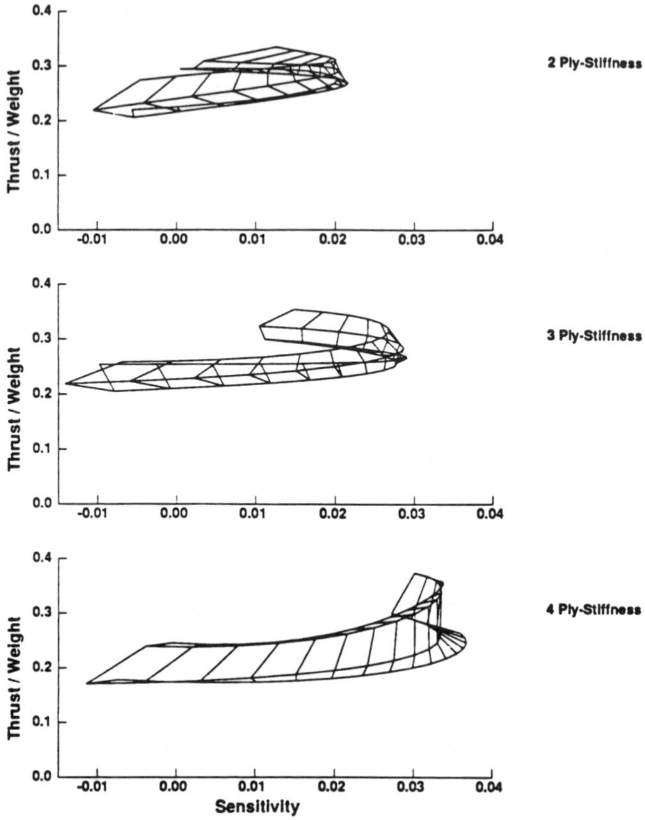

FIG. 13—*Experimental solutions for three different stiffness skis sliding on the 9-mm fiber length Astroturf.*

The force along the bottom of the ski is assumed to be perpendicular to the ski, and no frictional forces are considered. Frictional forces may have an impact on skiing mechanics; however, it should be smaller than the impacts produced by the momentum balance forces.

Carving is initiated at an arbitrarily defined angle, C_{init}. The existence of a transition range between skidding and carving forces is a primary assumption of the model. As C_{init} is decreased, transition carving occurs at lower sensitivities. The minimum thrust levels are unaffected by choice of C_{init}. Increasing C_{init} delays the onset of carving. $C_{init} = 80°$ represents a best guess of when carving might begin.

The skier is assumed to be a rigid body fixed to the ski. The boundary conditions of the ski flexure and torsion at the boot are those of a cantilever beam, and substantial moments at the boot are generated. A continuous deflection and first derivative of deflection through the boot are imposed. It is assumed that this reasonably reflects the nature of the ski deflection at the boot.

Although the model and the experiment are similar, they are not identical. Several features of the model do not appear in the experiment: (1) there is no skier mass; (2) the ski/skier mass does not accelerate centripetally through the turn; and (3) Astroturf is used rather than snow or ice. However, the balance between the vertical and circumferential force generated on the deflecting ski is an essential component of the model and is the basis of the comparison between the model results and the experiment.

Finally, it should be noted that many observations of common skiing wisdom are reproduced by this model. Skis with stiffer tails are faster although more difficult for beginning skiers to turn; skis with a soft flexural stiffness are easier to turn but are relatively inefficient and slow in turns; carving is initiated by pressing the tail of the ski into the ski; and so forth. Such general concurrence between the model and common skiing wisdom increases the credibility and potential usefulness of the model.

Conclusions

1. Three types of turns are described by the snow/ski model: skidding turns, carving turns, and turns in the transition between skidding and carving. When a section of the ski skids, the snow forces are proportional to those required to machine ice. Carving occurs on a section of the ski when that section follows a track in the snow already cut by a preceding section of the ski. The force generated by the snow on a carving section is that necessary to maintain the curvature of the ski and is smaller than the force required to machine the snow surface. The carving mechanism is the principal modeling assumption.

2. Many solutions exist for a specified turn radius and speed. The efficiency of these different solutions is characterized by two indices. These indices are the circumferential thrust required to maintain the steady-state turn, and the sensitivity of moment equilibrium of the snow forces to changes in tilt of the boot. Minimizing the required thrust minimizes energy losses from machining the snow surface. Low sensitivity predicts easier skier control of the equilibrium moment through fore–aft tilting of the boot.

3. When equilibrium solutions are plotted on the thrust–sensitivity plane, the *skidding solutions* show that an increased sensitivity accompanies decreasing required thrust, while the *carving solutions* show a simultaneously decreasing sensitivity and thrust. The required thrust of all carving solutions is smaller than those of skidding solutions.

4. The behavior between required thrust and sensitivity in skidding and carving solutions provides insights on the physics of skiing and may provide quantitative benchmarks for comparing different ski designs and testing ski design strategies.

APPENDIX A

Rotation Matrices

Two coordinate systems are used to describe the position and orientation of the skier, one being fixed in the snow, the other in the skier. The system fixed in the snow, the X–Y–Z coordinate sysem, is fixed with the Z-axis normal to the snow with the snow surface spanning the X–Y plane. The system fixed at the skier, the x–y–z system, is initially coincident with the X–Y–Z system with the skier facing in the y direction, and z vertical. The origin of the x–y–z system is at the skier center of mass. The x–y–z system is first rotated about the Z-axis, then the Y-axis, and then the X-axis. The rotation matrix relating the x–y–z system to the X–Y–Z system through the angles α_Z, α_Y, and α_X is given by:

$$\underline{R} = \begin{bmatrix} 1 & 0 & 0 \\ 0 & \cos\alpha_X & -\sin\alpha_X \\ 0 & \sin\alpha_X & \cos\alpha_X \end{bmatrix} \begin{bmatrix} \cos\alpha_Y & 0 & \sin\alpha_Y \\ 0 & 1 & 0 \\ -\sin\alpha_Y & 0 & \cos\alpha_Y \end{bmatrix} \begin{bmatrix} \cos\alpha_Z & -\sin\alpha_Z & 0 \\ \sin\alpha_Z & \cos\alpha_Z & 0 \\ 0 & 0 & 1 \end{bmatrix} \tag{A1}$$

$$= \begin{bmatrix} (\cos\alpha_Z \cos\alpha_Y) & (-\cos\alpha_Y \sin\alpha_Z) & (\sin\alpha_Y) \\ (\sin\alpha_X \cos\alpha_Z \sin\alpha_Y + \sin\alpha_Z \cos\alpha_X) & (-\sin\alpha_X \sin\alpha_Z \sin\alpha_Y + \sin\alpha_X \cos\alpha_Y) & (-\cos\alpha_Y \sin\alpha_X) \\ (-\cos\alpha_X \cos\alpha_Z \sin\alpha_Y + \sin\alpha_X \sin\alpha_Z) & (\sin\alpha_X \cos\alpha_Z + \sin\alpha_Z \sin\alpha_Y \cos\alpha_X) & (\cos\alpha_X \cos\alpha_Y) \end{bmatrix}$$

The skier is then translated to the point ($X = R$, $Y = 0$, $Z = Z$). In addition to rotating the skier from an initially upright position, this rotation matrix is used to convert the angular velocity expression $\underline{\dot{\theta}}$ (measured in $X-Y-Z$) to $\underline{\omega}$ (measured in $x-y-z$):

$$\underline{\omega} = \underline{R}\dot{\theta} \tag{A2}$$

Before rotating with the skier as a rigid body, the ski pivots at the boot through angles ε_t and ε_r. Positioning of the ski relative to the skier is achieved by a premultiplication matrix:

$$\underline{P} = \begin{bmatrix} 1 & 0 & 0 \\ 0 & \cos\varepsilon_t & \sin\varepsilon_t \\ 0 & -\sin\varepsilon_t & \cos\varepsilon_t \end{bmatrix} \begin{bmatrix} \cos\varepsilon_r & 0 & -\sin\varepsilon_r \\ 0 & 1 & 0 \\ \sin\varepsilon_r & 0 & \cos\varepsilon_r \end{bmatrix} = \begin{bmatrix} \cos\varepsilon_r & 0 & -\sin\varepsilon_r \\ \sin\varepsilon_r \sin\varepsilon_t & \cos\varepsilon_t & \cos\varepsilon_r \sin\varepsilon_t \\ \sin\varepsilon_r \cos\varepsilon_t & -\sin\varepsilon_t & \cos\varepsilon_r \cos\varepsilon_t \end{bmatrix} \tag{A3}$$

Hence, the normal to the bottom of the undeflected ski is given by

$$\hat{n} = \underline{R\ P} \begin{bmatrix} 0 \\ 0 \\ -1 \end{bmatrix} \tag{A4}$$

References

[1] Schultes, H., *Principles of Modern Alpine Ski Design*, Olin Ski Company, Middletown, CT.

[2] Sakata, T., "Considerations on Mechanical Properties of Skis," in *Skiing Trauma and Safety: Sixth International Symposium, ASTM STP 938*, C. D. Mote, Jr. and R. J. Johnson, Eds., American Society for Testing and Materials, Philadelphia, 1987, pp. 86–99.

[3] Lieu, D. K. and Mote, C. D., Jr., "Mechanics of the Turning Snow Ski," in *Skiing Trauma and Safety: Fifth International Symposium, ASTM STP 860*, R. J. Johnson and C. D. Mote, Jr., Eds., American Society for Testing and Materials, Philadelphia, 1985, pp. 117–140.

[4] Lieu, D. K. and Mote, C. D., Jr., "Experiments in the Machining of Ice at Negative Rake Angles," *Journal of Glaciology*, Vol. 30, No. 104, 1984, pp. 77–81.

[5] Mote, C. D., Jr. and Louie, J. K., "Accelerations Induced by Body Motions During Snow Skiing," *Journal of Sound and Vibration*, Vol. 88, 1983, pp. 107–115.

Education and Behavior

Victor M. G. Damoiseaux,[1] *Anna M. L. de Jongh,*[1] *Lex M. Bouter,*[2] *and Harm Jan Hospers*[1]

Designing Effective Health Education for Downhill Skiers: Results of a Randomized Intervention Study

REFERENCE: Damoiseaux, V. M. G., de Jongh, A. M. L., Bouter, L. M., and Hospers, H. J., **"Designing Effective Health Education for Downhill Skiers: Results of a Randomized Intervention Study,"** *Skiing Trauma and Safety: Eighth International Symposium, ASTM STP 1104*, C. D. Mote, Jr. and Robert J. Johnson, Eds., American Society for Testing and Materials, Philadelphia, 1991, pp. 241–248.

ABSTRACT: This article presents the results of a randomized intervention study among Dutch downhill skiers of 18 years and older. The objective of the study was to find an effective method to convince skiers that they have to adjust their ski bindings adequately. Literature study revealed that adequate adjustment of bindings (that is, by an expert and by means of a test device) is the most important behavior that can be manipulated to decrease the occurrence of ski injuries.

Three conditions were varied: when (the "moment") information materials were sent to skiers (one week versus three weeks before departure on a ski vacation), the medium (cassette versus leaflet), and the approach (fear-arousing versus neutral information). In this way, eight experimental groups were composed. In addition, a control group was formed that did not receive any information. The effects of the three conditions on the following factors were measured: attention, comprehension, intention, and behavior.

The cassette received a higher degree of attention than the leaflet, irrespective of time or degree of fear. The level of comprehension was higher in all experimental groups than in the control group. The information sent long before departure and with a high degree of fear produced the most effect on the level of comprehension. As for the factors intention and behavior, no differences were found between the experimental groups and the control group. Differences in intention and behavior did appear among the distinctive experimental groups. The information sent shortly before departure as well as the information with a low degree of fear proved to have the least effect on intention. Behavior was most affected by information with a high degree of fear, irrespective of time and medium.

KEY WORDS: downhill skiing, ski bindings, health education, prevention, injury, evaluation

Only ten years ago in the Netherlands, skiing was primarily practiced by sports fanatics and people with heavy purses. Today, almost one million Dutch tourists every year travel to Austria, Switzerland, and France to go skiing, proving that the sport has developed into a national sport. Although it is believed that, in general, sports participation has a favorable effect on health, there are also some drawbacks: sports injuries constitute a serious demand

[1]Associate professor, research assistant, associate professor, and research assistant, respectively, Department of Health Education, University of Limburg, P.O. Box 616, 6200 MD Maastricht, the Netherlands.

[2]Department of Epidemiology and Health Care Research, University of Limburg, P.O. Box 616, 6200 MD Maastricht, the Netherlands.

on the financial resources of national health care and they often disturb social and economic functioning (for example, absenteeism).

Health education can focus on influencing human behavior to prevent such injuries. By intentional interventions, health education tries to eliminate those behaviors that threaten health and to promote factors that have favorable effects on health. Effective health education depends on systematic planning and evaluation [*1*]. This study deals with the design of health education for downhill skiers that aims at reducing the injury incidence. The results of this study will constitute the basis of a national campaign in the Netherlands.

There are numerous causes and risk factors of ski injuries. Most risk factors are relatively constant and hard to influence and therefore inappropriate as an object for health educational intervention. The only behavioral factor proven to be related to ski injury is the adjustment of ski bindings. Several authors stress the importance of good information on adequate adjustment of ski bindings [*2–6*]. In the past decades, the incidence of ski injuries has decreased, which is probably due to an increased attention to extrinsic causes, in particular technical improvements of skiing gear [*2,4*].

As early as 1976, Johnson observed a relation between binding adjustment and occurrence of ski injuries [*7*]. Evaluation of a Swedish intervention [*8*], in which skiers were given the opportunity to adjust their ski bindings adequately on the ski run, revealed that well-adjusted bindings increase by 50% the chance of release at the right moment, resulting in a decrease of more than 10% of lower extremity injuries. Several authors have confirmed these findings [*5,9*].

Only one study [*3*] dealt with determinants playing a role in behavior concerning adjustment of ski bindings. The real problem seems not to be the actual adjustment of the bindings—a majority of the bindings are adjusted—but rather the lack of knowledge of adequate and individual adjustment [*3*]. The best way to adjust the bindings adequately is with the help of experts and a test device [*10*]. Therefore, this study focuses on the design of effective health education with this message.

To find the most effective health education intervention, we varied three conditions:

1. *Medium*: leaflet versus cassette.

Little is known about the results of auditory information materials because they are rarely used. A majority of Dutch skiers travel to their winter sports destinations by car equipped with a cassette recorder, and, therefore, it is possible to play the cassette during the journey. Music, played at intervals during the message, was meant to increase its attractiveness.

2. *Moment of receiving*: one week versus three weeks before departure on ski vacation.

One important reason why information is not effective is that the message reaches the receiver at the wrong time. In this study, we varied the moments at which the information was conveyed, at an interval of two weeks, in order to detect the moment at which the receiver is the most receptive to the message.

3. *Approach*: fear-arousing versus neutral.

In our study, we varied the degree of fear-arousing information. In the version that aims specifically to arouse fear, we emphasized the seriousness of injuries and the vulnerability of the skier. In the other version, we tried to be as neutral as possible, giving information about ski risks without working on the persons's feelings (for example, "Do not be fooled, your own arms, legs, ribs, purse and vacation are at stake" versus "Do not be fooled, it is your own safety that is at stake").

Material and Methods

The central message of our intervention was: "Have your ski bindings adjusted in a ski shop with the aid of a test device." In composing the message, we aimed at a terse, brief, and comprehensible formulation. We have, therefore, chosen items that are directly related to the adjustment of bindings:

- Effectiveness of adequate adjustment,
- Functioning of bindings and the necessity of individual adjustment,
- Disposal of possible misconceptions (for example, "rented skis are already adjusted"),
- Precautionary measures to profit optimally from the adjusted bindings (maintenance, transport),
- Possible barriers to the desired behavior (for example, cost of adjustment), and
- Inevitable risks of skiing.

The message was written by professional copywriters, subsequently pretested in the target audience, and criticized by communication experts and subject experts (ski instructors, ski shop employees, national ski federation members, and so forth).

To find the most effective communication method, we used a quasi-experimental study design [*11*]. By manipulating three independent variables on two levels, eight experimental groups were formed (Table 1):

- Medium (cassette versus leaflet),
- Moment (one week versus three weeks before departure), and
- Approach (fear-arousing versus neutral).

We also formed a control group of skiers who did not receive any information.

The study population included persons of 18 years and older who were recruited at ski fairs. Visitors of ski fairs were asked to take part in a telephone survey on the subject of skiing and safety. Adjustment of ski bindings was not mentioned. The 1380 people who agreed to take part in the survey were all planning to practice downhill skiing during the winter of 1987/1988.

Seventy respondents were pretested; 22 skiers did not comply with the inclusion criteria (for example, they were younger than 18 years or they were not going skiing) and were left out. Thus, the sample consisted of 1288 people; 136 were listed under the control group and the rest were divided into eight experimental groups, an average of 145 per group. These skiers were distributed at random among the conditions medium, moment of receiving, and approach, and subsequently received a leaflet or cassette before their departure.

TABLE 1—*Study design.*

Experimental Groups					
		Medium			
		Cassette		Leaflet	
	Time	1 week before departure	3 weeks before departure	1 week before departure	3 weeks before departure
Fear	high low	message 1 message 2	message 1 message 2	message 1 message 2	message 1 message 2
Control Group					
		no message			

The telephone survey was done after the skiers received a cassette or leaflet and after their ski vacations with the aid of an interactive computer-controlled interview system. The interviews were conducted over 22 days, in the afternoon and evening. The results were analyzed with the SPSS-X program [*12*].

Results

Response was very high (91.5%), which can be explained by the fact that the respondents had promised beforehand to cooperate in the survey. The response is well divided among the different groups, although the mean response for the experimental groups was higher (92.3%) than for the controls (83.8%). In comparing demographic and personal factors (for example, sex, age, and skiing experience) in response and nonresponse, and in the experimental groups and the controls, no differences can be found.

A majority of the respondents were male (56% versus 44% female), and a substantial proportion were younger than 35 years (58%), whereas only 3% were older than 55 years.

Most of the respondents have practiced downhill skiing before; only 8% were going to ski for the first time. More than half of the respondents were fairly experienced, having already skied during six seasons or more. However, having skiing experience does not mean that one is an advanced skier. A better means to indicate skill might be the level of difficulty of the ski runs. The more experienced the skiers, the more often they choose more difficult ski runs. Of the respondents in this study, 42% skied on easy ski runs, 54% on medium ski runs, and only 4% on difficult ski runs. Many of the surveyed skiers (70%) never ski on runs that are too difficult for them. More than a quarter (28%) do so now and then, while only 2% often does so. Skiers who go skiing more often are less inclined to ski on too difficult ski runs.

Respondents were asked about their physical preparation (ski gymnastics, fitness training) and their weekly number of hours of sports participation. One quarter of the respondents do not practice sports at all and did not prepare themselves physically for winter sports. Respondents were also asked to give an estimation of their own condition: 8% think their condition is bad, 60% think they are in reasonable to normal shape, and 33% think they are in good condition. No significant differences were found in physical preparation, number of hours of sports participation, and estimation of physical condition between skiers who adjusted their bindings and those who did not. The same holds for differences between the injured and the uninjured skiers in our study.

Approximately half of the respondents report to be aware of certain risks involved with skiing, and the more experienced the more aware one seems to be. As a rule, only those people who go on a ski vacation more often ski at higher altitudes. They are, in general, less afraid of accidents than people skiing at a lower altitude.

We found that three quarters of the respondents would check any advice on safety and health on its reliability and effectiveness before following such advice. Skiers showing a positive attitude toward observance of advice, indeed, did have their bindings adjusted more often. It is remarkable that more than half of the skiers have never been explicitly informed about how to prevent ski injuries. Almost 40% of the respondents had ever received such information from their ski instructor. On the other hand, some two thirds of the population said they had read, heard, or seen something, sometime about prevention of ski injuries by other media (newspaper, magazine, radio, television).

Injuries and Adjustment of Bindings

Almost 8% of the respondents had been injured during this (skiing) season (9.3 per 1000 skiing days); half of them were not seriously hurt, and their injuries did not withhold them

TABLE 2—*Kind and location of injuries (*N *= 89) (percentages).*

Kind		Location	
Bruise, strain, sprain	55.1	knee	29.2
Fracture	7.9	leg	15.7
Ruptured muscle	6.7	chest/shoulder	15.7
Dislocation	5.6	thumb	12.4
Ruptured ligament	3.4	neck/head	3.4
Cut	3.4	other	23.6
Unknown	18.0		

from skiing. About one third had to stop skiing for a couple of days. Table 2 shows the kind and location of the injuries. In more than 40% of the cases, the injuries were caused by a fall or a collision. Bindings are mentioned as a cause in only 7% of the cases. It is possible, however, that these figures are somewhat biased. For example, when a skier falls and the bindings do not release, the cause will probably be described as "fall" when, in fact, the injury was the result of unreleased bindings.

In our study, 83% of the population adjusted their bindings. A vast majority had them adjusted in a ski shop, and 35% of the whole population tested the settings of their bindings with a test device.

Differences Between the Groups

By analysis of variance (ANOVA), we examined the effect of the three conditions (medium, moment, approach) on changes in attention, comprehension, intention. and behavior.

An average of over 75% of the experimental groups remembers having received information materials. The cassette made the strongest impression. Of the respondents who received a cassette, 95% remembered it; only 55% of the respondents who received a leaflet remembered it. No differences in effect on remembrance are noticed between the varying periods of receiving the information before departure (one versus three weeks) nor between the varying approaches (high versus low degree of fear). Table 3 shows the differences among the experimental groups with respect to attention, operationalized as reading or listening to the message.

Only the "medium" condition appears to produce a main effect ($F(1, 784) = 5.5$; $p < 0.05$). Where the cassette has a higher score in remembrance, the leaflet scores higher in attention (measured in terms of reading and listening). A large part of the respondents (88%) kept the information materials. Almost two thirds of the respondents discussed the

TABLE 3—*Attention (mean scores) among respondents remembering having received information (*N *= 785).*[a]

		Time	
Medium	Fear	Short Period	Long Period
Cassette	high	2.62	2.68
	low	2.70	2.71
Leaflet	high	2.79	2.77
	low	2.78	2.79

[a]1 = Not read or listened to; 2 = partly read or listened to; 3 = read or listened to.

TABLE 4—*Comprehension (mean knowledge scores) among respondents in the experimental groups (N = 1040).*[a]

Medium	Fear	Time: Short Period	Time: Long Period
Cassette	high	2.55	2.47
	low	1.90	2.42
Leaflet	high	2.51	2.21
	low	1.85	2.53

[a] −5 = all questions wrong; +5 = all questions correct.
Mean knowledge score in the control group (N = 110) was 1.70.

contents of the materials with other people. Those who received a cassette spoke with others (75%) about the content more often than those who received a leaflet (56%).

In summary, the cassette made a stronger impression on the respondents than the leaflet.

To measure the respondents' "comprehension" of the message, we asked a number of questions concerning the contents, added up on a knowledge scale (Cronbach's alpha = 0.56). After comparing the knowledge of the controls to the knowledge of all receivers of any information, a significant higher level of knowledge can be noticed in the experimental groups ($t(1019) = 2.34$; $p < 0.05$). The effects of the different conditions on the level of knowledge are presented in Table 4.

There is a significant interaction between moment of receiving and fear ($F(1, 1040) = 6.9$; $p < 0.05$). In other words, a combination of both conditions (high fear and long time) produces the maximum effect on the level of knowledge. The "medium" condition does not have a particular effect on knowledge.

There were no significant differences between the experimental groups and the controls in intention or behavior. Effects of the varying conditions on the intention to adjust the bindings are represented in Table 5.

With respect to intention, there appears to be a main effect of both time and fear ($F(1, 953) = 4.3$; $p < 0.05$; $F(1, 953) = 6.7$; $p < 0.01$). The information received shortly before departure produces the least effect on intention concerning adjustment of bindings. The same holds for information with a low degree of fear.

The effect of the different conditions on adjustment behavior is presented in Table 6. From this table we can conclude that the condition "fear" has a significant effect on the

TABLE 5—*Positive intention*[a] *(percentages) towards adjustment of bindings among respondents in the experimental groups*[b] *(N = 954).*

Medium	Fear	Time: Short Period	Time: Long Period
Cassette	high	84	88
	low	76	87
Leaflet	high	94	88
	low	79	87

[a]Including those who actually adjusted their bindings.
[b]Percentage with positive intention in the control group (N = 91) was 82.

TABLE 6—*Adjustment behavior (mean scores) among respondents in the experimental groups (N = 940).*[a]

Medium	Fear	Time: Short Period	Time: Long Period
Cassette	high	2.94	3.06
	low	2.76	2.97
Leaflet	high	3.05	3.08
	low	2.83	2.94

[a]1 = not adjusted, 2 = adjusted by themselves or by friends, 3 = adjusted in a ski shop, and 4 = adjusted in a ski shop and tested with a test device.

Mean score for adjustment behavior in the control group (N = 89) was 2.86.

adjustment behavior ($F(1, 939) = 5.6$; $p < 0.05$). A high degree of fear scores significantly higher than a low degree of fear, irrespective of time and medium. And these groups score significantly higher than the controls.

Discussion and Conclusions

This study served as a prototype for a national campaign to reduce ski injuries. However, it is difficult to prove that health education intervention can minimize the number of injuries. There are two reasons for this. First, one cannot expect that an occasional leaflet or cassette will have a permanent effect on the behavior of skiers. These mediums are primarily expected to increase the level of knowledge and to incite a process of consciousness. Second, considering the incidence of ski injuries, our study population is too small to detect a reduction in ski injuries. Furthermore, it is questionable whether the results of the study provide sufficient material for a mass media campaign. One characteristic of such a campaign is the undifferentiated target audience. In our study, we specifically asked for participation and we sent the information materials to specific addresses. This probably explains the high response to the study.

Basically, the problem consists of two related questions. The first is whether health education interventions can minimize ski injuries. Before the intervention we had to be certain that behavior is (partly) the cause of the problem. The available literature [*2–5*] convinced us that this is true. Furthermore, we assumed that it is very likely that intention and behavior concerning adjustment of ski bindings can be influenced and changed. We concluded that health education interventions can induce the desired changes.

The second question is which method is the most suitable to use in a campaign. This question is more difficult to answer. The present study shows that fear-arousing information materials produce the most effect. Such information emphasized mainly the seriousness of the injuries and the vulnerability of the skier. However, fear-arousing information materials are not recommended in every health problem. It can only be used adequately when the message gives precise directions, in terms of behavior, about how to prevent the health problem at issue. In the case of ski injuries, fear-arousing information turned out to be very suitable. Differences between leaflet and cassette are relatively small. The cassette makes a strong impression and has a clear after-effect because it stimulates listeners to discuss the contents with other people. But the high attention value of this medium can probably be explained by the fact that the cassette is rarely used to pass information. If it were used more often, this effect would probably be less evident. Where the main effects on knowledge, intention, and behavior are concerned, the leaflet gives about the same results as the cassette. For practical reasons, therefore, the leaflet is recommended.

Although we are convinced that the moment at which the message reaches the target population is essential in the information process, we could not prove this assumption empirically in this study. It seems very likely that the information materials sent shortly before departure on a ski vacation produce the least effect: the receivers probably do not have enough time to adjust the bindings adequately. It is therefore important to allow the target audience enough time to perform the desired behavior.

To produce effects on the level of knowledge, on intention, and on behavior, health education interventions have to be worked out methodically, systematically, and purposively. The message constitutes an essential part of the campaign. Messages of advice to prevent ski injuries have to be brief, comprehensible, and easy to carry out. Before implementation of an intervention, it has to be established beyond reasonable doubt that the advice actually leads to the desired change of behavior.

References

[*1*] Bouter, L. M. and Kok, G. J., "Planning Health Education for Downhill Skiers," in this volume, pp. 249–256.

[*2*] Johnson, R. J., Ettlinger, C. F., Campbell, R. J., and Pope, M. H., "Trends in Skiing Injuries," *American Journal of Sports Medicine*, Vol. 8, 1980, pp. 106–113.

[*3*] Rosen, J. C., Johnson, R. J., Lefebre, M. F., and Pope, M. H., "Behavioral Determinants of Skiers' Failure to Adjust Release Bindings," *Clinics in Sports Medicine*, Vol. 1. 1982, pp. 209–215.

[*4*] Hauser, W. and Gläser, H., "Verletzungen beim alpinen Skilauf: Veränderungen und Trends," *Deutsche Zeitschrift für Sportmedizin*, Vol. 38, pp. 191–198.

[*5*] Bouter, L. M., *Injury Risk in Downhill Skiing: Results from an Etiological Case-Control Study Conducted Among Dutch Skiers*, De Vrieseborch, Haarlem, 1988.

[*6*] Bouter, L. M. and Knipschild, P. G., "Causes and Prevention of Injury in Downhill Skiing," in *The Physician and Sports Medicine*, Vol. 17, 1989, pp. 80–94.

[*7*] Johnson, R. J. et al., "The Interrelationship between Ski Accidents, the Resultant Injury, the Skier's Characteristics and the Ski Boot Binding System," *Orthopedic Clinics of North America*, Vol. 7, No. 1, 1976, pp. 11–12.

[*8*] Johnson, E., "Does it Pay to Test Bindings Used in Downhill Skiing? A Cost–Benefit Analysis of a Ski Safety Campaign," *Konsument Verket*, Vol. 3, 1983, pp. 1–13.

[*9*] Caldwell, F., "Bindings: A Critical Role in Downhill Ski Safety," *The Physician and Sports Medicine*, Vol. 12, No. 1, 1984, pp. 148–162.

[*10*] Nagel, A. and Mösch, S., "Test Devices for Ski Bindings Sold in Sport Shops: State of the Art and Future Development," in *Skiing Trauma and Safety: Sixth International Symposium, ASTM STP 938*, C. D. Mote Jr. and R. J. Johnson, Eds., American Society for Testing Materials, Philadelphia, 1987, pp. 217–224.

[*11*] Cook, T. D. and Campbell, D. T., *Quasi-Experimentation: Design & Analysis Issues for Field Settings*, Houghton Mifflin Company, Boston, 1979.

[*12*] SPSS, Inc., *SPSS-X User's Guide*, 2nd ed., McGraw-Hill Book Company, New York, 1986.

Lex M. Bouter[1] *and Gerjo J. Kok*[1]

Planning Health Education for Downhill Skiers

REFERENCE: Bouter, L. M. and Kok, G. J., "**Planning Health Education for Downhill Skiers,**" *Skiing Trauma and Safety: Eighth International Symposium, ASTM STP 1104*, C. D. Mote, Jr. and Robert J. Johnson, Eds., American Society for Testing and Materials, Philadelphia, 1991, pp. 249–256.

ABSTRACT: The planning of health education to prevent ski injuries is often incomplete and not stated explicitly, while the evaluation of health education is executed only partially or not at all. This article presents a theoretical framework for planning and evaluating health education for downhill skiers. Systematic planning consists of an analysis of the magnitude of the problem, an analysis of the behavioral risk factors, a study of the determinants of the behavior at issue, the design of an optimal intervention, and the implementation of this intervention. The evaluation phase deals with the effects of the planning on these five levels (implementation, intervention, determinants, behavior, and injury risk). Some common pitfalls are mentioned, and special attention is given to the study of determinants of behavior and to the design of the intervention. Furthermore, the importance of pretesting health education material is underlined. There seems to be a strong need for further research on the etiology of ski injury and its determinants of behavior before prevention can be realized.

KEY WORDS: downhill skiing, injury, health education, determinants of behavior, pretesting, evaluation

While most people agree that participation in recreational downhill skiing is conducive to health, the negative consequences in the form of injuries generally attract less attention. Available data on the incidence of ski injuries indicate that the problem is a substantial one in terms of morbidity, medical consumption, and absence from work and sport [*1*]. Health education is often advocated as a solution and a means of prevention. The planning of these health education activities is often incomplete and not stated explicitly. Furthermore, the evaluation usually is executed only partially or is altogether nonexistent, although at least some work is done in this field [*2*].

This article presents a theoretical framework for planning and evaluating health education for downhill skiers. The specific examples given from the ski injury literature are only to provide an illustration of the theoretical considerations. Most of them are simplistic generalizations and could be criticized easily. For a more realistic overview of the etiology of ski injuries in general, and of behavioral risk factors in particular, the reader is referred to other publications [*3,4*].

The central thesis of this paper is that the effectiveness of health education for downhill skiers is determined by the quality of the planning process [*5,6*]. A thorough evaluation of the health education intervention is a condition *sine qua non* for establishing this effective-

[1]Associate professor of epidemiology, Department of Epidemiology and Health Care Research, and professor of health education, Department of Health Education, respectively, University of Limburg, P.O. Box 616, 6200 MD Maastricht, the Netherlands.

ness. Therefore, this paper presents an overview of the several phases of the process of planning and evaluating health education aimed at the prevention of ski injuries. Several common pitfalls are also mentioned. Special attention is given to the study of the determinants of behavior and to the design of the behavioral intervention. Finally, a number of conclusions are drawn, and some priorities for future research are mentioned.

Planning Health Education

A model for explicit planning and evaluation of health education is presented in Fig. 1. Planning and evaluation each have five related steps. These ten steps in total can be indicated by their central questions. These questions are presented below, and as an example, the prevention of ski injuries as a result of inadequate binding adjustment will be taken.

Step 1: How Serious Is the Problem?

Most authors agree on an incidence of 2 to 4 medically treated ski injuries per 1000 ski person days [*1*,*3*]. About 50% of these are lower extremity equipment-related (LEER) injuries [*7*]. This certainly does not mean that this subgroup of injuries can be fully attributed to the failure of the ski bindings to release in time. There are reasons to believe that only lower leg injuries (about 12% of all injuries [*8*]) are likely to be amenable to prevention by current binding systems.

Step 2: What Behavior is Involved?

In the literature, an abundance of putative behavioral risk factors for ski injury are mentioned [*1*,*3*]. However, studies adequately establishing and quantifying the etiological role of these factors are very sparse. While clearly not all LEER injuries can be prevented by an optimal adjustment of the current ski bindings, it still appears to be possible to lower injury rates further by promoting proper binding adjustment procedures [*9*]. A recent German preventive trial shows (again) that bindings generally are adjusted far above the recommended setting and that readjustment by an expert may even lower the incidence of LEER injuries by a factor of three [*10*], although this large effect could be doubted on biomechanical grounds and might be specific to the particular population of skiers included in this study.

PLANNING

Step 1——>Step 2——>Step 3————> Step 4————>Step 5

PROBLEM - BEHAVIOR - DETERMINANTS - INTERVENTION - IMPLEMENTATION

Step 10<——Step 9<——Step 8<———— Step 7<————Step 6

EVALUATION

FIG. 1—*Model of planning and evaluating health education.*

Step 3: What Are the Determinants of the Behavior?

A limited study of the behavior determinants [*11*] indicated that one of the most frequently observed mistakes is that skiers adjust their binding much too high after a fall that the skier interpreted to be due to inadvertent release. In this study, the belief that adequate adjustment can prevent injury and can also prevent inadvertent release appeared to be an important determinant of the desirable behavior. Furthermore, it turned out that skiers are more likely to have their bindings adjusted if they think that experts favor taking this action [*11*]. Of course, determinants of other identified behavioral risk factors should be studied as well.

Step 4: What Options Are There for Change?

Health education intervention could stress the opinion of experts on the subject of the health education and, for example, make clear what the relation is between suboptimal binding adjustment and injury risk. Special attention might be given to explaining that adequately adjusted bindings almost never release inadvertently. These are several ways to formulate this message. A recent study [*12*] revealed that phrasing the information in a mildly fear-arousing way was more effective for this purpose than a more neutral formulation.

Step 5: How Can That Be Implemented?

Next the channel and the moment of the health education intervention have to be decided on. In the Dutch study mentioned above [*12*], postal delivery of an audio cassette about one week before the beginning of the winter sports holiday appeared to be relatively effective compared to brochures and to earlier delivery.

Step 6: Has the Implementation Been Carried Out as Planned?

This step is designed to ensure that the defined population of skiers at risk for injury actually received the health education intervention. This is a necessary, although not a sufficient, condition for effectiveness.

Step 7: Has the Intervention Been Released as Planned?

This step determines whether the skiers understood the message contained in the health education intervention. Failure to make fully clear which preventive behavior (for example, adjustment by an expert) is expected to reduce risk can be another source of ineffective prevention of ski injury.

Step 8: Have the Determinants of the Behavior Changed?

This phase is concerned with establishing whether the prevalence of the determinants of the desired behavior has risen satisfactorily. In our example, this part of the evaluation should focus primarily on the perceived advantages of adequate adjustment and the perception of the opinion of experts.

Step 9: Has the Behavior Changed?

Health education aims at modifying behavior. Therefore, quantifying behavioral change is important in the evaluation process. For the skiers from our example, this entails the question whether the target population engages in optimal binding adjustment more often.

Step 10: Has the Problem Been Lessened?

Of course, this is the ultimate measure of efficacy; Steps 6 to 9 can be considered the intermediary steps. In the example, the postintervention incidence of injury, more specifically of LEER injury, indicates the overall effectiveness of the health education intervention. For methodological reasons, this straightforward measure is often not presented. Unfortunately, it can be calculated that even a 50% decrease in incidence from 4 to 2 injuries per 1000 ski person days fails to reach statistical significance (at $\alpha = 0.05$) in a study involving 500 skiers, each skiing 10 days, half of them receiving the intervention and the other half being the control group [*13*].

Pitfalls

Unfortunately, the ten steps mentioned above are often not given the appropriate attention. The most common mistake is that people jump from the problem to the intervention without answering the planning questions in between. Furthermore, because evaluation is rare, the ineffectiveness of such interventions remains hidden. Evaluation is necessary for testing previous decisions and for making corrections to improve the intervention. Careful planning can avoid a number of potential pitfalls that we will describe and illustrate with examples.

Pitfall 1

Development of an intervention for a problem that does not exist. In our example, ski injuries are clearly a substantial problem, especially when analyzed in terms of incidence figures and severity of the injuries. However, it can be argued that the focus on LEER injuries is not justified because the proportion of them that would be preventable by optimally adjusting bindings might be much smaller than suggested by some authors [*4,10*].

Pitfall 2

Development of an intervention addressing behavior lacking a clear relationship with the problem. An example would be a program aimed at reducing levels of alcohol consumption during skiing. In contradiction to population opinions on this subject, empirical data show that detectable levels of alcohol in blood and breath among injured as well as among uninjured skiers have a prevalence of only a few percent [*1,14*]. So clearly there would be no need for an intervention because the behavior is not related to the problem. As another example, Bouter [*1*] showed that participation in ski gymnastics has probably no relation to the risk of having an injury. So an intervention advising skiers to participate in ski gymnastics can be *successful* if it has a high participation rate, but it may not be *effective* because no injuries are prevented. This possible pitfall is, in our opinion. currently the predominant threat to effective prevention of sports injuries. Valid knowledge about most putative behavioral risk factors contributing to the etiology of ski injury is still lacking [*1,3,4*].

Pitfall 3

Development of an intervention that is based on a misconceived idea about behavior determinants. An example is the educational programs on warming up for downhill skiers, based on the idea that people do not know how to perform the warming up exercises. The majority of people may know very well how to warm up but they do not want to do it, because, for instance, they think it ineffective or ridiculous. A general finding in health education research is that when a relation is shown between a health problem and behavior, knowledge about that relation is enough for some people to change their behavior. For a substantial group, however, knowledge is not enough. We elaborate on this point later when we describe models of behavior determinants.

Pitfall 4

Development of a wrong intervention, for instance, an intervention aimed at the wrong group. An example of this would be school health education with the message that children ought to wear close-fitting ski boots not made of thermoplastic material [*1*,*14*]. This could be ineffective because usually parents make the final decisions in buying ski equipment.

Pitfall 5

Development of a potentially effective intervention with a wrong implementation. For example, facilities for adequate and nonprofit binding adjustment may be made available to the subscribers to a ski magazine. The information about this service would probably not reach the majority of beginner skiers who may not subscribe to a ski magazine, who are generally more accident prone, and who often have badly adjusted bindings [*1*,*3*,*4*].

Pitfall 6

Unjustified satisfaction about the intervention. This concerns the failure to evaluate the intervention thoroughly. For instance, it could take the form of satisfaction about the large number of brochures on injury prevention handed out to skiers waiting for the ski lifts, with no notice taken of whether the number of injuries has been reduced.

Determinants of Behavior

In general, health educators have to rely on the epidemiological literature identifying the magnitude of the problem and the behavior that is (causally) involved (Steps 1 and 2 in Fig. 1) [*13*]. When such behavior is identified, the next step for the health educator consists of the clarification of its determinants. Figure 2 presents a recently developed model of behavior determinants [*15*]. This model states that external variables can influence behavior along three different pathways.

1. An *attitude* is the weighing of all the advantages and disadvantages of performance of the behavior, as seen by the individual. Health is only one of the possible considerations and often an unimportant one. When health is a part of the attitude, we may suppose that health motivation is a combination of the perceived severity of the health risk, the perceived

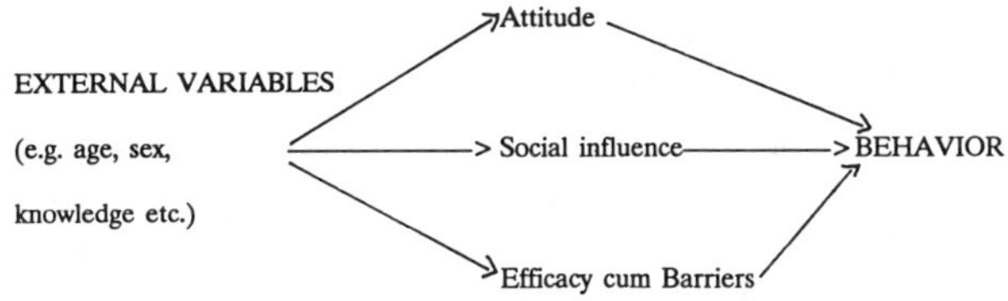

FIG. 2—*Model of behavior determinants adapted from DeVries et al.* [15].

susceptibility to the health risk, and the effectiveness of the preventive behavior. But, again, health considerations are mostly not dominant and other considerations like costs, (dis)like, status, and so forth, are often more important. For downhill skiers, risky behavior may even have a pleasant, stimulating effect. Skiers appear to have a relatively high sensation-seeking score, although predicted differences between injured and uninjured skiers could not be confirmed [*16*]. As said before, knowledge about risks is, for most people, not enough. A painful example is the unhealthy lifestyle of many physicians.

2. *Social influence* is the influence of others: directly by what others expect or indirectly by what others do (modeling). Social influence is often underestimated as a determinant of behavior. Social psychological studies show that social influence can lead to behavior that conflicts with previous attitudes, and most sport situations are social situations. The basis for social influence lies in two principles: people like to have the right information and the ideas of other people are sources of information, and people like to be socially rewarded, like getting compliments from others and belonging to a group. An example of the latter would be the often described situation of beginners taking much too difficult ski runs as a result of persuasion by more advanced members of the same ski party [*14*].

3. *Efficacy cum barriers* determines whether one is able to perform the (desirable) behavior. Efficacy is a person's estimation of his or her ability to perform the behavior; barriers are the real problems inside or outside the person that they face in actually behaving (inside: insufficient knowledge, skill, or endurance, and so forth; outside: resistance from others, time and money not available, conflicting lifestyle, and so forth). There is a logical relation between (perceived) efficacy and (real) barriers, but there is also an important relation between efficacy and success in performing the behavior. People with a higher efficacy have a higher chance of succeeding, independent of the existing barriers. But the discrepancy between (perceived) efficacy and (real) barriers should not become too large. Health educators can try to increase the efficacy to motivate people to adopt the preventive behavior. At the same time, however, they should help people to overcome barriers to performing that behavior. An example of a barrier to adequate adjustment of ski bindings is the limited availability of ski shops equipped with the appropriate test device [*9*]. Perceived inefficacy among beginning skiers often seems to focus on their inability to control velocity while descending a slope. Taking ski lessons might increase perceived efficacy [*1*,*4*].

We have described in theory the three determinants of behavior. To our knowledge, there are no systematic empirical studies on the determinants of desired and undesired behavior with respect to most putative behavioral risk factors for ski injuries. This is clearly an omission in research, and the gap needs filling urgently. Assuming that in the near future this kind of research will be conducted and specific determinants of behavior will be known, how do we get from determinants to interventions?

Behavioral Intervention

Changing by health education means changing by communication. Therefore, the first goal is to get attention and comprehension. Having achieved this and, subsequently, a change in determinants, the third and last goal is the maintenance of the behavior change. A once-only change is not enough; we want the desired behavior to become a habit. The major problem in achieving maintenance of behavior change is the possible negative experiences people have when performing the desired behavior. Health educators should always be realistic about the experiences after the change to the desired behavior. Mostly these experiences are not very positive in the short run.

Sometimes it is possible to present "organized" positive experiences, for instance, by presenting data about the number of ski injuries prevented related to the year before. In our example, this would mean informing downhill skiers of the number of LEER injuries prevented by the optimal binding adjustment. The best moment for this communication would seem to be shortly before the next winter sports season.

Figure 3 shows the three health education goals combined with four communication variables in the so-called health education matrix adapted from that devised by McGuire [*17*]. The cells of this matrix indicate decisions that have to be made, for example, which source attracts the most attention, which channel is able to change social norms, which group of receivers should be specially prepared for negative experiences, and so forth. In the literature [*17*], a rich quantity of empirical data can be found with respect to every possible decision.

Educational materials must be pretested to check whether they have the intended effect on the receivers, especially with respect to attention and comprehension [*18*]. It is not enough that all kinds of specialists on ski injuries agree that the information in the materials is correct. The next step is to have communication specialists judge the materials, and a final step is to try out the materials on a sample of the target group [*18*]. Only then is it possible to prevent all kinds of possible unwanted side effects that have not been recognized by the health educators themselves.

Pretesting should be integrated in the materials development process. To our knowledge, only one study deals with pretesting health education material for downhill skiers [*12*]. In this example, pretesting indeed led to major changes in the material.

Conclusion

Until now, prevention of ski injuries have been dominated by medical and technical experts. To be effective, these efforts should be supplemented by health education specialists. This cooperation may achieve a further reduction of ski injuries within the next 10 to 20 years. Health education can be an effective way of preventing ski injuries, but the effectiveness of health education depends on the quality of the planning. That means a careful analysis of the problem, the behavior, the determinants, the intervention, the implemen-

	Source	Message	Channel	Receiver
Attention & comprehension				
Change in attitudes, social influence, efficacy cum barriers				
Maintenance of behavior change				

FIG. 3—*Health education matrix adapted from McGuire* [17].

tation, and of the strength of the relationship between these five aspects. It is our opinion that, with respect to the prevention of ski injuries, we have not yet reached the stage that we know what to advise people. Epidemiological studies on the etiology followed by research on the determinants of the behavior at issue are necessary to fill in the gaps in our knowledge.

References

[*1*] Bouter, L. M., *Injury Risk in Downhill Skiing; Results from an Etiological Case-Control Study conducted among Dutch Skiers*, De Vrieseborch, Haarlem, 1988

[*2*] Danielson, K., Eriksson, E., Jonsson, E., Lind, E., and Lundkvist, S., "Attempts to Reduce the Incidence of Skiing Injuries in Sweden," in *Skiing Trauma and Safety: Fifth International Symposium, ASTM STP 860*, R. J. Johnson and C. D. Mote, Jr., Eds., American Society for Testing and Materials, Philadelphia, 1985, pp. 326–337.

[*3*] Bouter, L. M. and Knipschild, P. G., "Causes and Prevention of Injury in Downhill Skiing," *The Physician and Sportsmedicine*, Vol. 7, No. 11, 1989, pp. 80–94.

[*4*] Bouter, L. M. and Knipschild, P. G., "Behavioral Risk Factors for Ski Injury: Problem Analysis as a Basis for Effective Health Education," in this volume, pp. 257–264.

[*5*] Green, L. W., Kreuter, M. W., Deeds, S. G., and Partridge, K. B., *Health Education Planning: A Diagnostic Approach*, Mayfield, Palo Alto, 1980.

[*6*] Green, L. W. and Lewis, F. M., *Measurement and Evaluation in Health Education and Health Promotion*, Mayfield, Palo Alto, 1986.

[*7*] Johnson, R. J., Ettlinger, C. F., Campbell, R. J., and Pope, M. H., "Trends in Skiing Injuries," *American Journal of Sports Medicine*, Vol. 8, 1980, pp. 106–113.

[*8*] Johnson, R. J., Ettlinger, C. F. and Shealy, J. E., "Skier Injury Trends," in *Skiing Trauma and Safety: Seventh International Symposium, ASTM STP 1022*, R. J. Johnson, C. D. Mote, Jr., and M.-H. Binet, Eds., American Society for Testing and Materials, Philadelphia, 1989, pp. 25–31.

[*9*] Bouter, L. M., Knipschild, P. G., and Volovics, A., "Binding Function in Relation to Injury Risk in Downhill Skiing," *American Journal of Sports Medicine*, Vol. 17, No. 2, 1989, pp. 226–233.

[*10*] Hauser, W., "Experimental Prospective Skiing Injury Study," in *Skiing Trauma and Safety: Seventh International Symposium, ASTM STP 1022*, R. J. Johnson, C. D. Mote, Jr., and M.-H. Binet, Eds., American Society for Testing and Materials, Philadelphia, 1989, pp. 18–24.

[*11*] Rosen, J. C., Johnson, R. J., Lefebvre, M. F., and Pope, M. H., "Behavioral Determinants of Skiers' Failure to Adjust Release Bindings," *Clinics in Sports Medicine*, Vol. 1. 1982, pp. 209–215.

[*12*] Damoiseaux, V. M. G., de Jongh, A. M. L., Bouter, L. M., and Hospers, H. J., "Designing Effective Health Education for Downhill Skiers: Results of a Randomized Intervention Study," in this volume, pp. 241–248.

[*13*] Knipschild, P. G. and Bouter, L. M., "Risk Factors for Ski Injuries: A Crash Course of Epidemiologic Methods with Emphasis on Comparability in Experiments and Case-Control Studies," in *Skiing Trauma and Safety: Seventh International Symposium, ASTM STP 1022*, R. J. Johnson, C. D. Mote, Jr., and M.-H. Binet, Eds., American Society for Testing and Materials, Philadelphia, 1989, pp. 9–17.

[*14*] Ziegler, W. J., Jung, H., Matter, P., and Meier, P., *Skiing Conscious of Risks* (in German), Habegger Verlag, Derendingen, 1987.

[*15*] Vries, H. de, Dijkstra, M., and Kuhlman, P., "Self-Efficacy: The Third Factor Besides Attitude and Subjective Norm as a Predictor of Behavioral Intentions," *Health Education Research*, Vol. 3, 1988, pp. 273–282.

[*16*] Bouter, L. M., Knipschild, P. G., Feij, J. A., and Volovics, A., "Sensation Seeking and Injury Risk in Downhill Skiing," *Personality and Individual Differences*, Vol. 9, 1988, pp. 667–673.

[*17*] McGuire, W. J., "Attitudes and Attitude Change," in *Handbook of Social Psychology*, Volume II, G. Lindsay and E. Aronson, Eds., Guilfort, New York, 1985.

[*18*] Damoiseaux, V., *The Necessity of Pretesting Written Information Materials*, Internal Report, University of Limburg, Maastricht, 1989.

Lex M. Bouter[1] *and Paul G. Knipschild*[1]

Behavioral Risk Factors for Ski Injury: Problem Analysis as a Basis for Effective Health Education

REFERENCE: Bouter, L. M. and Knipschild, P. G., "**Behavioral Risk Factors for Ski Injury: Problem Analysis as a Basis for Effective Health Education,**" *Skiing Trauma and Safety: Eighth International Symposium, ASTM STP 1104*, C. D. Mote, Jr. and Robert J. Johnson, Eds., American Society for Testing and Materials, Philadelphia, 1991, pp. 257–264.

ABSTRACT: A problem analysis dealing with the importance of behavioral risk factors for ski injuries is based on the results of a case–control study conducted among Dutch skiers. In this study, cases (N = 572) were a sample of those who filed insurance claims for medical costs incurred as the result of a ski injury that prevented them from skiing for more than one day. Controls (N = 576) were a sample of uninjured skiers who filed insurance claims for nonmedical reasons.

Not taking ski lessons appeared to be a risk factor among beginners (odds ratio [OR] = 2.5; etiologic fraction [EF] = 12%). Failure of bindings to release is associated with a higher risk (OR = 3.2) for lower extremity injury, indicating that optimal binding adjustment can have a substantial preventive effect. Surprisingly, binding adjustment in the Netherlands more often involved the use of a test device compared to the ski resorts involved. In the latter case, the injury risk was higher (OR = 1.6; EF = 17%). From our data and the available literature, it can be concluded that alcohol consumption is probably not an important risk factor for ski injury. Several findings from our study seem to indicate that risk underestimation may be a risk factor for ski injury, but further study is necessary on this point. Taken together, the empirical basis for behavioral risk factors other than those mentioned above is still rather weak and thus a restrictive policy with respect to health education for downhill skiers would seem appropriate.

KEY WORDS: downhill skiing, injury, etiology, health education, ski lessons, binding adjustment, alcohol, risk underestimation

Downhill skiing has been gaining enormous popularity in the Netherlands over the last few decades. Some 700 000 Dutch skiers actively participate in downhill skiing in other European countries (70% in Austria) for an average of about 10 days a year [*1*]. Unfortunately, skiing is not without risk. Some 2 to 4 injuries needing medical treatment occur every 1000 skier days [*2,3*]. Consequently, the annual number of Dutch casualties ranges from 14 000 to 28 000. Resulting medical costs are substantial, as well as the number of days of restriction from work and sports participation.

Prevention of ski injuries should be based on sound knowledge of the etiology of these injuries. Epidemiological studies that identify and quantify the contribution of putative risk factors by comparing injured and uninjured skiers are essential for this purpose [*4*]. Preventive factors can be divided into technical improvements in equipment and ski run, safety regulations, and individual behavior. This article, based on data on behavioral risk factors

[1]Epidemiologists, Department of Epidemiology and Health Care Research, University of Limburg, P.O. Box 616, 6200 MD Maastricht, the Netherlands.

from our case–control study conducted among Dutch skiers [1], will focus on the last category.

Health education aimed at prevention of ski injuries should concentrate on behavioral factors that contribute to the incidence of injury [4]. Systematic problem analysis of the available etiological evidence should form the basis of all health education intervention [5]. These behavioral factors must be able to be modified in the desired direction by means of health education. Whether this is possible can only be answered conclusively in a preventive trial in which behavioral modification is attempted, although a study of the determinants of the behavior at issue can be very helpful [5].

The importance of a behavioral risk factor actually consists of two dimensions. First, there is the strength of the association between the factor and the incidence of injury. This is preferably expressed as a relative risk (RR), which can be estimated by using the odds ratio (OR) from a case–control study [6]. Table 1 illustrates this for the instance of a dichotomous risk factor. Second, the prevalence of the risky behavior at issue among the population is also of consequence for the maximal potential benefits of health education. In a case–control study, the prevalence in the population can be substituted by the prevalence in the control group. Dangerous behavior (high OR) that is very rare (low prevalence) will therefore not necessarily be the best focus for health education.

Both dimensions of the importance of a risk factor can be unified by the calculation of the etiologic fraction (EF). This is the fraction (percentage) of injuries that could be avoided theoretically by complete elimination of the risky behavior at issue in the population for which the EF is calculated [6]. Table 1 illustrates the calculation of the etiologic fraction for the instance of a dichotomous risk factor from case–control data. As an approximation of the prevalence (among the population) of the risk factor at issue, the prevalence in the control group is taken.

This article presents a problem analysis of the behavioral risk factors for ski injuries based on results from a case–control study conducted among Dutch skiers [1]. First, the design of this study will be described briefly. Second, behavioral risk factors will be presented—ski lessons, binding adjustment, alcohol consumption, and risk underestimation. Third, the consequences for health education aimed at downhill skiers will be critically discussed.

Methods

Cases (injured skiers) and controls (uninjured skiers) during the 1984/1985 season were obtained from the records of a company covering roughly one third of the market for ski insurance in the Netherlands. Most Dutch skiers are insured. The cases selected were skiers

TABLE 1—*Measures of association relevant for the assessment of the importance of a behavioral risk factor from a case–control study.*[a]

	I_1	I_0
RF_1	a	b
RF_0	c	d

$$OR = \frac{ad}{bc}$$

$$EF = \frac{P_1\,(OR - 1)}{P_1\,(OR - 1) + 1} \cdot 100\%$$

[a] RF_1 = risk factor present; RF_0 = risk factor absent; I_1 = injured; I_0 = uninjured; OR = odds ratio; EF = etiologic fraction; P_1 = prevalence of risk factor

who had filed claims for medical costs as a result of a ski injury that made skiing or other activities impossible for more than one day. An equal number of uninjured skiers was chosen by taking the next claim from an uninjured skier received by the insurance company for other reasons, for example, loss or theft. A postal questionnaire was sent shortly after the ski holiday to the population thus defined.

Methods of data analysis (bivariate, stratified, and multivariate) performed in our study are described elsewhere [*1*]. The same holds for the response, the nonbehavioral risk factors, and the discussion of the general aspects of the validity of the study [*1,7–9*]. The present article focuses on our findings with respect to putative behavioral risk factors and relates them to the available literature. The strength of the association between a factor and injury risk will be estimated by calculating the odds ratio (OR; cross product ratio) [*4,6*]. An OR greater than one indicates that the factor is a risk factor indeed, while an OR between one and zero suggests a preventive effect. An OR equal to one will be found when an association is absent. The 95% confidence interval (CI) of the OR gives an impression of the imprecision of the point estimate. A 95% CI not including the null-value (OR = 1) is equivalent to a *p*-value smaller than 0.05 in a two-sided significance test. Besides OR and 95% CI, a global estimation of the etiologic fraction (EF) will be provided where appropriate (see Table 1 for the method of calculation).

Behavioral Risk Factors

Ski Lessons

Our data confirm the existing consensus [*3,10*] that beginners have twice the injury risk of intermediate or advanced skiers (OR = 2.1; CI = 1.5 to 2.9). Ski lessons are supposed to improve the skill of the skier and might thus reduce the injury risk for beginners especially. In the literature [*3,11,12*], no agreement is found on the overall safety effect of ski lessons. In our study, no overall effect of ski lessons was identified (OR = 1.0; CI = 0.8 to 1.4), although a protective effect was found among the subgroup of skiers who went only once or twice for a ski holidy (Table 2). For Dutch skiers, the number of ski holidays seems to be an acceptable measure of experience, because usually no skiing is done between these holidays (which last on average ten days [*1*]).

The small group (9%) of beginners who refrain from taking ski lessons have a substantially higher (2.5 times) risk compared to beginners who do take lessons. Consequently, this subgroup of beginners contrasts noticeably unfavorably with intermediate or advanced skiers

TABLE 2—*Adjusted percentages[a] and odds ratios[b] comparing skiers who had taken ski lessons to those who had not, stratified for experience.[c]*

	Injured, %	Not Injured, %	OR	CI
	FIRST OR SECOND SKI HOLIDAY (*N* = 157)	(*N* = 132)		
Ski lessons	78	91	1.0	
No ski lessons	22	9	2.5	1.1–5.0
	THIRD SKI HOLIDAY OR MORE (*N* = 366)	(*N* = 432)		
Ski lessons	36	35	1.0	
No ski lessons	64	65	0.9	0.6–1.4

[a]After direct standardization for age and gender.

[b]Weighted average over six stata for age and gender (Mantel-Haenszel) followed by a test-based 95% confidence interval (CI).

[c]Operationalized as the number of the current ski holiday.

(OR = 2.1 · 2.5 = 5.3). Health education that persuades all Dutch beginners to take ski lessons would possibly lower the incidence of injury among beginners by roughly 12% (EF = 12%; this etiologic fraction can be calculated by using the formula from Table 1 and the data from the upper part of Table 2: OR = 2.5 and P_1 = 0.09). Some caution is warranted in generalizing this to skiers of other countries, because Dutch beginners probably lack ski experience completely, while, for instance, in alpine countries, beginners might already have some basic skill in skiing. On the other hand, the prevalence of not taking lessons among Dutch skiers is probably very low compared to beginners from other countries.

In contrast to what might be expected, we could not detect a protective effect of ski gymnastics lessons before the ski holiday (OR = 1.1; CI = 0.7 to 1.6). One fifth (19%) of the Dutch skiers prepare by means of a course in ski gymnastics, but it would be premature to advocate this as a risk-reducing measure.

Binding Adjustment

Ski bindings are constructed and individually adjusted to release when the forces on the bones and ligaments of the lower extremities get dangerously high. Substantial improvements have been made in this field within the last few decades [*13–15*]. The question is whether binding adjustment is still an important risk factor. Binding release in our study was indeed less frequent before lower extremity injury compared to other injuries (Table 3). The latter percentage can be looked on as a rough estimation of binding release during a randomly chosen fall among the control group, assuming that binding release has no bearing on the origin of (isolated) nonlower extremity injury. Following the same line of reasoning, completely avoiding the failure of the bindings to release during a fall would reduce lower extremity injury roughly by 22% among men and by 39% among women (etiologic fractions calculated as explained above).

These etiologic fractions clearly form a theoretical and unrealistic maximum of the benefits of health education achieving optimal adjustment for every skier. First, not all lower extremity injuries can be considered (theoretically) preventable by a timely release of the bindings. Johnson et al. [*13*] assume that the proportion of lower extremity equipment-related (LEER) injuries among the lower extremity injuries is 80%. Second, optimal ad-

TABLE 3—*Adjusted percentages[a] and odds ratios[b] comparing the release of only one or no binding to the release of both bindings within the injured population, stratified for gender.*

	Lower Extremity Injury, %	Other Injuries Only, %	OR[c]	CI
	MALES (N = 136)	(N = 129)		
Both bindings released	30	50	1.0	
One binding released	27	23	2.1	1.0–4.1
No release	33	13	3.2	1.6–6.5
Unknown	10	13		
	FEMALES (N = 204)	(N = 103)		
Both bindings released	18	34	1.0	
One binding released	29	22	2.7	1.3–5.7
No release	46	28	3.3	1.7–6.5
Unknown	7	17		

[a]After direct standardization for age and gender.
[b]Weighted average over six strata for age and gender (Mantel-Haenszel) followed by a test-based 95% confidence interval (CI).
[c]Odds ratios are given for the category at issues compared to the release of both bindings.

justment of the current ski bindings probably cannot prevent all LEER injury, because the design of the binding may cause it to release too late or not at all under certain circumstances [*9*]. From a recent German study [*2*], it appears that the bindings of uninjured skiers are adjusted on average 50% above the recommended setting of the binding release force, while the average deviation for the bindings of injured skiers with knee sprains is 85% and for tibia fractures even 150%. Hanft et al. [*16*] report that only the population suffering tibial shaft injuries as a result of bending and twisting has a distribution of release values that is substantially higher than the control population. Taken together, it seems that regular and adequate adjustment of ski bindings is indeed an important preventive measure on which health education should focus. However, knee injuries can probably not be prevented very effectively by adequate adjustment of ski bindings currently available.

Control of the right binding setting with a test device is widely advocated [*17*], but not always performed [*18*]. From our data it appears that two thirds of the ski shops in the Netherlands use such a device, while only one third of the shops at the ski resorts at issue actually test the binding setting. These observations are consistent with the fact that binding adjustment abroad at the ski resorts was associated with a 60% higher risk (OR = 1.6; CI = 1.2 to 2.2) compared to adjustment in the Netherlands [*9*]. Adjustment before traveling abroad could theoretically lower the incidence of injury among Dutch skiers by 17% (etiologic fraction based on OR = 1.6 and prevalence of adjustment at ski resort = 34%).

Alcohol Consumption

Alcohol consumption can increase the risks of skiing theoretically by both acute and long-term mechanisms. On the acute level, alcohol could influence reaction time, accuracy of movements, and the perception of risk [*19,20*]. The long-term effect may consist of a lowering of the intake of carbohydrates, thus hampering the glycogen resynthesis and thereby possibly increasing risk due to exhaustion and decreased movement control [*21*]. In contrast to what might be expected, perceptible blood or breath levels of alcohol are very rare both among injured and uninjured skiers [*2,19,22*]. Our study confirmed the relatively low prevalence of alcohol consumption during the breaks when skiing (Table 4). Those who did drink during the breaks took usually one or two drinks.

TABLE 4—*Adjusted percentages*[a] *and odds ratios*[b] *for different levels of alcohol consumption compared to no consumption during the breaks and during the ski holiday.*

	Injured, % (N = 572)	Not Injured, % (N = 576)	OR[c]	CI
	ALCOHOL CONSUMPTION DURING BREAKS			
Never	79	67	1.0	
Sometimes	18	28	0.6	0.4–0.8
Every day	3	6	0.5	0.3–0.9
	DAILY AVERAGE ALCOHOL CONSUMPTION[d]			
0 consumptions	28	22	1.0	
1 or 2 consumptions	33	31	0.8	0.5–1.1
3 or 4 consumptions	25	23	0.8	0.5–1.1
5 or more consumptions	15	23	0.5	0.3–0.7

[a]After direct standardization for age and gender.

[b]Weighted average over six strata for age and gender (Mantel-Haenszel) followed by a test-based 95% confidence interval (CI).

[c]Odds ratios are given for the category at issue compared to the first category ("never" and "0 consumptions," respectively).

[d]Expressed in standard glasses containing the same amount of alcohol for all alcohol beverages.

Surprisingly, it appears that alcohol consumption during breaks protects against injury. The same appeared to hold for the average daily consumption during the ski holiday (Table 4). Elsewhere [*1*] it was argued that this apparent acute and long-term protection by alcohol was not to be considered as causal. Our findings could originate (partly) from selective underreporting by injured skiers or in differences in personality between teetotalers and other skiers. Therefore, the etiologic fraction for converting teetotalers must be considered meaningless and is not calculated for this reason. Our overall impression is that alcohol is neither a substantial risk factor nor a protective factor for ski injury.

Risk Underestimation

Individual risk-taking behavior could be an important determinant of ski injury. Excesses in risk taking (relative to the circumstances and the skill of the skier) could be due to a sensation-seeking tendency or to risk underestimation. Although often mentioned in the popular literature [*22*] on downhill skiing, these factors are very difficult to operationalize. In a second study [*23*] among the respondents of our original case–control study, we used the Sensation-Seeking Scale [*24*] for this purpose. Skiers appeared to score relatively high on this scale, especially on the subscale indicating a desire to engage in risky activities. But contrary to what might be expected, injured skiers appeared to have a lower score on this personality trait than uninjured skiers [*23*].

Besides the possibility that the Sensation-Seeking Scale offers no valid operationalization of the risk-taking behavior of skiers, there seems to be the alternative explanation that underestimation of the actual risks is the crucial factor. Sensation seekers could be relatively skilled in assessing risks and performing at the limit of their individual capacities. In this perception, especially the skiers who underestimate the risk of certain situations or activities are at risk. This explanation finds some support in our result that skiers who reported that they had been rather afraid of having an accident leading to injury before their holiday, appeared to have a 40% lower injury risk (Table 5). Assuming that this mild fear represents a realistic assessment of the risks of skiing, health education focused on this point may decrease the incidence of injury (as indicated by the etiologic fraction) by a maximum of 35%. Of course, this is only a very tentative conclusion and further studies on the role of risk underestimation are needed before health education intervention can be reasonably based on this idea. Additional support for the role of risk underestimation comes from the general finding [*8,19,25*] that the injury risk is higher under favorable circumstances (cloudless, not cold, and good visibility).

Health Education for Skiers

In both our study and other studies mentioned above, the odds ratios calculated do not necessarily point to causality and may suffer from major or minor biases for a number of reasons [*1*]. For most variables, more precise measurement would be better, for example, binding adjustment, while sometimes external sources of data would seem to be preferable, for example, recklessness. Furthermore, a prospective instead of the usual retrospective design would be more informative about the effects of some factors, for example, physical condition. All doubts about the causal interpretation of the odds ratios have consequences for the interpretation of the etiologic fractions as well. Furthermore, the etiologic fractions are based on the debatable assumption that the prevalence of the behavioral risk factor among the control group is the same as in the population considered for the health education intervention. Because elimination of the risk factor at issue usually will not be total, the real effect on the incidence of injury will be considerably smaller than the etiologic fraction

TABLE 5—*Adjusted percentages[a] and odds ratios[b] for fearing an accident compared to not being afraid before the ski holiday.*

	Injured, % (N = 572)	Not Injured, % (N = 576)	OR	CI
Not afraid	87	80	1.0	
Slightly afraid	13	19	0.6	0.4–0.8
Very afraid	0	1		

[a]After direct standardization for age and gender.
[b]Weighted average over six strata for age and gender (Mantel-Haenszel) followed by a test-based 95% confidence interval (CI).

indicates. Addition of etiologic fractions is still a rather common mistake [*6*]. Risk factors are often strongly associated and act together in the causation of a ski injury. Summation of etiologic fractions would start from the unrealistic assumption that the risk factors at issue act completely independently of one another [*6*]. Also, the external validity of the data presented above can be questioned. Dutch skiers differ substantially from skiers in, for instance, alpine countries, which may hamper the generalizability of our data.

Let us assume that the problem analysis has yielded valid knowledge on the importance of some behavioral risk factors. This would only be a first step toward effective health education [*5*]. Further research would be necessary to study the determinants of the behavior at issue, so that the design of the intervention can be made optimal. The next step would be the execution of a preventive trial in which behavioral change and the reduction of the incidence of injury can be assumed [*15*]. Until now, only the optimal adjustment of ski bindings has been investigated in such a preventive trial [*26*].

Taken together, the empirical basis for the importance of most putative behavioral risk factors for ski injury is still rather weak. Exceptions to this rule are inadequate binding adjustment, the failure of beginners to take ski lessons and, to a lesser extent, underestimation of the actual risks. As far as the many other putative behavioral risk factors are concerned, we feel that a very restrictive policy with respect to health education is appropriate. We do not agree with the habit of smothering the skiers in an avalanche of well-meant preventive remarks; we think that effective prevention is impossible if education is handled in such a loose, aspecific way. Furthermore, we do not like the idea that some skiers might feel guilty about certain aspects of their behavior, for example, moderate alcohol consumption, prematurely decreed as being dangerous by health educators.

References

[*1*] Bouter, L. M., *Injury Risk in Downhill Skiing: Results from an Etiological Case-Control Study among Dutch Skiers*, De Vrieseborch, Haarlem, 1988.

[*2*] Hauser, W. and Gläser, H., *Alpine Skiunfälle und Verletzungen: Häufigkeit, Risicofactoren, Ursachen*, DSV, München, 1985.

[*3*] Shealy, J. E., "Overall Analysis of NSAA/ASTM Data on Skiing Injuries for 1978 through 1981," in *Skiing Trauma and Safety: Fifth International Symposium, ASTM STP 860*, R. J. Johnson and C. D. Mote, Jr., Eds., American Society for Testing and Materials, Philadelphia, 1985, pp. 302–313.

[*4*] Knipschild, P. G. and Bouter, L. M., "Risk Factors for Ski Injuries: a Crash Course of Epidemiologic Methods with Emphasis on Comparability in Experiments and Case-Control Studies," in *Skiing Trauma and Safety: Seventh International Symposium, ASTM STP 1022*, R. J. Johnson, C. D. Mote, Jr., and M.-H. Binet, Eds., American Society for Testing and Materials, Philadelphia, 1989, pp. 9–17.

[5] Kok, G. J. and Bouter, L. M., "On the Importance of Health Education: Prevention of Ski Injury as an Example," *American Journal of Sports Medicine*, Vol. 18, No. 6, 1990, pp. 600–605.
[6] Rothmann, K. J., *Modern Epidemiology*, Little, Brown & Company, Boston, 1986.
[7] Bouter, L. M., Knipschild, P. G., and Volovics, A., "Ability and Physical Condition in Relation to Injury Risk in Downhill Skiing," in *Skiing Trauma and Safety: Seventh International Symposium, ASTM STP 1022*, R. J. Johnson, C. D. Mote, Jr., and M.-H. Binet, Eds., American Society for Testing and Materials, Philadelphia, 1989, pp. 94–102.
[8] Bouter, L. M., Knipschild, P. G., and Volovics, A., "Personal and Environmental Factors in Relation to Injury Risk in Downhill Skiing," *International Journal of Sports Medicine*, Vol. 10, No. 4, 1989, pp. 298–301.
[9] Bouter, L. M., Knipschild, P. G., and Volovics, A., "Binding Function in Relation to Injury Risk in Downhill Skiing," *American Journal of Sports Medicine*, Vol. 17, No. 2, 1989, pp. 226–233.
[10] Jaffin, B., "An Epidemiologic Study of Ski Injuries: Vail, Colorado," *Mount Sinai Journal of Medicine*, Vol. 48, No. 4, 1981, pp. 353–359.
[11] Garrick, J. G. and Requa, R., "The Role of Instruction in Preventing Ski Injuries," *Physician and Sportsmedicine*, Vol. 5, No. 12, 1977, pp. 57–59.
[12] Shealy, L. E., Geyer, L. H., and Hayden, R., "Epidemiology of Ski Injuries: Effect of Method of Skill Acqusition and Release Binding Accident Rates," *Human Factors*, Vol. 16, No. 5, 1974, pp. 459–473.
[13] Johnson, R. J., Ettinger, G. F., Campbell, R. J., and Pope, M. H., "Trends in Skiing Injuries," *American Journal of Sports Medicine*, Vol. 8, No. 2, 1980, pp. 106–113.
[14] Kuriyama, S. and Fujimaki, E., "Current Trends in Ski Injuries and Their Relationship to Recent Changes in Ski Equipment," in *Skiing Trauma and Safety: Sixth International Symposium, ASTM STP 938*, C. D. Mote, Jr. and R. J. Johnson, Eds., American Society for Testing and Materials, Philadelphia, 1987, pp. 263–270.
[15] Tapper, E. A., "Ski Injuries from 1939 to 1976: The Sun Valley Experience," *American Journal of Sports Medicine*, Vol. 6, No. 3, 1978, pp. 114–121.
[16] Hanft, S., Ettlinger, C. F., and Shealy, J. E., "A Study to Determine the Variability in Release Characteristics of New Alpine Ski/Boot/Binding Systems," paper presented at the Eighth International Symposium on Ski Trauma and Safety, Riksgräsen, Sweden, 15–21 May 1989.
[17] Delouche, G., "Bindings' Release Setting in Alpine Skiing," in *Skiing Trauma and Safety: Sixth International Symposium, ASTM STP 938*, C. D. Mote, Jr. and R. J. Johnson, Eds., American Society for Testing and Materials, Philadelphia, 1987, pp. 202–211.
[18] Nagel A. and Mösch, S., "Test Devices for Ski Bindings Sold in Sport Shops: State of the Art and Future Development," in *Skiing Trauma and Safety: Sixth International Symposium, ASTM STP 938*, C. D. Mote, Jr. and R. J. Johnson, Eds., American Society for Testing and Materials, Philadelphia, 1987, pp. 217–224.
[19] Biener, K. and Fassler, S., *Sportsunfälle*, Verlag Hans Huber, Bern, 1978.
[20] Bernett, P. and Schöffel, U., "Ursache and Prophylaxe von Skiverletzungen," *Münchener Medizinischen Wochenschrift*, Vol. 124, 1982, pp. 178–182.
[21] Brouns, F., Saris, W. H. M., and Hoor, F. ten, "Nutrition as a Factor in the Prevention of Injuries in Recreational and Competitive Downhill Skiing," *Journal of Sports Medicine*, Vol. 26, 1986, pp. 85–90.
[22] Ziegler, W. J., Jung, H., Matter, P., and Meier, P., *Risikobewust Skifahren*, Habegger Verlag, Derendingen, 1987.
[23] Bouter, L. M., Knipschild, P. G., Feij, J. A., and Volovics, A., "Sensation Seeking and Injury Risk in Downhill Skiing," *Personality and Individual Differences*, Vol. 9, 1988, pp. 667–673.
[24] Zuckerman, M., "Sensation Seeking and Sport," *Personality and Individual Differences*, Vol. 4, 1983, pp. 285–293.
[25] Biener, K., Freihofer, B., and Schwarzenbach, F., "Wetter und Skiunfälle," *Münchener Medizinischen Wochenschrift*, Vol. 12, 1979, pp. 427–430.
[26] Hauser, W., "Experimental Prospective Skiing Injury Study," in *Skiing Trauma and Safety: Seventh International Symposium, ASTM STP 1022*, R. J. Johnson, C. D. Mote, Jr., and M.-H. Binet, Eds., American Society for Testing and Materials, Philadelphia, 1989, pp. 18–24.

Author Index

Subject Index